OPHTHALMIC ASSISTANT

OPHTHALMIC ASSISTANT

PK Mukherjee MS

Consultant Ophthalmologist
Former Professor and Head
Upgraded Department of Ophthalmology
Pandit Jawahar Lal Nehru Memorial Medical College
Raipur, Chhattisgarh, India

JAYPEE BROTHERS MEDICAL PUBLISHERS (P) LTD

New Delhi • London • Philadelphia • Panama

Jaypee Brothers Medical Publishers (P) Ltd

Headquarters
Jaypee Brothers Medical Publishers (P) Ltd
4838/24, Ansari Road, Daryaganj
New Delhi 110 002, India
Phone: +91-11-43574357
Fax: +91-11-43574314
Email: jaypee@jaypeebrothers.com

Overseas Offices

J.P. Medical Ltd
83, Victoria Street, London
SW1H 0HW (UK)
Phone: +44-2031708910
Fax: +02-03-0086180
Email: info@jpmedpub.com

Jaypee-Highlights Medical Publishers Inc.
City of Knowledge, Bld. 237, Clayton
Panama City, Panama
Phone: + 507-301-0496
Fax: + 507-301-0499
Email: cservice@jphmedical.com

Jaypee Brothers Medical Publishers Ltd
The Bourse
111 South Independence Mall East
Suite 835, Philadelphia, PA 19106, USA
Phone: + 267-519-9789
Email: joe.rusko@jaypeebrothers.com

Jaypee Brothers Medical Publishers (P) Ltd
17/1-B Babar Road, Block-B, Shaymali
Mohammadpur, Dhaka-1207
Bangladesh
Mobile: +08801912003485
Email: jaypeedhaka@gmail.com

Jaypee Brothers Medical Publishers (P) Ltd
Shorakhute, Kathmandu
Nepal
Phone: +00977-9841528578
Email: jaypee.nepal@gmail.com

Website: www.jaypeebrothers.com
Website: www.jaypeedigital.com

Inquiries for bulk sales may be solicited at: jaypee@jaypeebrothers.com

Ophthalmic Assistant

First Edition: **2013**

ISBN: 978-93-5090-425-1

Printed at Repro India Limited

Dedicated to

All those paramedics, who work assiduously
in the anteroom of the consultant and go unrecognized.

Preface

There are many books written superbly for undergraduate students for whom ophthalmology is a separate subject that they must clear to obtain medical degree. There is no dearth of books for postgraduates as well. In contrast to this, books for paramedical ophthalmic assistants, who form the backbone of health services in ophthalmology both in government services and private sectors, are really few.

The present trend in training centers for paramedical ophthalmic assistants is to prescribe them to books meant for MBBS students. Naturally, these books are beyond comprehension of paramedical ophthalmic assistants. Their inability to understand these books lies in the fact that there is no uniform educational prerequisite for admission to these courses. Only a few pass class 12th with physics, chemistry and biology, rest may have arts/commerce as subjects for their high school examination. It is very difficult for these students to understand even the basics of human biology, chemistry and elementary physics.

To overcome these difficulties, the present book has been written. The book has outline of ocular anatomy, physiology and ophthalmic optics in simple language and terminology that can be understood by above-mentioned students. The book has separate chapters on disorders of different parts of the eye. The clinical features have been discussed in simple language. Only the outline of treatment has been given. No attempt has been made to give steps of surgery which are out of domain of paramedical ophthalmic assistants.

The book is well-illustrated by drawings and photographs. Hope this will be of use to paramedical ophthalmic assistants.

PK Mukherjee

Acknowledgments

I am thankful to Professor Dr SL Adile, Director, Medical Education, Government of Chhattisgarh; Dr AK Chandrakar, Professor and Head of the Department; Dr ML Garg, Professor of Ophthalmology, and Dr Nidhi Pandey, Associate Professor of Ophthalmology in Upgraded Department of Ophthalmology, Pandit Jawahar Lal Nehru Memorial Medical College, Raipur, Chhattisgarh, India, for their help, suggestions and constructive criticism during writing this book. They kept me supplied with their books, journals, notes whenever required.

Young Doctor Santosh Singh Patel, the dynamic Assistant Professor of Ophthalmology, deserves special mention and thanks for keeping me abreast with latest development in ophthalmology. He also supplied me photographs from his unending stocks of clinical photographs.

Dr Manik Chatterjee, Professor of Anatomy, re-freshened my knowledge of anatomy of the eye and their applied importance.

My sons-in-law, Shri Satyadeep Sahukar, Dr Abir Bandyopadyay and my daughters, Dr Protibha Mukherjee Sahukar and Dr Preeti Bandyopadyay, helped me to find out references from the Internet and drawing the figures on computer. Their efforts are duly acknowledged with thanks.

My wife, Protima, has been an inspiration personified in writing this book.

I am thankful to all my patients, who have permitted me to use their photographs in the book.

Shri Maneesh Dandekar of Hypersoft, Shantinagar, Raipur, Chhattisgarh, India, was never tired of typing and retyping the manuscript and giving the final shape to the flow charts and diagrams. His efforts are acknowledged with thanks.

I am thankful to all the members of M/s Jaypee Brothers Medical Publishers (P) Ltd, New Delhi, India, for their cooperation.

I am specially thankful to Shri Jitendar P Vij (Group Chairman), Mr Ankit Vij (Managing Director) and Mr Tarun Duneja (Director-Publishing) and Ms Samina Khan (PA to Director-Publishing) of M/s Jaypee Brothers Medical Publishers (P) Ltd, New Delhi, India, for all the help they have extended to me.

Contents

CHAPTER

1

Anatomy of the Eye

Human beings are placed at the peak of the evolution pyramid with five senses, i.e. vision, hearing, smell, taste and touch. Out of these the vision is most developed in human beings because they have precise distant vision, near vision, color vision, field of vision, depth perception and contrast sensitivity. Though human far vision is good yet it does not surpass the distant vision of may birds and animals. Some birds have near vision so well developed that they can pick up useful tiny food particles from grass or sand. Almost all animals have sharp night vision (scotopic vision) but most of the day flying birds have almost no night vision. Humans too have poor night vision. The color vision is unique among humans, animals and birds either have very poor color sense or they lack it altogether.

Theoretically a person with normal eye should have enough vision to see up to infinity provided the object is large and bright enough. An infant can see the smallest point from less than 5″ but have poor distant vision.

The human beings have been endowed with a pair of almost identical eyes. Each capable of functioning independently but are coordinated with each other neurologically. The advantage of having two coordinated eyes are: Increased field of vision, increased depth of focus and improved vision. A person who can read two lines on Snellen's chart in one eye and three lines in the other separately, will be able to read five or six lines when both eye are used. Loss of vision in one eye does not strain the other eye. The only drawback is loss of field on the affected side. An one eyed man may have good depth sense.

To have such a versatility and diversity human eyes must have elaborate focusing system, highly developed neural coordination between two eyes, large range of vision, highly developed color sense.

The focusing system comprises of:

1. Cornea
2. Aqueous
3. Vitreous

4. Lens
5. Faculty of accommodation and convergence
6. Normal binocular movements

The neural coordination is brought about by:

1. Various reflexes
   - Light
   - Accommodation
   - Convergence

Which are governed by

1. Neural centers and tracts
2. Supra nuclear path
3. Coordinated binocular movement
4. Accommodation and convergence

ANATOMY OF THE EYE

The anatomy of the eyes can be broadly divided into:

1. The orbit and its contents
2. The eyeball (globe)
3. The adnexa of the eye
4. The intraocular structures

Orbits

The orbits are two irregular spaces placed one on each side of the midline of the face, under the forehead (frontal bone) above the cheek bone (maxilla) below. The nasal cavity lies in between the two orbits. The orbits are surrounded all-round by bones except on the outer side.

The orbits are two irregular pyramids. The apex of each pyramid is directed backwards. The sides are formed by thin bones. The walls are neither of equal length nor thickness. The medial wall of one side is parallel to the medial wall of the other side. The lateral (outer) wall is inclined towards the apex. The base of the pyramid is formed by a large circular opening in front. There are three apertures of unequal size and shape in each orbit. They are—Apex, superior orbital fissure and inferior orbital fissure. The first two communicate with the brain and transmit important nerves and vessels. Through the apex pass the optic nerve and the ophthalmic artery (Fig. 1.1).

The superior orbital fissure transmits the third, fourth and sixth cranial nerves along with lacrimal, frontal and nasociliary branch of the fifth nerve. The superior and inferior ophthalmic veins also pass through the superior orbital fissure (Fig. 1.2).

The inferior orbital fissure communicates with the maxila. It transmits few branches of inferior ophthalmic vein and maxillary division of the fifth nerve.

The orbit is lined by periorbita that continues with periosteum of skull and face. Besides there are various fascias in the orbit that divide the orbit in separate surgical space.

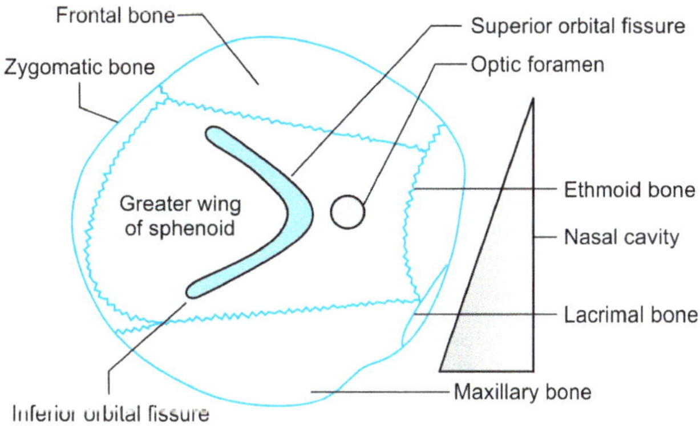

Fig. 1.1: Relative positions of bone forming the right orbit

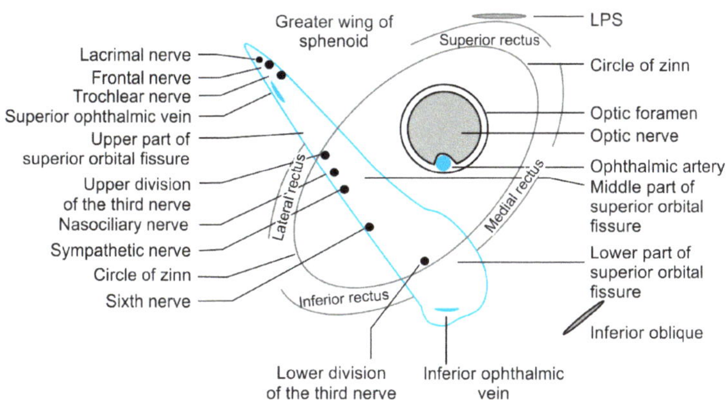

Fig. 1.2: Structures passing through superior orbital fissure and optic foramen

The orbital contents are:

1. The globe
2. The muscles
3. The cranial nerves: The second, third, fourth nerves, branches of fifth nerve and the sixth nerve
4. The branches of ophthalmic artery
5. The superior and inferior ophthalmic veins
6. The branches of sympathetic chain
7. The ciliary ganglion
8. The orbital fat
9. The orbital fascia
10. There are no formed lymphatics in the orbit

The border of the base of orbital pyramid is called the rim of the orbit. It is formed by bones stronger than the walls.

The orbital fascia consists of:

1. **Tenon's capsule**—It covers the globe from limbus to optic nerve. The space between the Tenon's capsule and the globe is called Tenon's space.
2. **Coverings of the extraocular muscles**—They cover the extraocular muscle from all sides. Sheaths of adjacent recti are joined to each other by a thin membrane called intermuscular membrane. This form a conical space in between the muscles. The space between the bony wall and the inner conical space is called extraconal or peripheral space (Figs 1.3 and 1.4) respectively.
3. **The check ligaments**—They are two in number, one extend from the medial rectus to the medial orbital margin and the other from lateral rectus to lateral orbital margin. They prevent excess movement of the globe.
4. **The transverse suspensory ligaments** are also two. The first is called superior transverse ligament, the second is called inferior transverse

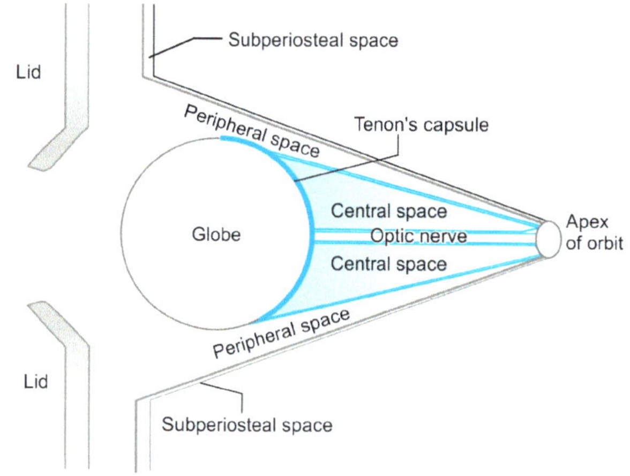

Fig. 1.3: Spaces of orbit—Lateral view

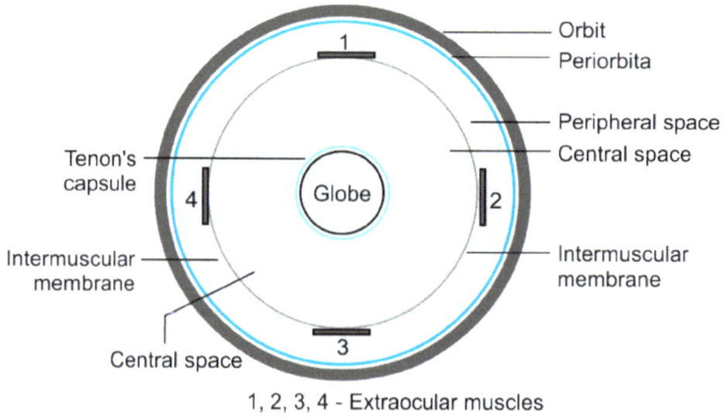

Fig. 1.4: Spaces of orbit—Front view

ligament. They prevent too much of up and down movement of the globe.

5. **The periorbita** is the periosteum of the orbit. It lines the inner surface of the orbital bones. It is continuous with periosteom of the skull and dura of the brain.
6. **Orbital septum**—It extends from the orbital margin to the tarsal plate. This divides the orbit into two unequal spaces:
   i. Small preseptal space
   ii. Large postseptal space

   It prevents infection from lid to pass into the orbit.

Extraocular Muscles

There are eight striated extraocular muscles and one plane muscle. Out of eight extraocular muscles, six are attached to the globe. They are:

1. Superior rectus
2. Medial rectus
3. Inferior rectus
4. Lateral rectus
5. Superior oblique
6. Inferior oblique

The recti are inserted in front of the equator and the oblique behind (Figs 1.5 and 1.6).

The remaining two, i.e. the levator palpebral superior and orbicularis are not attached to the globe.

The muscles that originate at the apex of the orbit are: Levator palpebral superior, the superior oblique, the superior rectus, the medial rectus, the inferior rectus and the lateral rectus.

The muscles that originate from the anterior part of the orbit are: Inferior oblique and orbicularis oculi (Table 1.1).

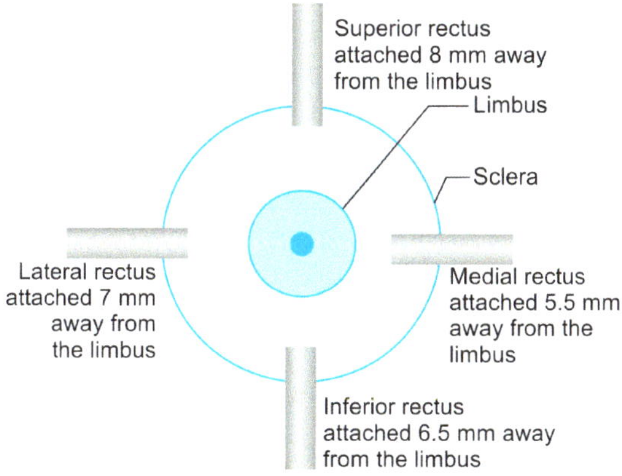

Fig. 1.5: Attachment recti to the sclera

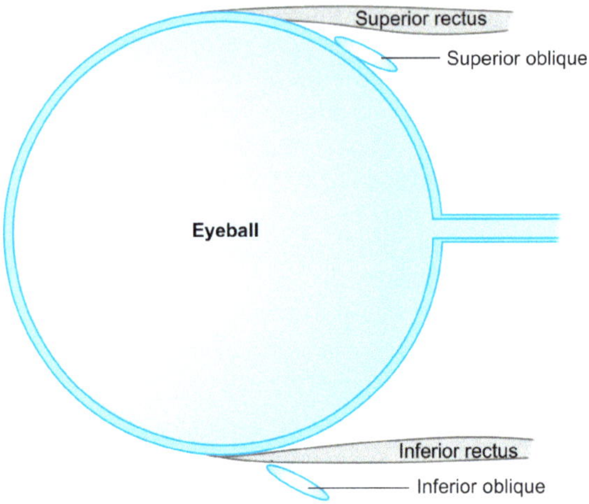

Fig. 1.6: Relation of the obliques to the recti

Table 1.1: Showing origin, insertion, nerves supply and action of cranial nerves

S.No.	Name of the muscle	Origin	Insertion	Nerve supply	Action
1.	Superior rectus	Annulus of zinn	8 mm behind the limbus	Third	Elevation adduction intorsion
2.	Medial rectus	Annulus of zinn	5.5 mm behind	Third	Adduction
3.	Inferior rectus	Annulus of zinn	6.5 mm behind the limbus	Third	Depression abduction extortion
4.	Lateral rectus	Annulus of Zinn	7 mm behind the limbus	Sixth	Abduction
5.	Superior oblique	Outside the Annulus of zinn	13.5–18.5 mm behind the limbus	Fourth	Intorsion depression abduction
6.	Inferior oblique	Medial side of the rim of the orbit	Behind the equator 16.5 mm from the limbus	Third	Extorsion elevation abduction
7.	Levator palpebral superior	Apex of orbit above the origin of superior rectus	Skin of the lid upper part of the tarsal plate upper fornix	Third	Elevate the upper lid
8.	Orbicularis oculi	Rim of the orbit	No definite insertion	Seventh	Closing the lids

The levator palpebral superior and orbicularis are not related to movement of the globe. They are concerned with opening and closing of the lids.

The above eight muscles are striated muscles (voluntary muscles) supplied by the cranial nerves.

The Muller's muscle is a non-striated muscle supplied by autonomic nervous system. It does not have a bony origin or insertion. It originates from the inferior surface of levator palpebral superior as a band and is inserted in the upper border of upper tarsal plate.

The cranial nerves in the orbit

The cranial nerves that pass through the orbit are:

1. Opticnerve (second nerve)
2. Oculomotor nerve (third nerve)
3. Trochlear nerve (fourth nerve)
4. Trigeminal nerve (fifth nerve)
   First and second division
5. Abducent nerve (sixth nerve)

The orbicularis is supplied by facial nerve (The seventh nerve) from outside the orbit.

Optic Nerve

It is the second cranial nerve responsible for vision, color vision. It also carries afferent fibers for light reflex and near reflex. It differs from other cranial nerves in the sense that it starts in the eye and ends in the brain, while other cranial nerves involved in eye start in the brain and end in the eye.

It starts in the ganglion cells of the retina and ends in the chiasma.

It is divided into four parts—(Fig. 1.7)

Intraocular
Intraorbital
Intracanalicular
Intracranial

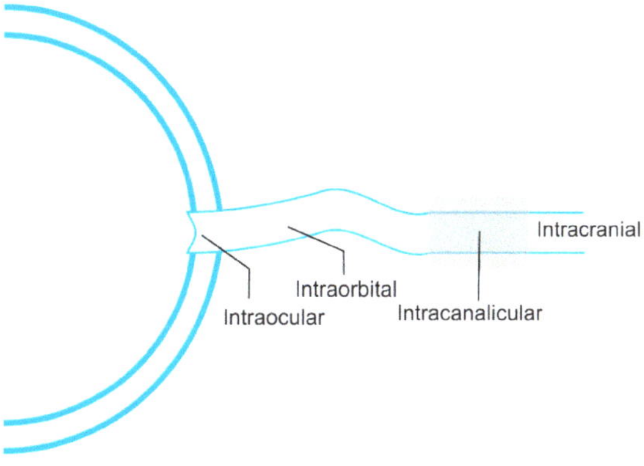

Fig. 1.7: Various parts of optic nerve

The intraocular part is called the **head of the optic nerve or papilla**. It is circular. Its diameter is 1.5 mm (It looks larger in direct ophthalmoscope due to 15 D magnification). It is slightly raised from the surface of the retina. It has a shallow depression in the center called the **cup of the optic disc**. The bottom of the cup is called the **lamina**. It has small holes in it. The central artery of the retina enters through the cup and the central vein of the retina leaves through the cup. The central retinal artery divides into four branches on the surface of the optic cup.

There is no vision on the optic nerve head, hence it represents the blind spot of the eye.

Intraorbital Part

Intraorbital part is the largest segment of the optic nerve. It extends from the back of the globe to the apex of the orbit, where it leaves the orbit through the optic foramen. It is covered by dura, arachnoid and pia which extend backwards in the brain. The cerebral fluid circulates between the arachnoid and pia (Fig. 1.8).

The central retinal artery which is a branch of ophthalmic artery enters the optic nerve from below 10 mm behind the globe. The central retinal vein leaves the optic nerve 12 mm behind the globe (Fig. 1.9).

The intraorbital part has a S shapes curve, it lies loose in the orbit hence not stretched during excessive movement of the globe.

The intracanalicular part is the part of the nerve that passes through the optic canal. The optic canal is a rigid bony canal formed by the lesser wing of the sphenoid bone. The anterior end forms the optic foramen. The optic canal joins the orbit to the brain. It also transmits ophthalmic artery.

The intracranial part of the optic nerve extends from the end of the optic canal to beginning of the optic chiasma.

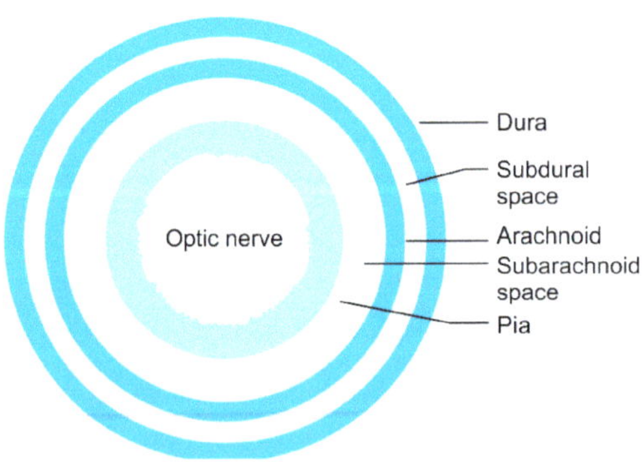

Fig. 1.8: Section of optic nerve showing its covering

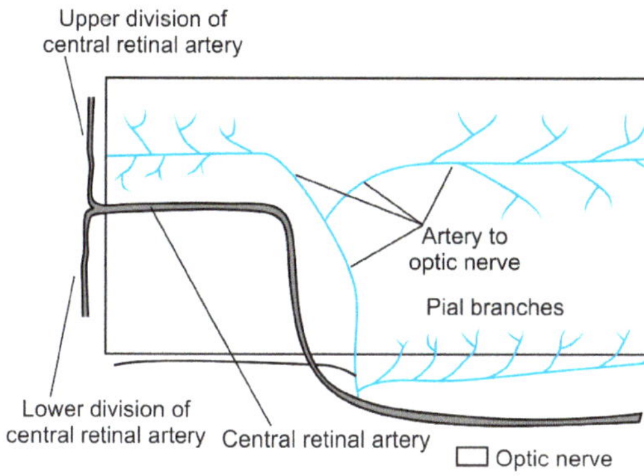

Fig. 1.9: Diagram showing origin of the central retinal artery and blood supply to the optic nerve

Oculomotor Nerve

The oculomotor nerve is meant for movement of the eyeball. It supplies all the muscles of the eyeball except the superior oblique and lateral rectus. It is also involved in constricting the pupil (miosis) and constricting the ciliary muscle (accommodation). The nerve starts in its nuclei in the midbrain, leaves the midbrain to form its basilar part then passes in the cavernous sinus after which it enters the orbit. Before entering the orbit it divides into two divisions, the upper division that supplies the superior rectus and the levator palpebral superior. The lower division supplies the medial rectus, the inferior rectus and the inferior oblique. It also gives a twig to the ciliary ganglion (Figs 1.10 and 1.2).

The ciliary ganglion is an important ganglion of the eye. It contains parasympathetic, sympathetic as well as pain fibers of internal structures of the eye. It is a pinhead sized structure situated inside the muscle cone in front the apex of the orbit between the optic nerve and the lateral rectus. It

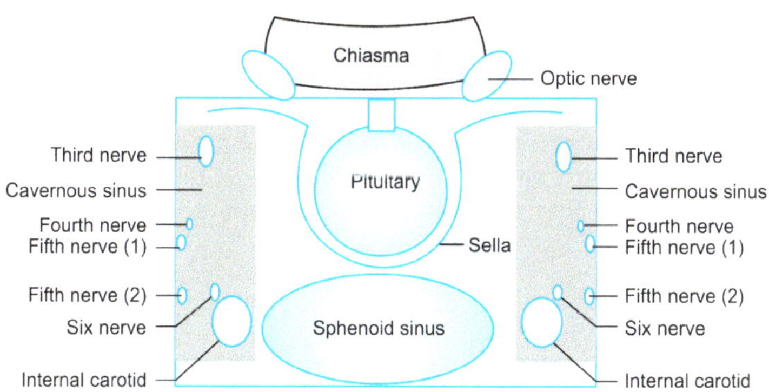

Fig. 1.10: Relative position of cranial nerves

lies 1.5 mm behind the globe. Paralysis of this ganglion leads to dilatation of the pupil and abolition of pain from uvea. This property is used to produce anesthesia by **retrobulbar injection** of anesthetic agent in the ganglion for intraocular surgeries (Fig. 1.11).

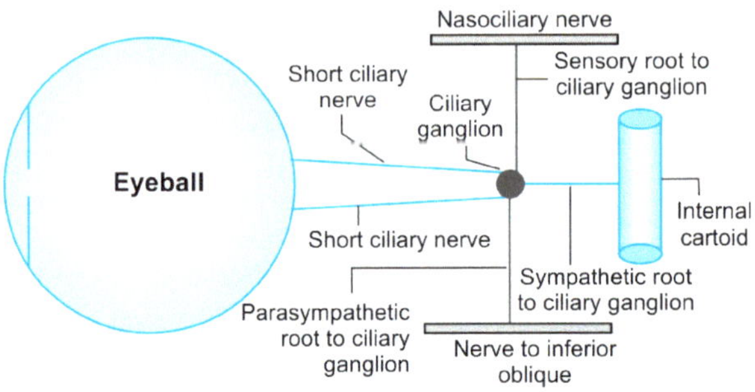

Fig. 1.11: Connections of ciliary ganglion

Trochlear Nerve

It is the fourth cranial nerve. It supplies only one muscle, the **superior oblique**. The nerve has a small nucleus in the midbrain. The fibers from one nucleus cross over to the other side to form the nerve of the other side. For example the fibers from the right nucleus forms the left trochlear nerve and the left for right nerve.

This is the only cranial nerve that come out of the midbrain on the back side (dorsal). After it leaves the midbrain it does not come near any other structure until it reaches the cavernous sinus. After the cavernous sinus the nerve enters the orbit through the superior orbital fissure outside the circle of zinn and remains outside the muscle cone. It is not paralyzed by usual retrobulbar block.

Abducent Nerve

It is the sixth cranial nerve. Like trochlear nerve it too supplies only one extraocular muscle, i.e. the **lateral rectus muscle**. It has a long intracranial course. The nucleus of the sixth nerve is situated in the lower part of the pons. The nerve comes out of the brain at the lower border of the pons. In the cavernous sinus it lies in the substance of the cavernous sinus and not the wall like the third and the fourth nerves. It enters the orbit through the superior orbital fissure inside the circle of zinn to supplies the lateral rectus of the same side.

Globe

This is also called the eyeball. It is a spherical structure but not a perfect sphere. Its circumference is not equally curved all over. The anterior one fifth which is called **cornea** is more curved than rest of the globe, which is called the **sclera** or the white of the eye. The anteroposterior diameter is more than other diameters. At birth the globe is smaller with a diameter of 16 mm. The diameter increases for first few years to reach 24 mm by tenth- year and remains so for rest of the life. If the diameter is less than 24 mm the eye becomes hypermetropic and if the diameter is more than 24 mm the eye becomes myopic (Fig. 1.12).

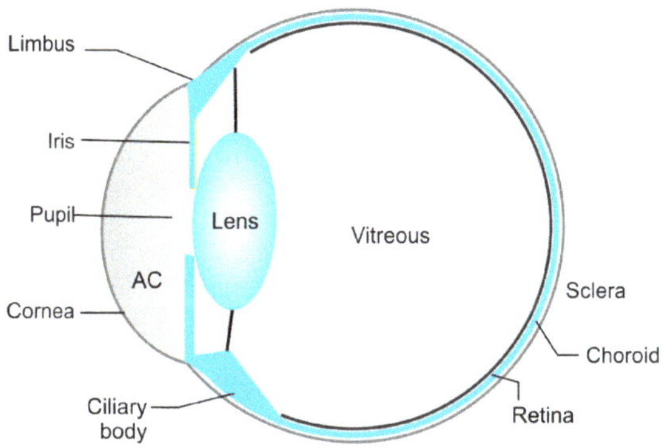

Fig. 1.12: Diagram of globe

The globe is divided into two parts:
1. A large white opaque part—**The sclera**
2. A smaller transparent parts—**The cornea**

Sclera

The sclera forms the posterior 5/6 of the globe. It extends from the optic nerve up to the cornea. The function of the sclera are:

1. Keep the inside of the globe dark.
2. Protect the intraocular structures.
3. Act as attachment for extraocular muscles.
4. Act as passage for nerves, arteries and veins to and from the inner structures.
5. It is not involved with vision.
6. It is less pain sensitive than cornea.
7. The thickness of sclera is not uniform through out. It is thickest round the optic nerve. It is almost equally thick at the junction of cornea with sclera. It is thinnest at the insertion of the recti muscles.
8. There are hardly any blood vessels in the sclera but long and short posterior ciliary vessels pass through the sclera.
9. The long and short ciliary nerves pierce the sclera to reach the uvea.
10. The sclera is covered by a loose vascular structure on the outer surfaces the conjunctiva which is separated from the globe by Tenon's capsule.

Cornea

The cornea forms the anterior one-fifth of the outer coat of the eye (globe). The main function of the cornea is **optical**. The other function is protective. The optical function of the cornea can be divided into two parts:

1. It acts as a strong convex lens of + 40 D when rays pass through the cornea (refracted). Its refractive index is 1.37.
2. It also acts as a convex mirror, when light rays are reflected from its surface. The reflected image formed by the cornea is small, erect and virtual.

Though the cornea looks circular, it is not so in fact its vertical diameter is less than horizontal diameter. The horizontal diameter is 12 mm and vertical diameter is 11 mm. This makes the vertical meridian more curved than the horizontal meridian.

The two surfaces of the cornea are not of the same curvature. The back (posterior) surface is more curved than the front surface. Thus, the cornea is thicker on the periphery and thin the center. Thus, the central cornea is weaker than the peripheral cornea.

The cornea is always wet. It is bathed in tear film in front and aqueous behind. The tear film supplies oxygen to the cornea and the aqueous gives other nutrients to the cornea.

The surface of the cornea is always bright. Loss of brightness is a sign of disease and cause fall of vision.

The cornea is almost devoid of blood vessels except near the limbus. Presence of blood vessels in the cornea denotes disease of the cornea.

The cornea is one of the most pain sensitive parts of the body. It is supplied richly by pain sensitive nerve endings which arise from the nasociliary branch of the trigeminal.

The cornea is five layered structure. The layers are (Fig. 1.13):

1. Epithelium
2. Bowman's membrane
3. Stroma
4. Descemet's membrane
5. Endothelium

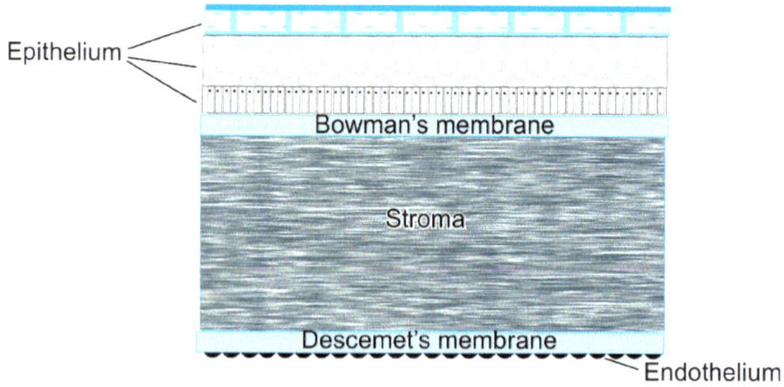

Fig. 1.13: Layers of cornea

1. Epithelium

The epithelium itself is three-layered. The epithelium is continuous with conjunctiva hence infection from conjunctiva can easily pass into the cornea. The epithelium is covered by tear film. The epithelium can be pealed off the cornea with ease. A breach in the epithelium heals quickly. A breach in epithelium can be demonstrated by instilling **fluorescein drop two percent** as bright green area. The diseased epithelial cells stain with other dyes also they are rose bengal one percent and lissamine green.

Tear Film

The eyes should always remain moist for clear vision. This is brought about by healthy tear film that covers not only cornea but also the conjunctiva. An abnormal tear film causes dryness of the cornea and conjunctiva. The condition is called **dry eye**. The tear film has three distinct layers each with special function.

The layers are—(Fig. 1.14).

1. Oily layer (lipid)
2. Watery layer (aqueous)
3. Mucus layer

The oily layer is most superficial. It is secreted by glands at the lid margin. It prevents evaporation of watery layer. The watery layer is the middle layer. It is thickest out of the other two layers. It is secreted by lacrimal and accessory lacrimal glands. It forms the greatest bulk of tear film.

The mucus layer is the innermost layer. It is secreted by goblet cells of the conjunctiva. Its function is to anchor the aqueous layer to the corneal epithelium.

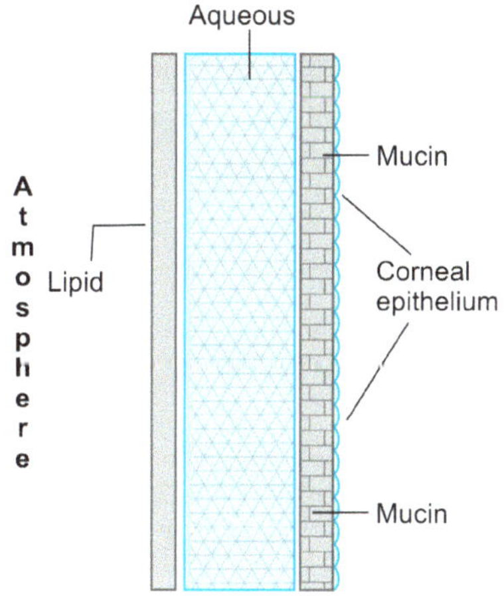

Fig. 1.14: Diagram showing various layers of tear film

The functions of the tear film are:

1. It keeps the cornea and conjunctiva wet.
2. It removes unwanted materials from the cornea and conjunctiva.
3. It forms an essential part of the optics of the cornea.
4. It provides oxygen to the cornea.
5. It provides some nutrition to the cornea.
6. It has mild anti-infective property.

Production of Tear

The main bulk of the tear is produced by the lacrimal gland. To this are added the oily secretion from the lids and mucus secretion from the goblet cell of conjunctiva. The tear is constantly produced and eliminated from the eye at a well regulated quantity. The tear production is brought by a delicate balance between the fifth nerve and the seventh nerve.

Drainage of Tear

The drainage of tear is brought about by constant blinking of the lids and pump action of the lacrimal sac. For this it is essential to have normal puncta, canaliculi, lacrimal sac and nasolacrimal ducts.

The quantity of tear present in the eye is roughly measured by a simple test called **Schirmer test**.

2. Bowman's Membrane

The **Bowman's membrane** is a thin membrane of uniform thickness. It is a strong membrane that prevents passage of infection and toxin to the deeper layer. It can not be repaired once it is destroyed.

3. Stroma

This accounts for ninety percent of bulk of cornea. It is formed by many lamellae made of collagen. They are very compact and are arranged in such a way that they do not obstruct passage of light through them. The stroma blends with the sclera hence inflammation from sclera can travel to cornea with ease.

4. Descemet's Membrane

It is a strong membrane under the stroma. It differs from Bowman's membrane in the sense that it has a capacity to regenerate.

5. Endothelium

Endothelium is the innermost layer of the cornea. The single-layered endothelium is attached to the Descemet's membrane. The endothelial cells have poor power of regeneration. The endothelial cells of the cornea are continuous with endothelial cells of the iris. The main function of the endothelium is to prevent the aqueous from getting into the stroma. The aqueous reaches the stroma when the endothelium is damaged. This results in swelling of the stroma.

Limbus

The limbus is also called **corneo scleral junction**. It is a meeting place of cornea on one side and conjunctiva and sclera on the other side. It is not well demarcated. It is roughly 1 mm wide area all around the cornea. The corneal epithelium which is four to five layered on the cornea becomes eight to ten layered on the limbus and becomes continuous with the bulbar conjunctiva. The Bowman's membrane does not reach up to the limbus but the stroma blends with the sclera. The Descemet's membrane stops as thickened band inside as Schwalbe's line. The endothelium does not reach the limbus. The limbus is highly vascular structure.

Conjunctiva

The conjunctiva may be considered as the mucous membrane of the eyeball. It spreads from the limbus to the lid margin. It is almost transparent. The sclera is visible through the normal conjunctiva. The conjunctiva is highly vascular. The vessels are very thin in normal eye. They become prominent in diseases of the conjunctiva and make the eye look red. The conjunctiva is moist. It is richly supplied by sensory nerves. It has rich lymphatic supply as well.

The conjunctiva can be divided into following parts (Figs 1.15 and 1.16):

1. Palpebral conjunctiva
2. Bulbar conjunctiva
3. Fornix

1. The palpebral conjunctiva extends from the lid margin up to the fornix. The conjunctiva that covers the lid margin is called **marginal conjunctiva**. It can not be separated from the lid margin. On the outer surface it is continuous with the skin of the lid margin.

The **tarsal conjunctiva** extends from the inner lid margin to the fornix. It is divided into two parts:

1. Tarsal conjunctiva
2. Orbital conjunctiva

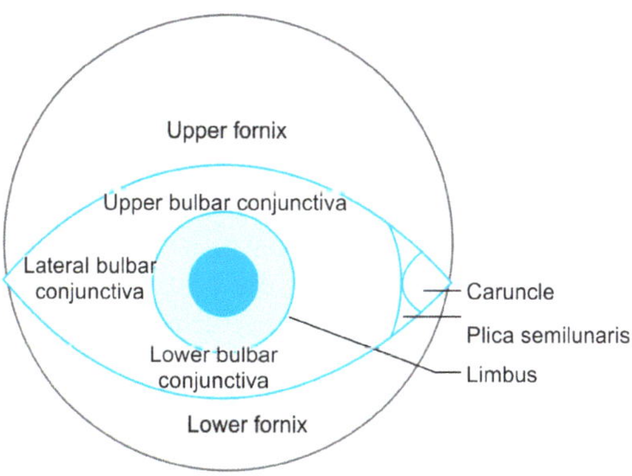

Fig. 1.15: Various parts of conjunctiva—Front view

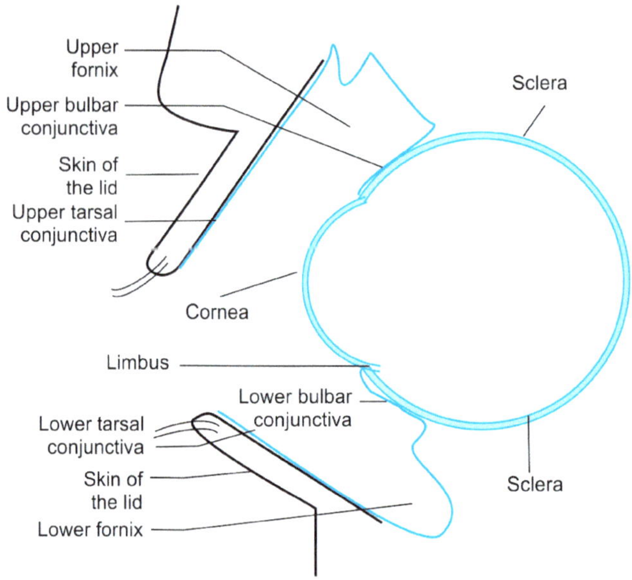

Fig. 1.16: Various parts of conjunctiva—Side view

The tarsal conjunctiva is firmly adherent to the tarsal plate. The attachment is so firm that the conjunctiva can not be separated from the tarsal plate. In normal conjunctiva the tarsal glands are visible as translucent lines. The tarsal glands are not visible in diseases of the conjunctiva. Tarsal conjunctiva is the place where papillae and follicles develop. It is a common site for fibrosis.

The orbital conjunctiva extends from the border of the tarsal plate to the fornix. The junction on either side is not well marked. It contains **Wolfring glands** that secrete mucus. The conjunctiva of the fornix is very loose. The upper fornix is larger and deeper than lower.

2. The **bulbar conjunctiva** is the largest and most visible part of the conjunctiva. It extends from the limbus to upper fornix above, to lower fornix below, medial canthus towards to nose and lateral canthus towards the ear. It can be moved over the sclera except 3 mm round the limbus, where it is firmly attached to the sclera. Due to its looseness lots of fluid can accumulate under the conjunctiva. The space under the conjunctiva is called **subconjunctival space,** where medicines can be injected. Like other parts of conjunctiva it is always moist. There are hardly any visible blood vessels in the bulbar conjunctiva unless it is diseased. The conjunctiva contains **goblet cells** that secrete mucus.
3. Fornix

The junction of the bulbar and palpebral conjunctiva form the fornices. There are four fornices, the two deep fornices and two very shallow fornices. The deep fornices are upper and lower fornix. The shallow fornices are medial and lateral. Out of two deep fornices, the upper is larger and deeper.

The conjunctiva here is thrown into folds. The conjunctiva in the fornix is very loose. The ducts of lacrimal glands and **Krause's gland** open in the upper fornix. Only Krause glands are present in the lower fornix. The upper fornix is not easily visible. It requires a special technique, i.e. **double eversion** of the upper lid to see the upper formix. The lower fornix can be examined just by pulling the lower lid.

Caruncle

The caruncle is an oval mass of fleshy tissue in between the two lids on the nasal side of the conjunctiva. It is covered by conjunctival epithelium. It contains hair follicles, sebaceous glands and sweat glands that are absent in the conjunctiva. It also contains accessory lacrimal gland, Krause's gland and goblet cells similar the conjunctiva. It does not have any definite function.

Plica Semilunaris

It is a vertical crescent shaped fold of conjunctiva between the caruncle and the limbus. It too does not have any definite purpose.

Ocular Adnexa

The ocular adnexa consists of lids with their lining and the lacrimal apparatus.

Lids

There are two lids on each side. A large upper lid and a small lower lid. The upper lid extends from the eyebrow above to the lashes of the lid up to the canthi. The lower lid extends from the cheek to the lashes at the level of canthi. When the eyes are open and looking straight, the upper lid covers upper 2 mm of the cornea and the lower lid just touches the lower limbus (Fig. 1.17). When the eyes are closed, the upper lid comes down up to the pupil and the lower lid goes up to meet the upper lid. The space between the two lids is called **interpalpebral aperture**. The junction of the two lids are called **canthi**. They are two in number one medial and one lateral canthus. The canthi are kept in place by two **canthal ligament** one on each side extending from the canthus to the orbital rim.

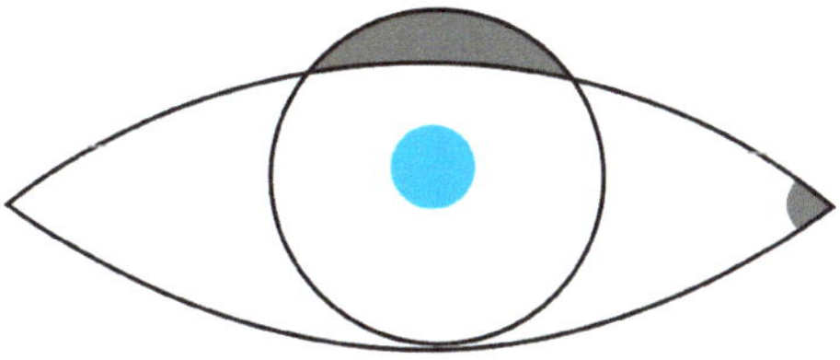

Fig. 1.17: Position of normal lid in relation to limbus and pupil

The lids act simultaneously in harmony. The upper lid covers more area than the lower lid. The main function of the lids is to protect the orbit, the eyeball and the conjunctiva. Its movement spreads the tear uniformly on the cornea and the conjunctiva. The closure of the lids forces the tear out of the conjunctival sac and drain in lacrimal sac.

The structure of both the lids are similar except the presence of a well developed **levator palpebral superior** and **Muller's muscle** in the upper lid.

Structures of the lid are (Fig. 1.18):

1. The skin
2. The fibromuscular layer
3. The conjunctiva
4. The lid margin

The skin of the lid is very thin and loosely attached to the underlying muscle **by areolar tissue**. The skin can be moved over the fibromuscular structure and lifted. The upper lid forms a well-marked horizontal crease. The skin blends with the marginal conjunctiva.

The lid margin is the transient zone between the skin in front and conjunctiva at the back. The front end is rounded, the back end is sharp. The front end contains the eye lashes. The lashes are arranged in three to four rows. The lashes of upper lid are more in number and larger than the those of the lower lid. The lashes of the upper lid are curved upwards while the lower lid lashes are curved downwards.

Two types of glands open at the root of the lashes, they are:

1. Gland of moll: These are sweat glands.
2. Gland of zeis: These are sebaceous gland.

A gray line lies between the anterior and posterior border of the lid margin just in front of the opening of the **meibomian glands**, which are modified sebaceous gland.

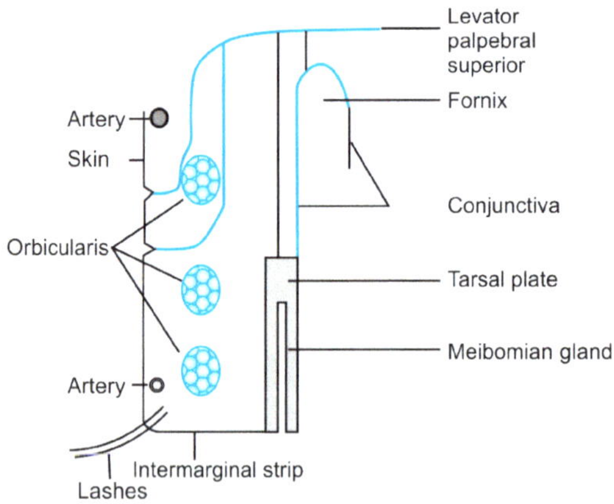

Fig. 1.18: Diagram showing vertical section of the upper lid

On the medial side of the lid margin, two millimeter from the medial canthus are two **lacrimal puncta** one in each lid.

Fibromuscular Layer of the Lid

The fibromuscular layer comprises of:

1. The septum orbitale and the tarsal plate
2. The muscles of the lid
   i. The orbicularis
   ii. The levator palpebral superior
   iii. The Muller's muscle

The **septum orbital** is a fibrous structure that extends from the periorbita of the orbit to the tarsal plate. In fact the tarsal plates are embedded in the septum orbitale. It divides the orbit in two un equal parts. A smaller **preseptal part** and a larger **postseptal part**. Its function is to prevent the contents of the orbit to bulge forward. It also gives support to the tarsal plate and prevents pre septal infection to pass into the orbit.

Tarsal Plate

Each lid in its posterior part has a fibrous structure called tarsal plate. The tarsal plate of the upper lid is larger than that of the lower lid. The function of the tarsal plate is to give firmness to the lid and support the lid. It also acts as attachment of **levator palpebral superior** in the upper lid. The tarsal plate contains the **meibomian glands**. The meibomian glands of the upper lid are larger and more in number than lower lid.

The **levator muscle in** the upper lid is attached to the top of the tarsal plate. To the lateral and medial side it is attached to lateral and medial palpebral ligament.

The posterior border of the tarsal plate is firmly attached to the tarsal conjunctiva.

Muscles of the Lid

1. **The orbicularis oculi**
   This is a striated muscle that lies in the front part of the orbit in a circular fashion. It has two parts:
   a. **Palpebral part**—This is placed in the lid and is used to close the lid lightly.
   b. **The orbital part**—This is placed mostly in the front part of the orbit and is used to close the lid tightly.
   The action of the orbicularis is to close the lids. This action is opposed by the levator palpebral which opens the lids. The orbicularis is supplied by the **seventh nerve**. Paralysis of this muscle prevents the lid from being closed and the condition is called **lagophthalmos**.
2. **The levator palpebral superior**
   This muscle is present in the upper lid. It is also a striated muscle. The function of it is to lift the upper lid. A delicate balance exist between the

levator and the orbicularis. When the orbicularis contracts, the levator relaxes and when the levator contracts the orbicularis relaxes.

The muscle takes origin from the apex of the orbit passes under the roof of the orbit in a fan shaped manner. The nasal end of the fan is attached to the medial palpebral ligament while the outer end in attached to the lateral canthal ligament.

The muscle is divided into **three parts**. The most anterior passes through the fibers of the orbicularis and is inserted in the skin of the lid.

The central part is attached to the top of the tarsal plate.

The posterior part is inserted in the conjunctiva of the upper fornix.

The muscle is supplied by the **upper division of the third nerve**. Its paralysis causes marked drooping of the upper lid. The condition is called **ptosis**.

The Muller's muscle is a small strip of unstriated muscle. It is better developed in the upper lid. It does not have any bony origin or insertion. It originates from under the surface of the levator and is attached to the orbital margin of the tarsal plate. In the lower lid it arises from the inferior rectus muscle. It is supplied by **cervical sympathetic** and not by any cranial nerve. Its paralysis causes mild drooping (ptosis) of the upper lid.

Lacrimal System

Lacrimal system consists of two parts (Fig. 1.19):

1. Structures producing tear
2. Structures draining tear

Structures producing tear consist of:

1. Main lacrimal gland
2. Accessory lacrimal glands

The main lacrimal gland is the main source of tear in the eye. It is situated at the superotemporal aspect of the orbit. It is neither visible nor can be felt by the finger. The main gland is divided into two parts—(1) orbital part, (2) palpebral part. The former is larger of the two. There are ten to twenty

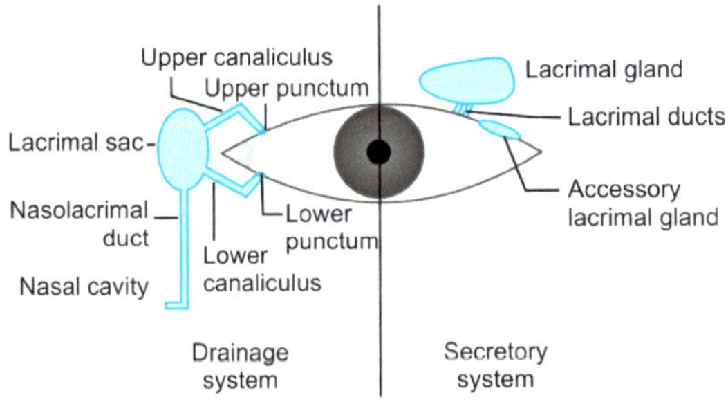

Fig. 1.19: Diagram showing lacrimal system

ducts that carry tear from the lacrimal gland to the conjunctiva. The ducts open in the conjunctival sac above the lateral end of the tarsal plate. The lacrimal sac is supplied by **trigeminal, facial** and **sympathetic nerves**.

The accessory glands play a minor role in producing tear. They are situated in the conjunctiva. They are

- Krause's gland
- Wolfring's gland
- Glands situated in the plica and caruncle
- Infraorbital glands

The structures draining the tears consist of:

1. The lids
2. Upper and lower puncta
3. Upper and lower canaliculi
4. The nasolacrimal duct

The lids by their regular blinking movements push the tear from upper fornix towards the medial canthus across the conjunctiva and the cornea. The sharp inner margin of the lower lid prevents the tear from flowing out, over the lid margin.

Puncta

There are two puncta, one in each lid on the nasal side in the lid margin about 6 mm away from the medial canthus. They are about 1mm in diameter. The lower puncta along with lower canaliculus drain 75% of tear.

Canaliculi

Each puncta has a corresponding canaliculus. Each canaliculus has a vertical and a near horizontal part, both meet at an angle. The canaliculi lie in the substance of the lid. They are not visible. The two canaliculi join each other before entering the lacrimal sac.

Lacrimal Sac

The lacrimal sac lies in the lacrimal fossa in the anterio medial part of the orbit. The upper part is dilated and rounded. The rounded area is called the **fundus of the sac**. The lower end of the sac opens in the **nasolacrimal duct**. The sac is 15 mm x 5 mm hollow structure. The sac is surrounded by bone on all sides except the front surface, which lies under the medial palpebral ligament. The normal sac is neither visible nor felt by finger unless distended.

The nasolacrimal duct is a tube that joins the lacrimal sac to the nasal cavity. It is surrounded by bones from all sides and can not be felt by fingers.

Intraocular Contents

The intraocular contents are (Fig. 1.20):
- Uvea—Iris, ciliary body, choroid
- Retina
- Vitreous
- Lens and suspensory ligament
- Aqueous

Out of the above five the first two are vascular and capable of inflammation and neoplasm. The remaining three do not have any blood supply hence are not inflicted by inflammation and new growth.

Arrangement of Intraocular Contents

The outermost layer of the eyeball is formed by the cornea and sclera, 5/6 by the sclera and remaining by the cornea. It is lined by uvea (choroid) that forms the middle coat. The innermost coat is formed by the retina. The space inside the retina filled by vitreous, **lens and the aqueous**. The lens along with its suspensory ligament divides the eyeball into two unequal chambers. A large **vitreous chamber** and a smaller **aqueous chamber**. The iris again divides the aqueous chamber into two unequal parts; one large **anterior chamber** and a **small posterior chamber**. The anterior and posterior chambers communicate through a central hole in the iris—the **pupil**. The anterior and posterior chamber are filled by a clean fluid called **aqueous humor**.

The uvea is the middle coat of the eye. It divides into three parts:
1. The iris
2. The ciliary body
3. The choroid

The iris is most anteriorly placed part of the uvea. It hangs like a curtain behind the cornea and in front of the lens. It is dark in color. Its surface is uneven with small pits in it. It divides the aqueous chamber into two parts, a large anterior chamber and small posterior chamber. They communicate with each other through circular hole in the center of the iris called the

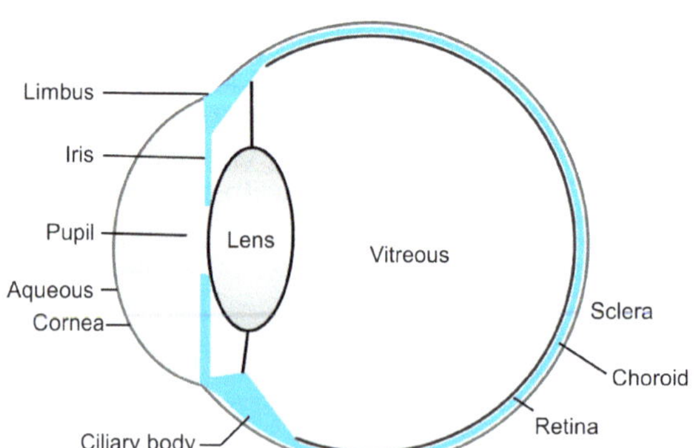

Fig. 1.20: Diagram of globe

pupil. The normal pupil is about 3.5 to 4 mm in diameter. It is smaller in children and in old age. The pupil is smaller in eyes with darker iris. It is small in hypermetropia. A pupil smaller than 2 mm is called **miotic pupil** and a pupil larger than 4 mm is called **mydriatic (dilated) pupil**. The pupil constricts in bright light and dilates in dark. The size of the pupil in both eyes in generally equal. If there is difference in size of the pupil it is called **anisocoria**. The size of the pupil can be changed by many drugs. The drugs that constrict the pupil are called **miotics**. Commonly used drug is **pilocarpine**. The drugs that dilate the pupil are called **mydriatics**. The commonly used mydriatics are **atropine**, **homatropine**, **cyclopentolate**, **tropicamide**, **adrenaline** and **phenylephrine**.

The function of the pupil are:
1. Regulate amount of light entering the eye.
2. Allow free flow of aqueous from posterior chamber to anterior chamber.

The iris arises from the ciliary body. The iris is thin at its origin from the ciliary body hence likely to be torn by injury. It is thicker at the pupillary border. The pupillary border is darker than rest of the iris.

The iris has a single-layered endothelium on its front surface. The endothelium is continuous with corneal endothelium. It is absent over the small pits seen on the front surface of the iris. They are called the **crypts of the iris**. They are the cause of roughness of the iris.

The structure behind the endothelium is called stroma. It is the thickest part of the iris. It contains blood vessels, connective tissue, iris pigment, **two nonstriated** muscle, the constrictor and the dilator muscles.

The constrictor muscle is situated round the pupil and meant to constrict the pupil. It is supplied by third nerve.

The dilator muscle is situated near the base of the iris. It is meant to dilated the pupil. It is supplied by the cervical sympathetic.

The innermost layer of the iris is the iris epithelium. It has two layers: one pigmented and the other nonpigmented. They are extension of pigmented and nonpigmented layers of the ciliary body. The pigmented layer lies behind the nonpigmented epithelium.

The reflexes that constrict the pupil are:
1. Light reflex
2. Near reflex
3. Accommodation
4. Convergence

Before going to understand pupillary reflex it is essential to understand visual path as it is intimately associated with pupillary reflex.

Visual Path

The visual path is a neural tract. It is not a reflex path. However, the afferent arm of the light reflex and the accommodation reflex pass through it (Fig. 1.21).

The visual path extends from the **retina** up to the **visual cortex**. The stimuli from the retina pass in the **optic nerve**; from there they pass in the **chiasma**. The retinal fibers arising from the temporal (outer side) pass

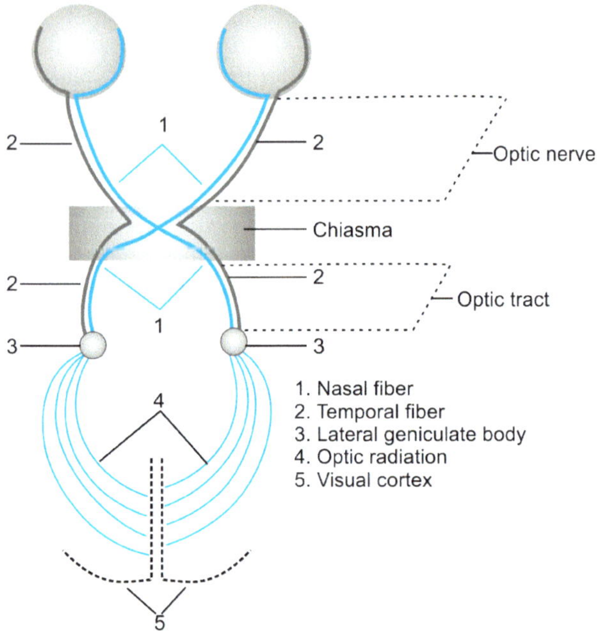

Fig. 1.21: Arrangement of retinal fiber in visual pathway

straight into the **optic tract** up to the **lateral geniculate body**, from there they pass into **optic radiation** and end in the **visual cortex** in the brain. The fibers arising from the nasal retina pass on the other side in the chiasma to pass to the optic tract, lateral geniculate body, optic radiation and visual cortex.

Thus the structures beyond the chiasma contain fibers from both the eyes.

Each reflex has **two paths**, one from the eye to the brain—this is called **afferent path** and the other is from the brain to the eye—this is called **efferent path**.

The afferent path of the light reflex (Fig. 1.22A) starts in the retina and passes through the **optic nerve—chiasma** and **optic tract**. From the optic tract it passes to the **third nerve nucleus**. In the chiasma some of the fibers cross over the other side. Thus each optic tract contains afferent fibers from both eyes. Hence when light is thrown in one pupil both the pupil constrict.

The efferent path starts in the third nerve nucleus, pass along lower division of the third nerve to the **ciliary ganglion**. From ciliary ganglion it pass into **short ciliary nerves** and end in sphincter pupillae.

Near Reflex

This consist of two reflexes: (1) the accommodation reflex, (2) the convergence reflex, which happen simultaneously but have different pathways.

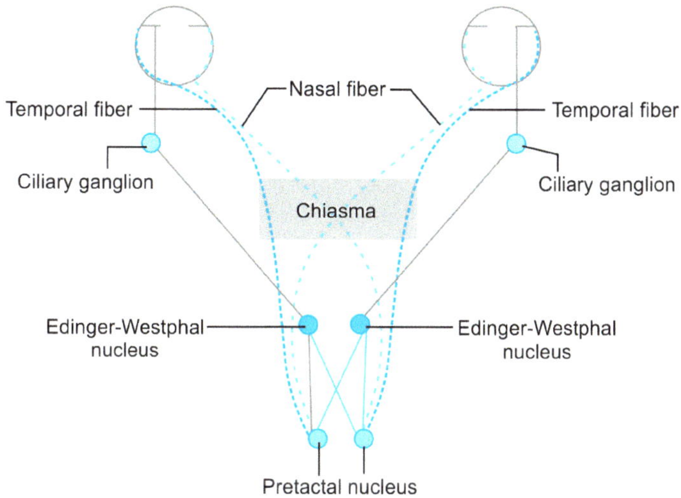

Fig. 1.22A: Path of light (Pupilary reflex)

Accommodation Reflex

The term accommodation means ability to see small objects at 30 cm. **The afferent path for accommodation** passes through optic nerve—chiasma—optic tract of the same side up to lateral geniculate body—striate cortex—para striate (Fig. 1.22B).

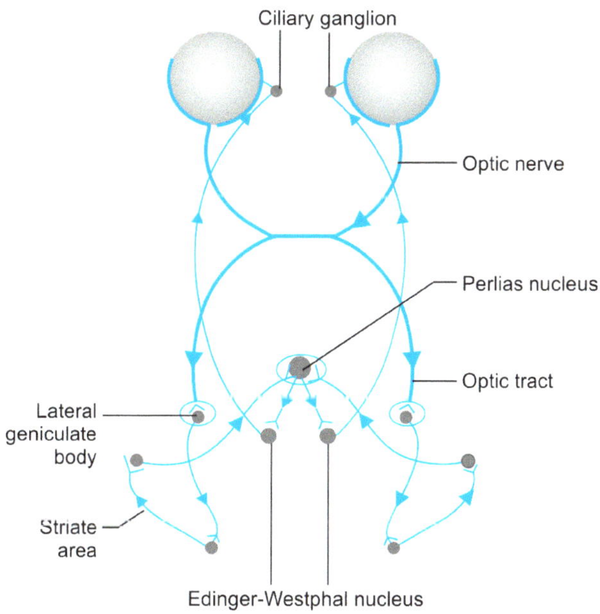

Fig. 1.22B: Pathway of accommodation

The efferent path starts in the third nerve nucleus, passes through the third nerve to the ciliary ganglion and ends in the ciliary body and iris.

Convergence Reflex (Fig. 1.22C)

The exact path of the convergence reflex is not well understood.

The **afferent path** most probably starts in the **medial rectus** from where it passes into the **third nerve** that takes it to the **mesencephalic nucleus** of fifth nerve from where it goes to the **convergence center** from there it goes to the **third nerve nucleus** and reaches the **ciliary ganglion**.

The three phenomenon: the constriction of pupil, accommodation and convergence go together when the eyes try to see small objects kept at near point, i.e. 30 cm

Ciliary Body

The ciliary body lies behind the iris and anterior to the choroid. In fact the iris arises from the ciliary body. The junction of the ciliary body to choroid is not well demarcated.

The ciliary body is triangular in shape with its apex towards the choroid and the base towards the lens. To the base are attached the suspensory ligaments of the lens. The outer wall of the triangle is parallel to the sclera with a potential space in between. The outer end of the base of the triangle is firmly attached to the sclera at **scleral spur**. The inner wall is divided into two parts—the **pars plicata** which contain **ciliary processes** and an avascular part called **pars plana**.

The ciliary body has a large stroma which is lined by epithelium on the inner side.

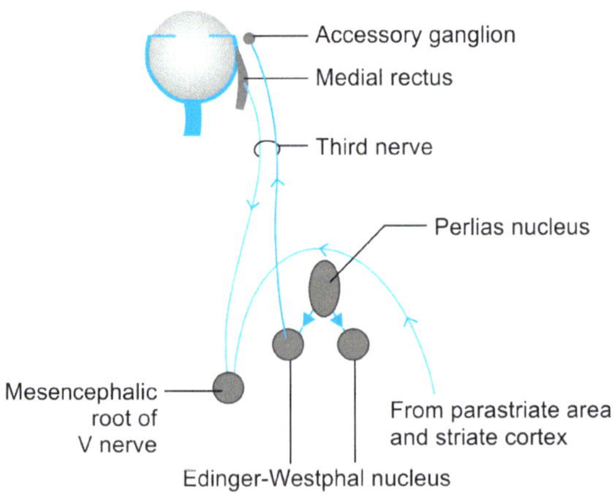

Fig. 1.22C: Path of convergence

The stroma is mostly made up of the ciliary muscles which are surrounded by connective tissue, vessels and nerves. The ciliary body is richly supplied by blood vessels. The ciliary muscles are unstriated. There are three types of muscles in the ciliary body:

1. The longitudinal muscles
2. The circular muscles
3. The oblique muscles

The ciliary muscles are supplied by parasympathetic via **short ciliary nerve**.

The ciliary body on its inner surface is covered by two layers of epithelium:

1. **The pigmented epithelium**: It is continuation of pigment epithelium of the iris in front and pigment epithelium of the retina behind.
2. **The nonpigmented epithelium** is continuation of nonpigmented epithelium of iris in front and sensory retina behind.

Ciliary Processes

These finger like projection arise from the pars plicata. Each process has a double-layered wall made up of ciliary epithelium. They are 60 to 70 in number. They contain a tuft of blood vessels. The main function of the ciliary processes is to form aqueous.

The functioning of the ciliary body are:

1. From its base arise
   a. The iris anteriorly
   b. The suspensory ligament of the lens in the middle.
2. It is responsible for accommodation.
3. It produces aqueous humor.

Aqueous Humor

The aqueous humor is a crystal clear fluid that fills both the posterior and anterior chamber, aqueous is formed in the ciliary processes at a constant rate in the posterior chamber from where it passes into the anterior chamber there it moves by convection current and leaves the anterior chamber via angle of anterior chamber (Fig. 1.23).

The function of the aqueous humor are:

1. Optical.
2. It provides nutrition to the lens and cornea.
3. It maintains intraocular tension.
4. It removes waste products.

Chambers of the Eye

As discussed earlier the lens along with its ligaments divide the interior of the eye in two unequal chamber—A large **vitreous chamber** and a small **aqueous chamber**. The former contains vitreous and the later contains

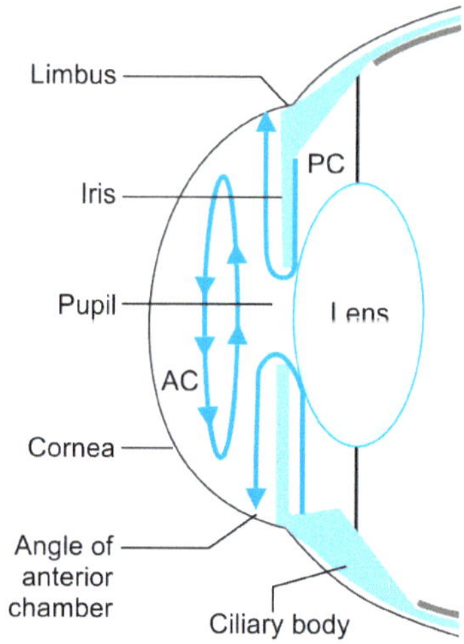

Fig. 1.23: Diagram showing circulation of aqueous

aqueous. The iris divides the aqueous chamber into two chambers agains a **large anterior chamber** (AC) and a **small posterior chamber** (PC) both are joined by the pupil.

The anterior chamber is a space bounded by the cornea in front and the iris, pupil and the lens behind. If the lens is absent the posterior boundary is formed either by anterior surface of IOL after cataract or vitreous as the case may be (see aphakia and pseudophakia). The two surfaces meet on the periphery to form the **angle of anterior chamber**. The angle is not impervious structure, it contains a sieve like structure called **trabecular meshwork** which opens in **canal of Schlemm** which in turn is joined to **episcleral vein** by a narrow **aqueous vein**. The anterior chamber does not have an uniform depth. It is deepest in center and is abolished at the angle of anterior chamber.

The posterior chamber is bound by iris, pars plicata of ciliary body, suspensory ligament and lens. The ciliary processes project in the posterior chamber and pour aqueous in the posterior chamber. The posterior chamber communicates with the anterior chamber through the pupil.

Formation of Aqueous Humor

There are three mechanisms involved in its production—**Secretion**, **ultra-filtration** and **diffusion**.

The aqueous is 99% water, remaining part is made up of solids dissolved in it. They are protein, ascorbic acid, sodium, potassium, urea and enzymes to name a few. The aqueous is formed constantly by the ciliary process at constant rate. The aqueous leaves the anterior chamber at a constant rate. There is a delicate balance between production and drainage of aqueous.

The production can be reduced by many drugs. The drainage can be reduced due to obstruction of the flow. The two common sites of obstruction are pupil and angle of the anterior chamber.

Choroid

The choroid is the largest part of the uvea. It extends from the pars plana to the optic nerve. It lies between the sclera, and the retina. There is a potential space between the choroid and the sclera it is called the **suprachoroidal space**. The choroid supplies blood to the retina specially the macula.

The choroid is very vascular. The vessels are held together by connective tissue. **There is no muscles in choroid**. The choroid is heavily pigmented hence black. The blood vessels of choroid are of three sizes, i.e. the large, medium and fine. The latter are called choriocapillaries which are responsible for blood supply to the retina. Between the retina and the choriocapillaries lies a thin membrane called **Bruch's membrane** which is attached to the pigment epithelium of the retina.

The function of the choroid are:
1. To supply nutrition to outer layers of the retina.
2. It keeps the inside of the eyeball dark.

Blood Supply of the Uvea

The uvea gets its blood supply from two sources:
1. Posterior ciliary arteries
2. Anterior ciliary arteries

Both are branches of **ophthalmic artery** which is the main source of blood supply to the eye and its adnexa.

Ophthalmic artery has twelve branches in the orbit. Out of which only two, the **posterior ciliary arteries** and the **muscular branches** supply the uvea. The twigs of the muscular branches that supply the uvea are called **anterior ciliary artery**.

The short posterior ciliary arteries are ten to twenty in number. They enter the sclera in a circular fashion round the optic nerve and divide to form choriocapillaries.

The long posterior arteries are two in number, one nasal (inner) and the other temporal (outer). They enter the sclera in front of short ciliary arteries one on each side and reach the ciliary body.

Anterior Ciliary Arteries

They enter the sclera 5 mm away from the limbus in front of the insertion of the recti muscles. They enter the ciliary body and join the posterior ciliary artery to form the **major circle of iris**. The major circle give branch to ciliary body, the ciliary process and recurrent branch. From the major circle of iris arise smaller branches that form the **minor circle of iris**. The venous drainage of the uveal tract is via four venae vorticosae.

Retina

The retina is the most developed neural part of the eye concerned with vision, color vision, vision in bright light (photopic), vision in dull light (night vision or scotopic vision) field of vision.

It is the innermost layer of the three coats of the eyeball and placed between the vitreous and the choroid. It extends from the optic nerve to the periphery of the choroid the **ora serrata**. The retina is firmly attached in these two places.

The retina is transparent but looks pink due to the pigments in the retinal pigment epithelium, visual purple in the rods and underlying choroidal blood vessels. The retina looses its transparency when diseased.

The retina develops from the two layers of the optic cup with a potential space in between. The retina can be divided into two parts, i.e. the layer of retinal pigment epithelium and sensory retina. The retinal pigment epithelium is attached to the Bruch's membrane.

The sensory retina has **three types of cells**:

1. Visual cells, the rods and cones
2. The bipolar cells
3. The ganglion cells

It has **two limiting membranes**, the external limiting and inner limiting membrane.

The **two nuclear layers**: The outer and inner nuclear layers.

The **plexiform layers**—The outer and inner and single layer of **ganglion cells** and nerve **fiber layer**.

Thus retina is ten-layered structured all over except at the macula and ora serrata. All the layers except the nerve fiber layer stop at the margin of the optic disc. The nerve fibers pass through the lamina to form the optic nerve. As there are no visual cells in the optic nerve head it has no visual sensation and forms the **blind spot**.

The retina is not uniformly thick all through. It is thinnest at ora serrata and thickest at the posterior pole.

The two visual elements too are not uniformly distributed. The **cones** which are concerned with central vision, day vision and color vision are maximum at the macula and scanty on the periphery. **The rods** which are concerned with night vision and peripheral vision are maximum on the periphery. The peripheral retina has very poor color sense.

The macula is an ill defined circular zone 5.5 mm in diameter, is the most sensitive part of the retina. It is situated in the posterior pole on the outer side of the disc. The central 0.35 mm is called **foveola**, it is surrounded by a zone 1.5 mm in diameter called **fovea**. The foveola is situated about 3 mm away from the temporal border of the disc. It is a small depression. It has only internal limiting membrane. All other layers are absent at foveola.

The retina has **double blood supply**. (1) The outer four layers get blood supply from the choriocapillaries. (2) The inner six layers get their blood supply from central retinal artery and its branches. The retinal arteries do not anastomose (mix) with each other (Fig. 1.24).

The central retinal artery is a branch of **ophthalmic artery**. It arises from the ophthalmic artery at the apex of the orbit and runs under the optic nerve. It enters the optic nerve from its under surface 10 mm behind the globe and takes central position in the nerve. It enters the globe at the center of the disc and divides into two branches—a superior branch and an inferior branch. Each divide into two branches again—one medial (towards nose) and other temporal (towards the ear) in curved fashion. Each keep on branching till it reaches the ora serrata. The temporal branches curve round the macula but do not give branches to the macula.

The retinal veins correspond with the artery at the places they cross the artery and the area is called **arteriovenous junction**.

Nerve Supply of the Eye

The uveal nerve supply can be divided into two parts:

1. Sensory via trigeminal—Nasociliary
2. Motor via oculomotor—Parasympathetic and sympathetic (iris and ciliary body)
   i. Of all the intraocular structure only iris and ciliary body are capable of movement.
   ii. The choroid and retina do not show any movement.
   iii. **The retina has no pain sensation**. The nerve supply to the eye can be divided into:
      a. Sensory supply to cornea and sclera by nasociliary

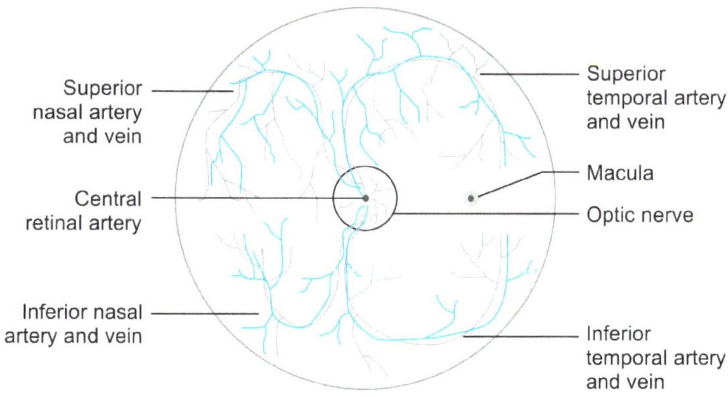

Fig. 1.24: Diagram showing retinal vessels

Note: Macula is not supplied by retinal vessels. The optic nerve gets blood supply partly from central retinal artery

b. Sensory supply to uvea by nasociliary
c. Motor supply to iris and ciliary process by:
   I. Parasympathetic
   II. Sympathetic

The nerves that supply the uvea are collectively called **ciliary nerves**. They are of two types:
1. Short posterior cililary
2. Long ciliary

The **short posterior ciliary nerves** are about 15 in number. They arise from the ciliary ganglion and carry both sensory as well as autonomic (motor) nerve. They enter the globe round the optic nerve. **The long ciliary** nerves are two in number. They arise from nasociliary nerve. They are mostly sensory. They are mostly parasympathetic in nature but have few sympathetic fibers as well.

The **long ciliary nerves are two** in number. They enter the globe one on each side of the optic nerve. They arise directly from the nasociliary nerve and carry mostly sensory fibers and few sympathetic fibers.

Lens

The adult normal lens is transparent structure that concentrates light rays on the retina. It is placed in front of the vitreous and behind the iris. The pupil allows the light to pass through it. It is suspended from the ciliary body. The lens when seen from front looks circular and when seen from sides it is elliptical and biconvex. At birth it is spherical. The diameter of the adult lens is 9 mm to 10 mm and thickness is 4.5 mm in the center. It has a front (anterior) and a back (posterior) surface. The anterior surface is less curved than the posterior surface. The place where the two surfaces meet is called the **equator of the lens** and is rounded. The center of the anterior surface is called **anterior pole**. This lies in the center of the pupil. The center of the posterior surface is called **posterior pole**.

The adult lens is semisolid. The lens of childhood is soft.

The structure of the lens are—(Figs 1.25 and 1.26):
1. Capsule
2. Epithelium
3. Fibers
   i. Cortex
   ii. Nucleus
4. Suspensory ligament

The **capsule** is single-layered structure that surrounds the lens on all the sides. It is not of equal thickness. It is thickest at the equator and thin at the poles. The posterior pole is thinnest. The overall thickness of the front capsule is more than the capsule at the back.

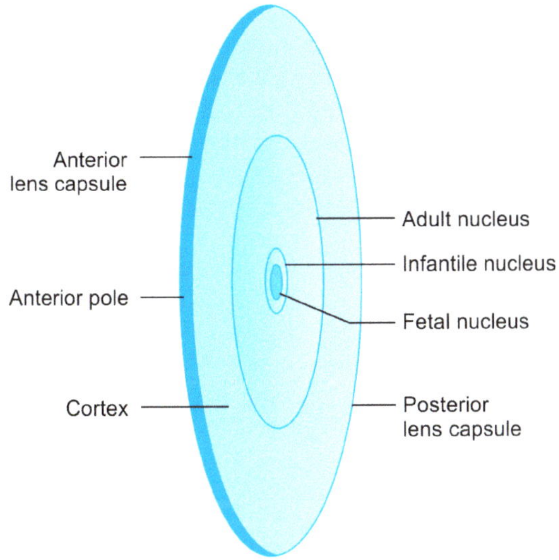

Fig. 1.25: Side view of the normal lens showing various parts

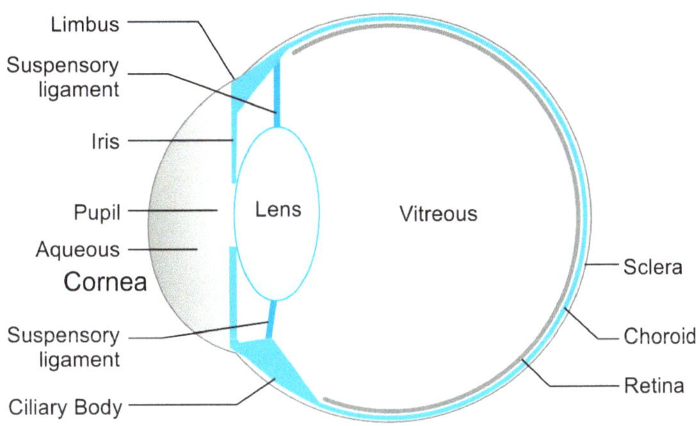

Fig. 1.26: Diagram of globe

Lens Epithelium

This comprises of single-layer of cubical cell. It is present only in the front surface under the capsule. The cells of the epithelium become long at the equator. They keep on increasing in length and multiply due to repeated division. The old elongated cells are pushed toward the center.

Fibers

The so called fibers are nothing but elongated epithelial cells. The old cells loose their nuclei. The process of elongation and division continue throughout the life. The oldest fibers become central most and compressed to form various zones of nucleus and each zone has a separate name according to time of their development. These are **embryonal**. They contain the oldest fibers laid down between one to three months of pregnancy. It is the smallest nucleus. The fibers laid over this between birth to puberty form the **infantile nucleus**. Nucleus formed after this is called **adult nucleus**.

The remaining part of the fibers that surround the nucleus from all sides is **called cortex**.

The suspensory ligament (zonules) are not true parts of the lens. There development is different from development of the lens. They originate in the ciliary body arising from both pars plana as well as pars plicata. They are inserted in the capsule at the equator. Their functions are to keep the lens in place. Suspensory ligament and lens form a barrier between the aqueous and vitreous chamber. Contraction of suspensory ligament change curvature of lens.

Action of the Lens

The lens has only one function that is to focus the rays of light on the retina from various distances by changing the curvature of the lens, thus changing the power of the lens. The ability to change the power of the lens is called **accommodation**. More is the curvature, more is the power. The other causes of increased power is increase in the refractive index of the lens. The refractive index of the transparent lens is 1.43. The total power of the lens is +15 to +16 D. The change in the refractive power can also be brought about if the water content of the lens is increased. This happens in diabetes and immature cataract.

Nutrition of the Lens

The adult **lens is avascular**. The sole nutrition of the lens comes from the aqueous after birth. During its development it gets its nutrition from a vascular envelop called **tunica vasculosa lens** that surrounds the lens from all sides.

The lens is 66% water and 33% protein. If the protein is denatured the lens fibers loose transparency.

Vitreous

Of all the intraocular structures the vitreous is largest in volume. It occupies two-thirds of the globe. It is an inert gel that extends from the back of the lens to the optic disc. It comes in contact with the retina from ora serrata to the margin of the disc. It is firmly attached to the ora serrata by a band of vitreous 4 mm wide. This is called the **vitreous base**. It has weak attachment at the macula. Its attachment to the back of the lens is very strong in children but gradually becomes loose. The bond between the lens and the vitreous is absent after 50 years of age. The vitreous does not have a formed capsule. Its periphery is more condensed than the rest and is called its capsule.

Rest of the vitreous is called cortex. The vitreous is 90% water to which are dissolved hyaluronic acid and polysaccharides.

The vitreous is a semisolid gel. It gets liquefied in disease and following injury. Its main function is optical. The other important function is to keep the retina in place. It also maintains the shape of the eye. It is avascular after birth. It has a low metabolism. It gets nutrition from the aqueous and the retina.

Development of the Eyes (Embryology)

The eye develops from the central nervous system that itself develops from neuroectoderm. The eye is not fully neuroectodermal in origin. The surface ectoderm and mesoderm also contribute in its development (Fig. 1.27).

The eyes start developing from very early stage of pregnancy when the embryo is only 2.6 mm in length, i.e. between second and third week of conception. The eyes grow out of the developing forebrain. Out of

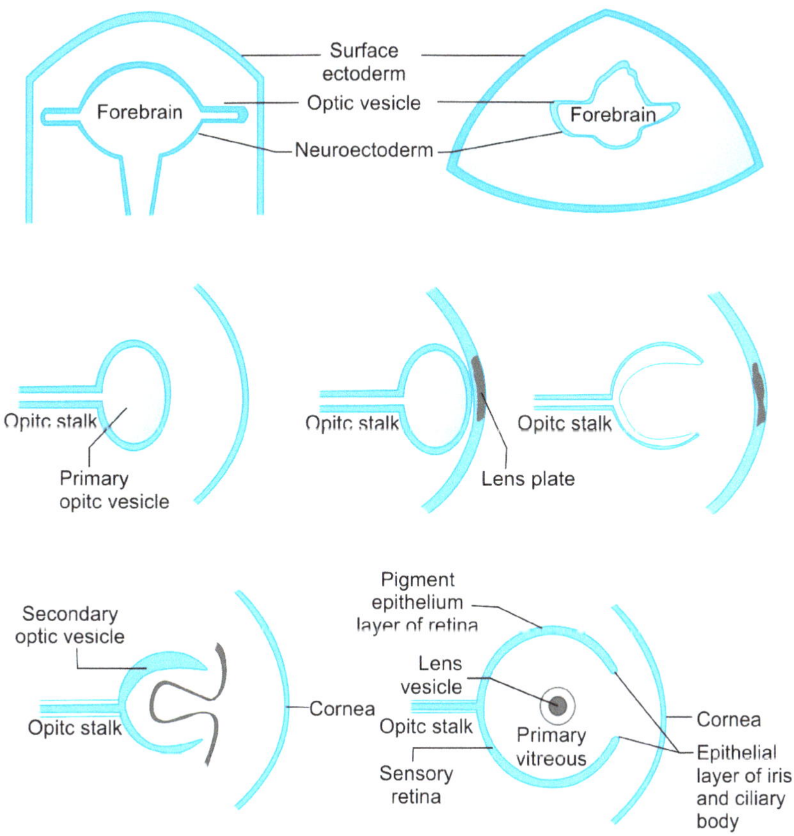

Fig. 1.27: Development of the eye

three germinal layers of the developing fetus (embryo): the ectoderm, the mesoderm and the endoderm, only the first two take part in development of the eyes. The ectoderm is divided into two types—the neuroectoderm and **surface ectoderm**.

To begin with the developing head of the embryo is two layered:

1. An outer covering of surface ectoderm.
2. A tube of neuroectoderm inside.

As the embryo grows the forebrain develops two pouches one on each side of the forebrain. The pouches are called **primary optic vesicles**. The primary optic vesicles is continuous with the forebrain by a narrow tube called the **optic stalk**, which is the future optic nerve.

As the primary optic vesicle grows it reaches the surface ectoderm. This starts two different type of changes (1) one in the primary optic vesicle and the (2) other in the surface ectoderm. The surface of the primary optic vesicle that comes in contact with the surface ectoderm becomes concave and grows backward making the primary optic vesicle two layered, at this stage it is called **secondary optic vescicle**, which ultimately develops into retina. From the outer wall develops the pigment layer while the inner layer gives rise to sensory retina. The structure is now called as **optic cup**. The two layers of the optic cup are continuous at the rim of the optic cup. From the tip of the cup develop the ciliary epithelium and pigment epithelium of the iris.

The primary optic vesicle undergoes the following changes:

Primary optic vesicle → Secondary optic vesicle → Optic cup → Retina, ciliary epithelium and pigment epithelium of the iris.

The surface ectoderm undergoes many changes.

The place where the primary optic vesicle touches the surface ectoderm thickness and the thickened area is called the **lens plate**. The lens plate rapidly grows and becomes concave and the structure is now known the **lens pit**. This deepens further, the two edges of the pit come together and join each other. Thus a hollow spherical structure is formed. This is called **lens vesicle**. This separates from the surface ectoderm and is pushed into the optic cup to be converted into a lens.

In the meantime the gap in the surface ectoderm disappears and from this surface ectoderm will develop the corneal epithelium, the conjunctival epithelium and the lid folds.

The optic cup closes from above downward and the gap between the two edges is called the **fetal fissure** through which the **hyaloid artery** enters the optic cup to supply nutrition to the lens before birth. The hyaloid artery extends from optic cup to the lens. Once the lens has developed and started getting its nutrition, the hyaloid artery gradually disappear. The vitreous develops from three sources, i.e. the surface ectoderm, the neuroectoderm and mesoderm in three stages, i.e. primary, secondary and tertiary vitreous. The mesoderm surrounding the optic cup given rise to sclera, extraocular muscles and part of the lower and outer walls of the orbit.

CHAPTER

2

The Physiology of the Eyes and Optics

THE PHYSIOLOGY OF THE EYE

The physiology of the eyes can be broadly divided into:

1. Physiology of vision
2. Binocular vision
3. Aqueous humor and intraocular pressure
4. Metabolism of the ocular structures
   1. The physiology of vision can further be divided into:
      - i. Optics of the eye
      - ii. Visual sensation
        - a. Light sensation
        - b. Form sensation
        - c. Color sensation
      - iii. Photochemical and electrical changes
      - iv. Neurology of vision
        - a. Visual path
        - b. Accommodation
        - c. Convergence

OPTICS OF THE EYE

The eye acts as an advanced form of camera.

In the camera an inverted small image is formed on the photographic film which retains the invisible image by a photochemical process. The image becomes visible by another set of chemical changes brought about by process called developing of the picture.

To have good picture, a camera requires an aperture, a lens system, a focusing system for various distance a timing system to suit the illumination and a film to retain the image.

The eye has all these properties. The aperture is the pupil. The dioptric system is the lens. The focusing system is accommodation, the timing system is provided by adaptation, the film is replaced by retina. The image formed on the retina is processed by the brain and the image is stored in the memory. All the images formed in the retina retain their original color.

Dioptric System of the Eye

The dioptric system of the eye consists of **cornea**, **aqueous**, **lens** and **vitreous**. All these when combined together act as a convex lens of +60 dioptre that has a focal length of roughly 24 mm which is equal to the distance between cornea and the retina. Thus parallel rays are brought to focus on the retina after they have been refracted by various media when accommodation is at rest.

The dioptre power of the eye can be divided into two parts:

1. Corneal dioptre
2. Combination of lens, aqueous and vitreous

Out of the two systems, the cornea contributes +43 D. The refractive index of the cornea is 1.37. The dioptric values of cornea can not be changed reflexly. It can be altered only by changing its curvature either due to disease (keratoconus), contact lens or by surgery. The remaining power is provided by combination of aqueous, lens and vitreous. The refractive index of aqueous is 1.33, the lens 1.43 and vitreous 1.33. The dioptric power of normal lens is +17 dioptre. Unlike cornea the dioptric power of the lens can be changed by a reflex process called accommodation.

> Dioptre (diopter) is an unit of measurement of converging power (positive or negative) of lens. It is reciprocal of—focal length in meters. A lens of one dioptre will have a focal length of 1 m and a lens of 10 dioptre will have focal length of 10 cm. Thus stronger a lens, shorter will be the focal length.

VISUAL SENSATION

The visual sensation are due to stimulation of the retina by light in the range of 400 to 800 nanometer (nm) commonly referred to as white light which is made up of seven colors of rainbow (VIBGYOR). Out of them only red, blue and green are involved in color vision. Wave length less than 379 nm (ultraviolet) and more than 720 nm (infrared) are not visible.

The light sensation is ability of the retina to feel its presence and intensity. It is evaluated by light minimum.

Light minimum is the smallest amount of light which can be felt by the retina to start the visual sensation. It depends on adaptation of the light. An eye can either be **dark adapted** or **light adapted**. An eye is said to be dark adapted when the eye can see an object in the dim lit area. Conversely ability to see in bright light is called light adapted. The vision in the light is called day vision (**photopic vision**) and in the dark is called night vision or (**scotopic vision**).

Form Sense

This is ability to appreciate the shape of an object. Ability of a person to correctly read the letters on Snellen's chart is an example of the faculty. This depends on the efficiency of the cones. It is best in the macula and is reduced on the periphery. The vision in the area 30° all-round the macula is called **central vision** and vision beyond 30° is called **peripheral vision**.

Color Sense

Color sense is most developed in humans. The animals are thought to have very poor color sense. The color sense is ability to differentiate between chemical response due to excitement of cones by light of different wave length.

The white light, i.e. the light without any visible color is in fact combination of seven different wave lengths ranging from 400 nm to 700 nm. They are violet, indigo, blue, green, yellow, orange and red.

Out of these red, blue and green are called **primary colors**. All colors are combination of these colors in different proportion. A color is said to be pure when it is not mixed with white. When all color receptors are stimulated the light looses all colors and the light is called white light. When none of the receptors are stimulated, the result is black color. Color receptors are present only in cones hence color vision is present only in photopic vision (day vision). In dark all the colors look gray of different shades.

There are two theories of color vision:

1. **Young-Helmholtz theory** states that three color perceiving elements in the cones, are red (570 nm), green (535 nm) and blue (455 nm).
2. **Hering theory**—This states that there are three visual substance which are responsible for all colors. They are:
   white—black, red—green and blue – yellow

Color Blindness

Abnormal color sense is called color blindness. It is not a type of blindness. It is better called **abnormal color sense**.

About 8% of male population has abnormal color sense. It is a hereditary condition, present at birth does not progress and there is no cure for the condition. There are many methods to screen color blindness. Commonest is Ishihara color plates see figure 4.24.

PHOTOCHEMICAL AND ELECTRICAL CHANGES THAT INITIATE VISION

Photochemical Changes

The **rods** and **cones** contain two different types of pigments. The rods contain **rhodopsin** and the cones contain **iodopsin**. The mechanism of action of both is the same (Flow chart 2.1).

The electrical changes are transmitted **through the bipolar and ganglion** cells to the optic nerve which transmits it through the visual path to visual cortex.

Flow chart 2.1: Mechanism of rhodopsin metabolism

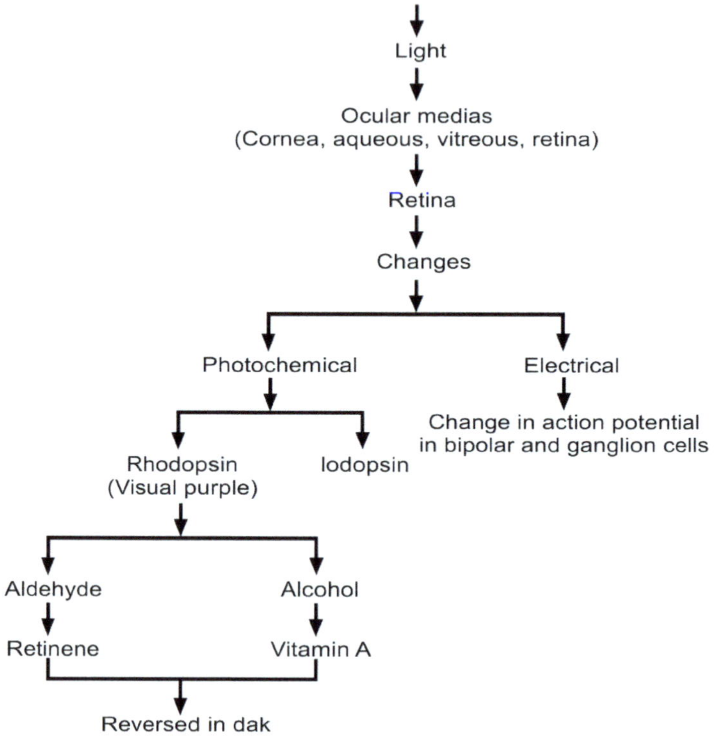

The electrical changes can be recorded on:

Electroretinogram (ERG)
Electrooculograph (EOG)
Visual evoked response

All the above are used to diagnose various types of blindness due to lesions of visual path at different levels.

Neurology of Vision

This consist of two pathways and three reflexes.

The pathways are:

1. Visual pathway
2. Pupillary pathway.

The reflexes are:

1. Light reflex
2. Accommodation reflex
3. Convergence reflex.

The visual pathway extends from the retina to the visual cortex in the brain. Part of the visual path is shared by the three reflexes.

Clinically the visual path is divided into following parts—(Fig. 2.1):

1. Retina
2. Optic nerve
3. Chiasma
4. Optic tract
5. Lateral geniculate body
6. Optic radiation
7. Visual cortex

The visual path consists of **three neurons**. (1) The first neuron starts in the rods and cones, and ends in bipolar cells of inner nuclear layer of the retina. (2) The second neuron starts from the ganglion cells and extends up to the lateral geniculate body. It has two synapses, one with the first neuron and second in the lateral geniculate body. (3) The third neuron starts from the lateral geniculate body to the visual cortex.

The distribution of the fibers in the tract varies from site-to-site. The position of fibers in the retina is shown in (Figs 2.2 and 2.3).

The retinal fibers enter the optic nerve. Each optic nerve contain **temporal**, **macular** and **nasal fibers**. Near the chiasma, the macular fibers become central. The temporal fibers occupy more space than the nasal. In the chiasma the temporal fibers pass straight to the optic tract of the same side but the nasal fibers cross over the optic tract of the opposite side. Thus, each optic tract contains temporal fibers of one side and nasal fibers of the other side. This arrangement continues in lateral geniculate body, optic radiation and optic tract. However, the relation between the fibers change.

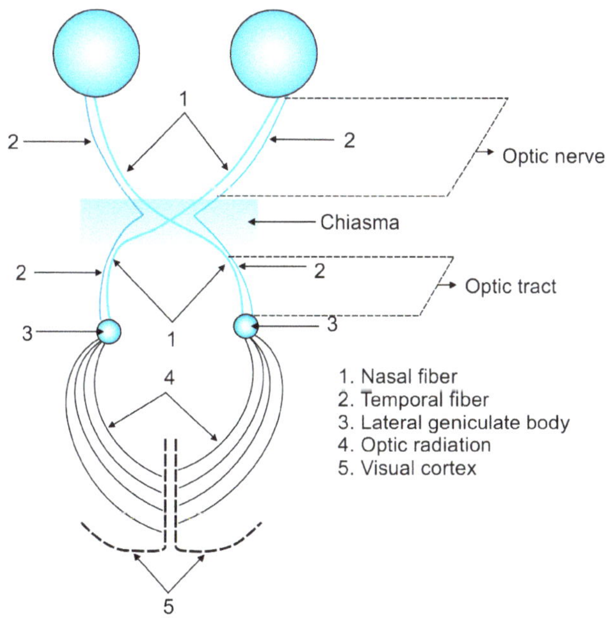

Fig. 2.1: Parts of visual pathway

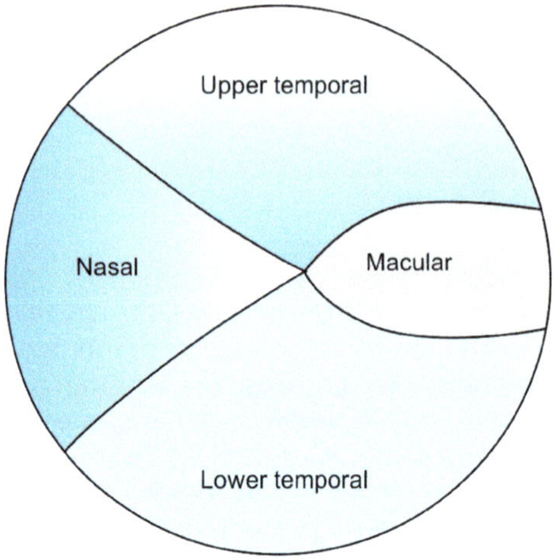

Fig. 2.2: Distribution of fibers at the back of the globe

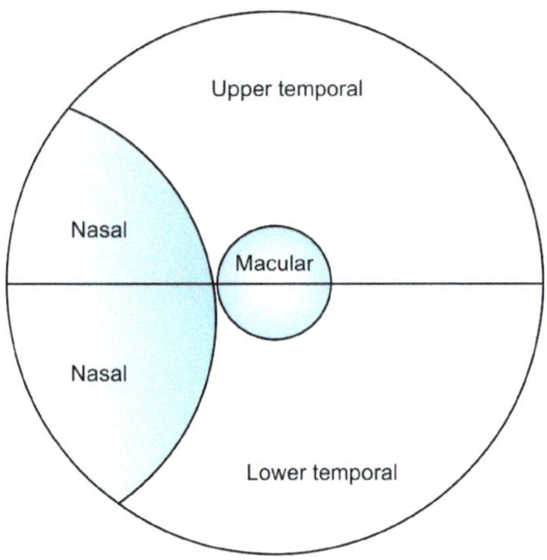

Fig. 2.3: Distribution of fibers near the beginning of the chiasma

Figure shows field changes due to disease at different levels (Figs 2.4 and 2.5).

Visual Fields

When a person looks at an object, he not only sees the object but also objects surrounding this object in three dimension. This area round the object of interest is the field of vision. Vision is not equal all-over the field. It is best at the point of fixation and gradually diminishes away form point of fixation. There is no vision outside the field of vision.

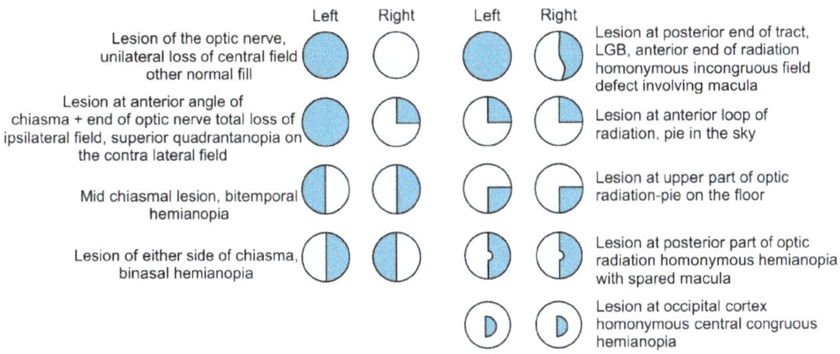

Fig. 2.4: Typical field changes at various levels of left visual path

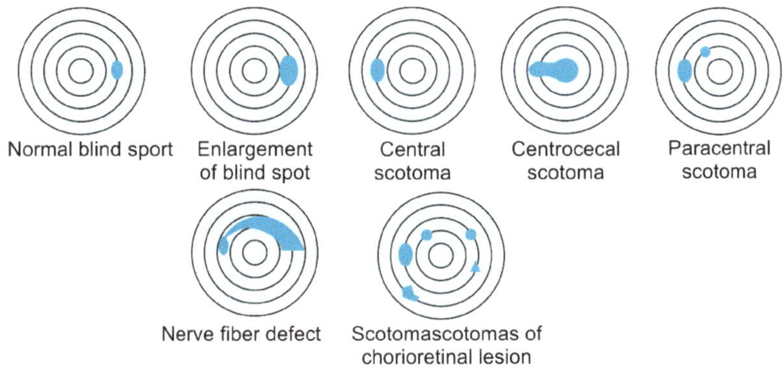

Fig. 2.5: Examples of central field changes

The **normal field of vision** is defined as "Island of vision surrounded by sea of blindness". In fact the island of vision is shaped as a hill which has best vision at the top (Fig. 2.6).

The normal field of vision of any eye is not a circle. It extends 60° above, 60° nasal, 75° below and 100 to 110° temporal from the point of fixation. The field of vision of both eyes is far larger than that of one eye.

Defects in field of vision are called **scotomas**. They have many shapes and sizes, depending upon the area of visual path involved.

> As the optic nerve has no vision, it acts as a natural scotoma and called the blind spot. It represents a deep well in the island of vision.

There are two types of fields:

1. Peripheral—This is 60° x 60° x 75° x 110° (Fig. 2.7)
2. Central—This is limited to 30° all-round the point of fixation (Fig. 2.8)

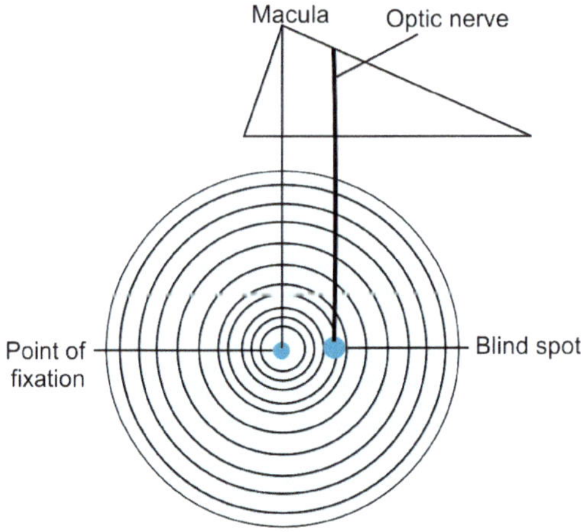

Fig. 2.6: Island of vision surrounded by sea of blindness. Hill of vision best vision at point of fixation. No vision in blind spot that represent optic nerve head

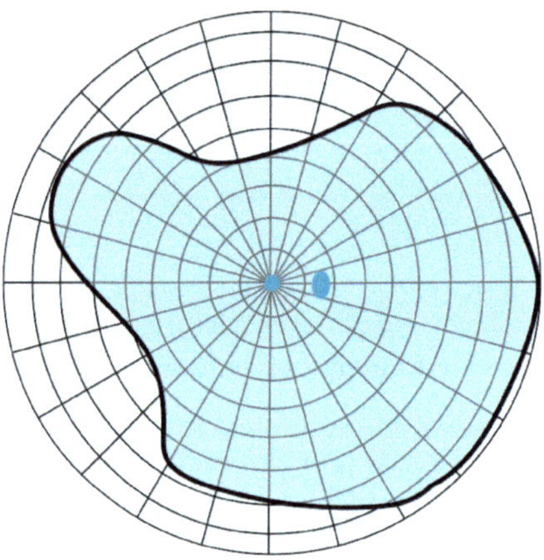

Fig. 2.7: Perimetry chart for peripheral field (right eye)

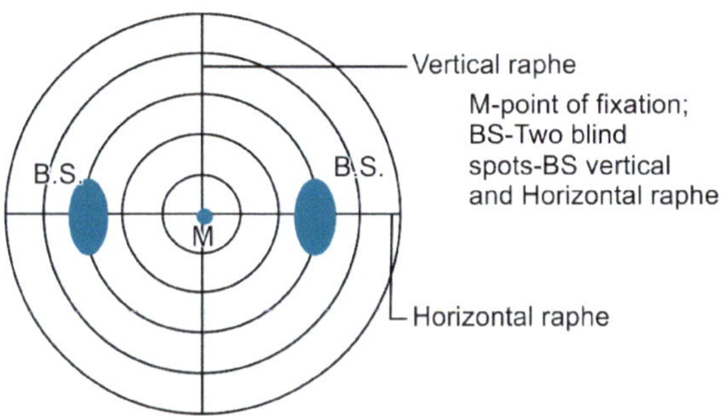

Fig. 2.8: Normal central field

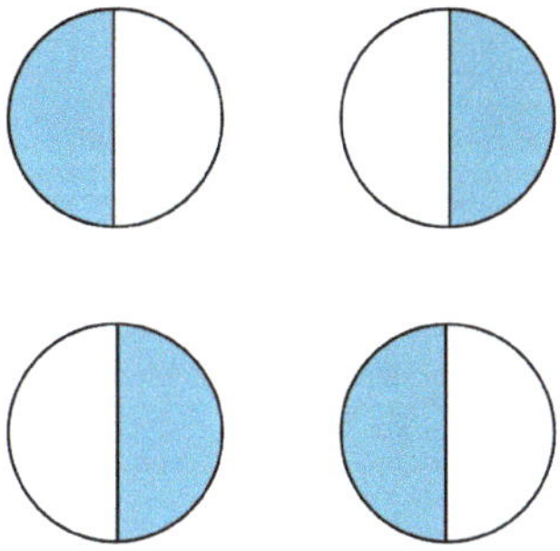

Fig. 2.9: Hemianopic field

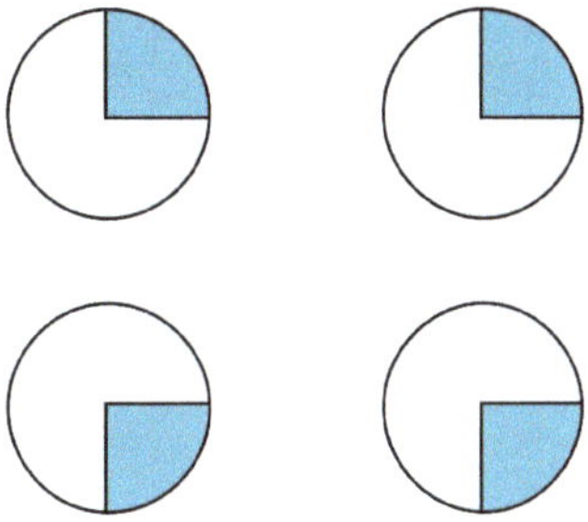

Fig. 2.10: Quadrantanopic field

Types of Scotoma

The shape and position of the scotomas according to location of lesions are:
1. Due to lesions of retina and optic nerve
2. Due to lesions from chiasma to optic radiation

1. Lesions of retina and optic nerve (Fig. 2.5):
   i. Central
   ii. Centrocecal
   iii. Paracentral
   iv. Arcuate
   v. Enlargement of blind spot
   vi. Peripheral constriction
   vii. Tube vision
   viii. Total loss of field
   ix. Altitudinal
2. Lesions from chiasma to optic radiation produce following field changes.

They are:
- Hemianopic (Fig. 2.9)
- Quadrantanopic (Fig. 2.10)

Hemianopia is loss of one-half of vertical field. It is bilateral.

Quadrantanopia is loss of one quadrant. The lesion between optic disc to chiasma are unilateral and on the same side.

Those in chiasma and beyond it are bilateral.

Methods of Charting Field of Vision

1. Central fields are charted on:
   i. Amsler grid at a distance of 30 cm (Figs 2.11A to D)
   ii. Bjcrrum screern.
2. Peripheral fields are charted by:
   i. Confrontation method
   ii. Perimeter
      - Listers perimeter
      - Goldmann's projection perimeter
      - Automated perimeter

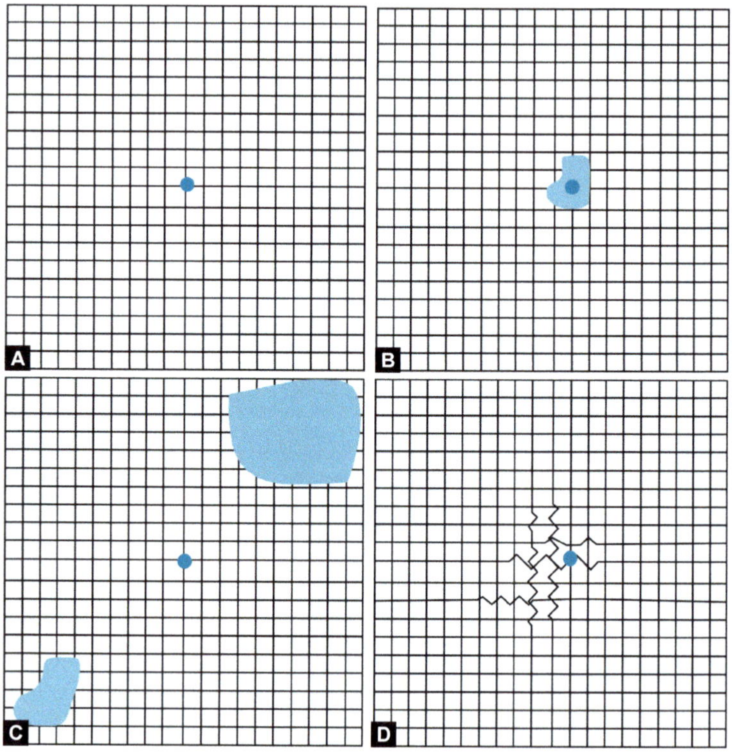
Figs 2.11A to D: (A) Normal Amsler grid; (B) Central scotoma on Amsler grid; (C) Scotoma away from the macula; (D) Metamorphopsia

Importance of Field Charting

They are useful in diagnosing lesions of:
- Retina
- Macula
- Optic nerve
- Glaucoma
- Localizing of lesions of optic path

Pupillary Pathway

This comprises two paths:
1. Parasympathetic
2. Sympathetic

The iris contains two involuntary muscle, the constrictor muscle which is situated round the pupil. The function of this muscle is to constrict the pupil. The muscle is supplied by **parasympathetic fibers** through the **inferior division of third** nerve via the **ciliary ganglion** and short **ciliary nerves**.

The dilator muscle is situated towards the periphery of the iris. It dilates the pupil and is supplied by **cervical sympathetic** through ophthalmic division of fifth nerve → Nasociliary nerve → Long ciliary nerves → the dilator of the pupil.

In normal life there is a delicate balance between the constrictor and dilator muscles and the pupil has a size of 3 to 4 mm. A pupil smaller than 2.5 is called **miotic pupil** and the process is called **miosis**. A pupil larger than 4.5 mm is called **mydriatic** pupil and the process is called **mydriasis**. The drugs that constrict the pupil are also called **miotics**. The commonly used miotics are—**Pilocarpine** and **carbachol**. The drugs that dilate the pupil are called **mydriatics**. The commonly used drugs are **atropine**, **homatropine**, **tropicamide** and **cyclopentolate**, **adrenaline**, **phenylephrine**.

Both the pupil constrict when light falls on any of the two pupils, if the optic nerve is normal on both the sides if the light is thrown on one pupil, the pupil on the side getting the light constrict.

This is called direct light reflex. At the same time, the pupil on the other side also constricts. The constriction of the other is called indirect reaction (see Fig. 1.22A).

Accommodation (See Fig. 1.22B)

Accommodation is a process by which small objects kept near the eye is made visible in an emmetropic eye (any eye that does not need glasses).

In an emmetropic eye, parallel rays from infinity are brought to focus on the retina after the rays have passed through the refractive media, i.e. cornea and lens. For all practical purposes rays arising from 6 m and beyond are considered to be parallel. As the object shifts from 6 m towards the eye, the rays become divergent. As the object nears the eye, the rays become more and more divergent.

The point from where the rays are parallel is called **farpoint** or **punctum remotum**. This is infinity for emmetropic eye, finite for myopic eye. A myope of –5 D has a farpoint of 20 cm in front of the eyes and does not require accommodation to see distant. In hypermetropic eye, it is an imaginary point behind the eye. The patient requires accommodation to see.

A point which is seen clearly when the eye is fully accommodated is called **near point** or **punctum proximum**. It is different at different ages in emmetropic eyes. In a child it is 7 cm, at 30 years it is 14 cm and at 40 years it is 25 cm. It is also influenced by error of refraction. The accommodation can be calculated by dividing 100 by near point so in a child it will be 100/7 = 14 D and at 30 years it will be 100/25 = 4 D. This is expressed in dioptre and called **dynamic refractive power**.

The difference between the farpoint and near point is called **range of accommodation**.

The difference between the refractive power at rest and when accommodated fully is called **amplitude of accommodation**.

When the eye is at rest, the lens capsule is relaxed, the front surface has a curvature of 10 mm and the posterior surface has a curvature of 6 mm. This is brought about by relaxing the suspensory ligament by contraction of ciliary muscle. This slackening of the suspensory ligament allows the front surface to relax and bulge forward. The curvature of the front surface is increased. The back surface does not change. The change in curvature is most marked in the pupillary area.

Accommodation is associated with **convergence** of the eyes and **constriction of the pupil**

As the person ages, his near point shifts away (recedes) from the eye. By 40 years of age the near point recedes more than 30 cm, the usual reading distance and this condition is called **presbyopia**.

Paralysis of accommodation is called **cycloplegia**, which can be brought about by drugs called **cycloplegics**. These are atropine, homatropine, cyclopentolate and tropicamide. All these drugs are not only cycloplegic but also dilate the pupil. Thus all cycloplegics are mydriatic but adrenaline, phenylephrine are only mydriatic but not cycloplegics.

Besides drugs some neurological conditions like **internal ophthalmoplegia** and **total third nerve paralysis** also cause cycloplegia. Accommodation in children is stronger than in adults and require strong drug like atropine to produce cycloplegia. Increased accommodation is called **cyclotonia**. This can happen by use of strong miotics as well as prolonged near work.

The near point of accommodation is measured by moving a small object from 33 cm towards the eye when the letters which were clear at 33 cm become blurred. This gives near point of accommodation. It should be tested for each eye separately.

Convergence (See Fig. 1.22C)

When the eyes are at rest, i.e. looking at infinity, they are not really parallel to each other but slightly divergent. To keep the eyes in primary position, the eyes are slightly moved towards the nose.

To see a near object, the eyes have to move more towards the nose. This movement is called **convergence**. This is associated with **accommodation** and **constriction of the pupil**. The three factors—convergence, accommodation and miosis are synkinetic (go together) and can not be separated in a normal eye.

The exact path of convergence is not as clearly marked as that of accommodation and pupillary reaction.

Like accommodation the convergence too has a **range** and **amplitude**. The **farpoint of convergence** is at infinity. The **near point of convergence** is about 8 cm in front of the eye. This is measured by moving a small target from 33 cm toward the eye till diplopia takes place. The range of convergence is the distance between the far and near point of convergence.

The amplitude of convergence is difference between the power of convergence at rest and when the eye is fully converged.

The convergence is measured in two units:

- Meter angle and
- Prism dioptre

The meter angle is the angle formed by each eye with a line perpendicular to the nose in front when the eyes are converging. When the eyes meet the median line as 1 meter, it is called 1 meter angle. When it meets at 2 mt, it is ½ ma, at ½ meter it is two meter angle.

The amount of accommodation in dioptres is equal to convergence in meter angles.

To see an object kept at 1 meter distance, it should accommodate 1 D and convergence 1 ma in a normal eye.

The strongest prism that is just sufficient to produce diplopia for near is the power of convergence.

Interaction Between Convergence and Accommodation

Though the near reflex is divided in two parts, i.e. accommodation reflex and convergence reflex, they are interlinked and can not be separated at will. Whenever the eyes accommodate, they converge as well. This is called **accommodative convergence** (AC). The accommodative convergence divided by accommodation in dioptre is called AC/A. Normal AC/A is 3:5.

Binocular Vision

When a person looks at an object, the image of the object is formed separately on each fovea. This should cause diplopia (seeing two) but in life this does not happen. The human brain is capable of converting the two separate images into one. This is a mental impression and called **binocular single vision**. Binocular single vision is not present at birth. It starts developing at very early age, i.e. first two to three months and is fully developed in first two to three years provided during this period (1) Eyes are straight (not squinting), (2) The eyes have equally sharp vision, (3) The brain can create mental impression of central vision. Failure of any of these will result in loss of binocular single vision and the child will have squint. The aim of treatment of squint is not only correction of squint but to give binocular single vision.

The binocular single vision has following grades:

1. Simultaneous macular perception
2. Binocular fusion
3. Stereopsis

Lack of any of the above will lead to squint. All the grades are tested on an instrument called **amblyoscope (synaptophore)**.

Simultaneous Macular Perception

This is ability of the two eyes to combine two different objects, one focussed on right fovea and the other on left fovea to complete one picture. Where a picture of a bird is projected in the right eye, at the same time, a picture of a cage is projected in the left eye. The patient is asked to see through the two tubes of the amblyoscope. What the patient sees is a bird inside the cage. There may be other pictures also like a lion and a cage, a sentry and his room.

Binocular Fusion

This is ability of the two eyes to superimpose two separate incomplete pictures to form a complete picture. For example the right eye sees a picture of a boy with a feather and his cap and no bird in hand. The left eye sees the boy with the bird in hand and no feather in cap. When the two pictures are superimposed, the patient sees a boy with a cap and the feather and a bird in hand.

Stereopsis

This is ability to feel the depth (distance between two objects in front of each other). This is a binocular feature. Stereopsis can be tested not only on synaptophore but also on other stereoscopes. The commonest being Titmus stereopscope (Fig. 2.12).

Advantage of Binocular Single Vision

1. Binocular vision is always more than uniocular vision. A person who can read three lines on vision chart in each eye separately will be able to read five or six lines with both eyes open.
2. Binocular field is larger than uniocular field.
3. Field defects of one eye is generally masked by intact field of other eye.
4. Binocular single vision has stereopsis which is not found in unilateral vision.

Aqueous Humor (See Fig. 1.23)

Aqueous humor is a crystal clear essential intraocular fluid found in anterior and posterior chambers. The main function of the fluid is to supply

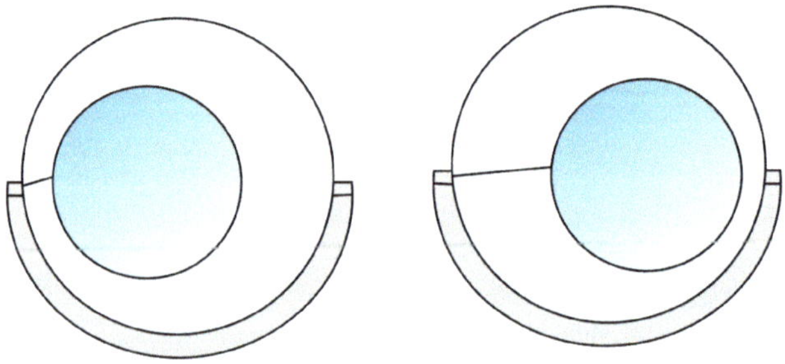

Fig. 2.12: Slide for stereopsis

nutrition to avascular structure of the eye, i.e. the lens and the cornea. The lens fully depends on the aqueous for its nutrition. The other functions are (1) maintaining intraocular pressure, (2) remove waste product (3) act as optical media with refractive index of 1.37 that is equal to that of cornea but less than that of lens.

The aqueous is formed in the ciliary processes of the ciliary body at a constant rate. It also drains at a constant rate. In a normal eye the volume of aqueous is only 0.26 ml at a given time. There are **three processes** by which the aqueous is formed. They are (1) Secretion, (2) diffusion (3) ultra filtration. **There is no method by which aqueous production can be increased**. There are many drugs that reduce its production. Aqueous production is greatly reduced in diseases of ciliary body.

(1) The aqueous after being produced in the posterior chamber passes through the pupil to the anterior chamber. (2) The iris at the pupillary border gives slight resistance to the flow of the aqueous from posterior chamber to anterior chamber. (3) If the resistance is more than normal as happens in many disease, the flow of aqueous from posterior chamber to anterior chamber decreases. (4) The pressure in the posterior chamber increases. (5) This pushes the iris forward and may block the angle of the anterior chamber. (6) From the pupil, the aqueous enters the anterior chamber and circulates in the anterior chamber supplying nutrition to the cornea and the lens. (7) The aqueous leaves the anterior chamber via the angle of anterior chamber.

The angle is formed by the sloping end of the cornea, the ciliary body and root of the iris. It is about 45° in normal eyes. It is narrow in newborn and hypermetropic eyes. The angle is not a solid structure. At its apex is **trabecular meshwork** which is like a many layered network. The trabecular meshwork opens in **canal of Schlemm**, which goes round the cornea. From the canal of Schlemm the aqueous passes into multiple venous channel, situated in the sclera to drain into **episcleral vein** from where the aqueous is absorbed by **conjunctival veins**. 90% of the aqueous drains through angle of anterior chamber, remaining part drain by uvea and sclera.

Obstruction at any of these structures slows down the flow of aqueous resulting into rise of intraocular pressure. Prolonged and sustained rise of intraocular pressure damages the retina and the optic nerve causing diminished vision and field changes. Persistent rise of intraocular tension with damage is called **glaucoma**.

The aqueous is 99% water, remaining part is made up of organic and inorganic matters like protein, enzymes, lactates, ascorbic acid and glucose. The normal protein content is only 0.02% which is very less than in blood but in inflammation of iris and ciliary body it rises and the aqueous is called **plasmoid aqueous**. The normal aqueous looks clear but the plasmoid aqueous looks hazy, when it becomes more hazy, the heavy particles (pus) settles down at the bottom of the anterior chamber and the condition is called **hypopyon**. It is a vision threatening condition.

Intraocular Pressure

To maintain its appearance and focusing, the eye must remain in a constant shape which is brought about by its firm wall, i.e. cornea and sclera and **intraocular pressure**.

The intraocular pressure is produced and maintained by aqueous humor. There is a delicate balance between production and drainage of aqueous.

The normal intraocular pressure ranges between 15 mm Hg to 21 mm Hg. Constant low pressure, i.e. less than 5 mm Hg is called **hypotony** while constant pressure higher than 21 mm Hg is called **glaucoma**. In severe glaucoma, this pressure may go as high as 80 mm to 90 mm Hg.

The intraocular pressure is not uniform throughout the day and night but the difference between lowest and highest pressure is generally not more than 7 mm. In glaucoma, this difference is more than 7 mm. The intraocular pressure is more in the morning than in the evening. Only few persons may have evening rise of tension. This difference in tension is called **diurnal variation**. A change more than 7 to 8 mm is suggestive of glaucoma. Generally intraocular tension in two eyes is equal. A difference more than 6 mm between the two eyes is also suggestive of glaucoma. If a puncture is made in the cornea, the aqueous will drain out fast and intraocular tension will fall to zero. The eyeball will become soft.

The intraocular pressure is measured by an instrument called **tonometer**. The commonly used tonometer is **Schiotz tonometer**.

The tonometers belong to two groups, i.e. (1) **Indentation tonometer** and (2) **Applanation tonometer**.

The commonly used Schiotz's tonometer is an indentation tonometer. The example of applanation tonometer is Goldmann tonometer. The applanation tonometer is an optical tonometer.

Metabolism of Ocular Structures

As far as metabolism is concerned, the structures of the eye can be divided into two broad groups:

1. The vascular structure, the retina and uvea
2. The avascular structure, the cornea and the lens

The vascular structures share the metabolic process of any other vascular structure in the body.

The fine vessels (capillaries) carry nutrients to all the vascular structures including retina and uvea. The walls of these have a two way path—(i) that carries nutrition to the tissue and (ii) that take away waste product from the tissue.

The **retina** is a very special fine structure that has a **high rate of metabolism**. The inner layers of the retina are supplied by the retinal vessels on the retina (They are visible for examination by ophthalmoscope). The outer layers are supplied by **choriocapillaries** (These are not visible by ophthalmoscope). If any of these two fail, the retinal cells die, leading to loss of vision.

The choroid is not as delicate as retina, has an elaborate blood supply by way of choriocapillaries and suffers less than retina if its nutrition is cut-off.

Avascular Structure

The two avascular structures of the eye, the **cornea** and the **lens** are the two major optical components of the eye. They allow the light to pass through them. For this property they have to remain **transparent**. Any loss of transparency lead to diminished vision.

Cornea

Out of the five layers of cornea, the two, i.e. (1) The epithelium and (2) the endothelium have more active metabolism than the stroma. Out of epithelium and endothelium, the epithelium is more active than endothelium but endothelium once damaged is lost forever. It can not be repaired. The epithelium is capable of regrowth (regeneration) and repair. The source of nutrition to the epithelium are:

1. **Oxygen** dissolved in the tear and the limbal capillaries
2. **Glucose** from aqueous and limbal capillaries

The endothelium gets its nutrition from the aqueous.

Corneal Transparency

The cornea should be able to pass visible light (ordinary light) in range of 380 nm to 760 nm for clear vision.

The light is partly **reflected** from the epithelial surface and the epithelial surface acts as a **convex mirror**. This does not interfere with remaining rays to pass through the cornea by refraction. The cornea as a whole acts as a **convex lens** of + 43 D. Any loss of transparency will result in development of opacity in the cornea which in turn will cause blurring of image on the retina.

The following factors keep the cornea transparent:

1. There are no vessels in the central area of the cornea. Development of vessels in the center of cornea will diminish vision.
2. The cornea is richly supplied by sensory nerves but the nerve fibers in the substance of cornea are transparent, hence do not interfere with vision.
3. There are no pigments in the cornea. Development of pigment reduce vision.
4. The corneal fibers, the epithelial cells and endothelial cells are arranged in regular fashion.
5. The endothelium prevents aqueous to enters the stroma. The cornea looses its transparency if aqueous finds its way in the stroma.
6. The corneal stroma remains dehydrated (dry) and not swollen.

Lens

The lens is **avascular**. It depends solely on aqueous humor for its nutrition. The three parts of the lens—the **capsule**, **cortex** and the **nucleus** have different metabolism. The nucleus has least metabolism. The cortex has more metabolic activity. The capsule is a semipermeable membrane through which the nutrient mostly carbohydrate passes to the cortex. The aqueous also supplies oxygen to the lens.

PHYSIOLOGICAL OPTICS

Though the light around us looks colorless, it is in fact a mixture of seven colors of different wavelength, i.e. VIBGYOR. The colors are not visible unless the light is passed through a prism. According to their wavelength, the violet has shortest wavelength of 397 to 424 nm (400 nm), the red has longest wavelength 647 nm to 723 nm (700 nm). The white light which is combination of these seven colors has a wavelength of 400 nm to 700 nm (Fig. 2.13).

The light travels in a straight line. When light strikes a surface, two things happen: (1) The light is **reflected** back as per law of reflection. (2) The light travels through the media and **refracted** as per law of refraction. Brighter the surface larger the reflection, i.e. mirror. Denser is the media, more is the refraction.

Law of Reflection

If a beam of light forms an angle on a reflecting surface (mirror), it will be reflected back. The light falling on the surface is called **incident ray** and the other is called **reflected ray**. They form an angle between them. The angles between the **normal** (90°) at point of incidence and the incidence ray are reflected ray are known as **angle of incidence** and **angle of reflection**. They are equal. **The incidence ray, the reflected ray and the normal are in the same plane** (Fig. 2.14).

There are two types of mirrors:

1. Plane mirror
2. Spherical mirror:
   i. Concave mirror
   ii. Convex mirror

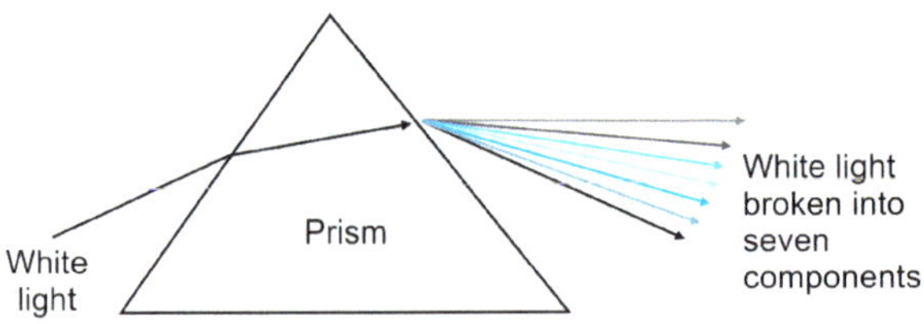

Fig. 2.13: Dispersion of light through prism

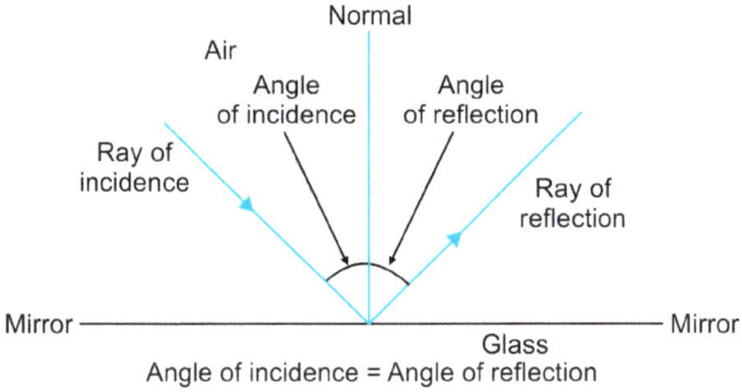

Fig. 2.14: Reflection on plane surface

Plane Mirror

When an object is kept in front of a plane mirror, an **erect**, **virtual**, **laterally rotated** image of the **same size is** formed at a distance equal to distance between the object and the mirror and mirror and the image **behind** the mirror. The image can not be projected on a screen (Fig. 2.15).

If a mirror is rotated through an angle say 20°, the image will rotate through 40°.

Uses of Plane Mirror in Ophthalmology

1. Testing vision in room less than six meters.
2. Plane mirror retinoscope.
3. As reflecting device in direct ophthalmoscope, indirect ophthalmoscope, slit lamp and amblyoscope.

Spherical Mirror

The spherical mirrors can be

- Concave
- Convex

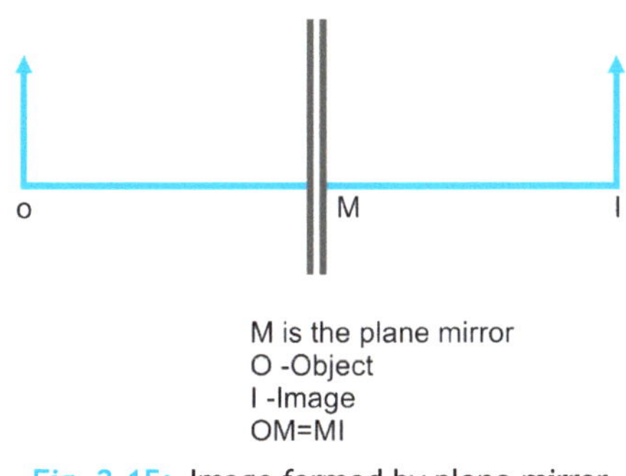

Fig. 2.15: Image formed by plane mirror

The law of reflection as in plane mirror is equally applicable to spherical mirror.

Each spherical mirror has **an arc**, a **center of curvature**, a **vortex** of the mirror. The center of the arc of the mirror is the vortex or pole of the mirror. The line joining the pole of the mirror to the center of the curvature is the **principal axis of the mirror**. The point where the parallel rays meet on the principal axis is **focus** point of the mirror (Fig 2.16 and 2.17).

Image formed by a spherical mirror depends upon the focal length of the mirror and distance of the object from the mirror.

The following are the position and type of the image when the object is kept at various distances from the concave mirror (Figs 2.16 and 2.17) (Table 2.1).

Uses of Concave Mirror in Ophthalmology

The concave mirror is used in **mirror retinoscope** and indirect ophthalmoscope. The posterior capsule of the clear lens acts as a concave mirror, giving a small inverted image that moves against the movement of torch. This is the **fourth Purkinje image**.

Convex Mirror

The image formed by convex mirror is virtual, erect and small, when placed at any distance from the mirror (Fig. 2.17).

Uses of Convex Mirror in Ophthalmology

Convex mirror has **no practical use in ophthalmology**. It is worth noting that the cornea and anterior lens capsule act as a convex mirrors and the

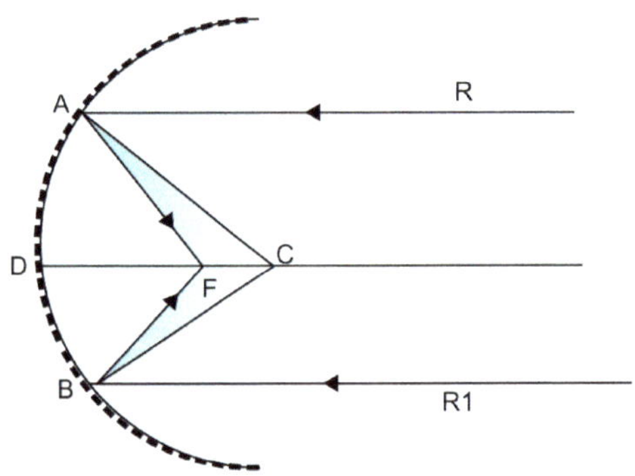

ADB is the concave mirror
DC is the principal axis of the mirror
AC and BC are the normals of the mirror
AR and BR1 are rays parallel to the principal axis and meet at F
F is the focal point
FD is the focal length

Fig. 2.16: Reflection in a concave mirror

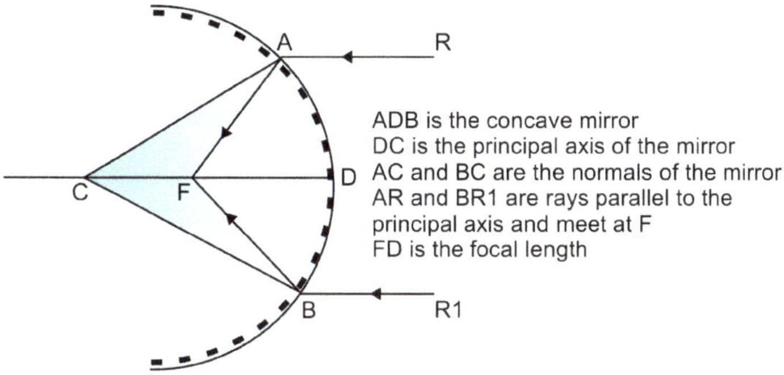

Fig. 2.17: Reflection in a convex mirror

Table 2.1 Characteristics of the images in relation to distance of object from the concave mirror

	Position of object	Characteristics of image
1.	At infinity	At the focus real and pinpoint (Fig. 2.18)
2.	Between center of curvature and infinity	Between the mirror and center of curvature—real, inverted, small
3.	Between focal point and mirror	Between the center of curvature and infinity, real, inverted magnified
4.	At the center of curvature	At the center of curvature—real, inverted, same size as object
5.	At the focal point	Real inverted image at infinity
6.	Between the focal point and the mirror	The image is virtual, erect, magnified, behind the mirror

images formed are small and move with movement of the torch placed in front of the eye (see Purkinje image). This property of cornea is the basis of two diagnostic instruments, i.e. the **Placido disc** and **keratometer**.

Refraction

When a ray of light passes through a homogenous medium:
1. It travels in straight line.
2. When it strikes another medium, it is partly reflected back and partly travels through the second media.
3. While travelling through the second medium, it deviates from its original path. **This deviation is called refraction**.

Refraction at Single Surface

When the ray passes from rarer to denser medium, it bends towards the normal. When the ray passes from denser to rarer medium, it bends away from the normal.

Like reflection, the light falling on the junction of two medium is called **ray of incidence**. The line perpendicular to the surface at a point where the ray of incidence meets, the second medium is the **normal**. The ray that changes its path is called **ray of refraction** (Fig. 2.18).

(1) If the incidence ray is at right angle to the interface, it is not refracted. (2) In case of angle of incidence that causes the angle of refraction to become 90°, the refracted ray will travel along the surface of the interface and this angle is called **critical angle** (Fig. 2.19).

If the angle of incidence is more than the critical angle, the ray is no more refracted but reflected back. This is called **total internal refraction**. This property is utilized to divert back the rays of light in ophthalmic instruments like microscope, slit lamp and ophthalmoscope.

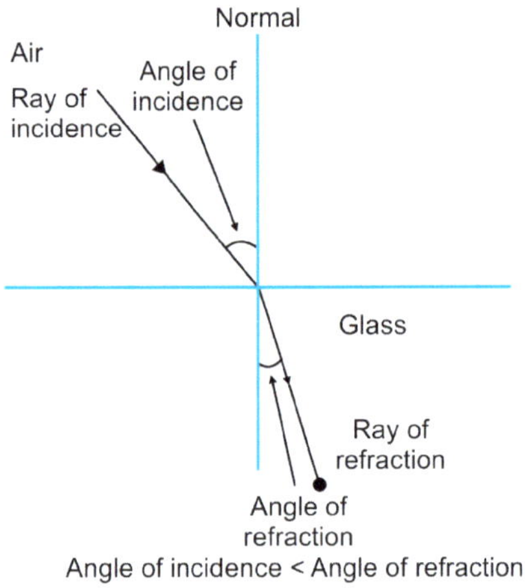

Fig. 2.18: Refraction on plane surface

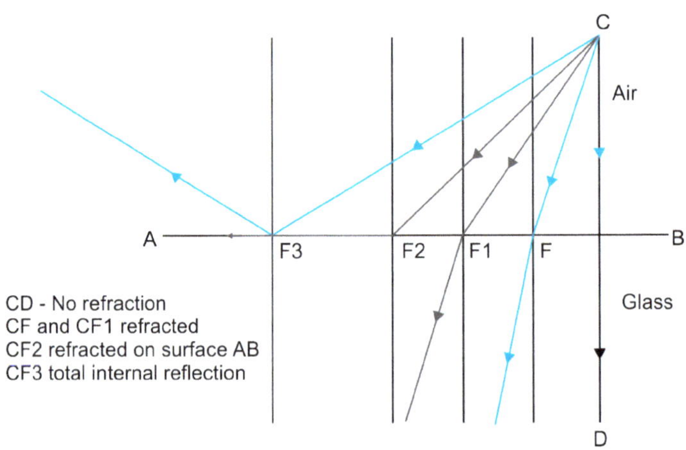

Fig. 2.19: Total internal reflection and critical angle

Refractive index is a constant that is arrived by dividing sin angle of incidence by sin angle of refraction. Sin angle of incidence/sin angle of refraction = Constant = Refractive index = μ

The refractive index of air is considered to be one.

Refraction at Two Parallel Surfaces

Lets consider ABDC to be a rectangle of glass with refractive index of 1.4 with air all-round with refractive index of 1.0.

N is point of incidence at interface, AB, i.e. between air and glass, NN1 is the normal at N. LN is the ray of incidence and angle LNN1 is the angle of incidence at surface AB. NN2 is the refracted ray and angle ENN2 is the angle of refraction at surface AB. The ray NN2, the refractive ray at surface CD meets the second surface at N2 and is refracted as N2O. The N3N2F is normal at N2. If the refracted ray N2O is traced back it becomes parallel to original ray LN and refracted back as OG. This forms the principle of refraction through a prism (Fig. 2.20).

A prism is a triangular optical device that is bound on two sides by two inclined surfaces that meet at an **apex**. The surface on the third side, i.e. opposite the apex is the **base of the prism**. When a beam of light strikes any of the inclined surfaces of a prism to pass through the substance of the prism, it is refracted twice: Once when it enters from air to glass and then again glass to air. The refracted ray deviates towards the base of the prism and when an eye receives this ray, it seems to come from the apical side. This deviation depends upon the **refractive index of the prism** and its **refracting angle** (Fig. 2.21 and 2.23).

The ray of light can be deviated by adjusting the direction of the ray in relation to the side of the prism. A ray can be rotated by 90° or may be reversed (Figs 2.22 and 2.23).

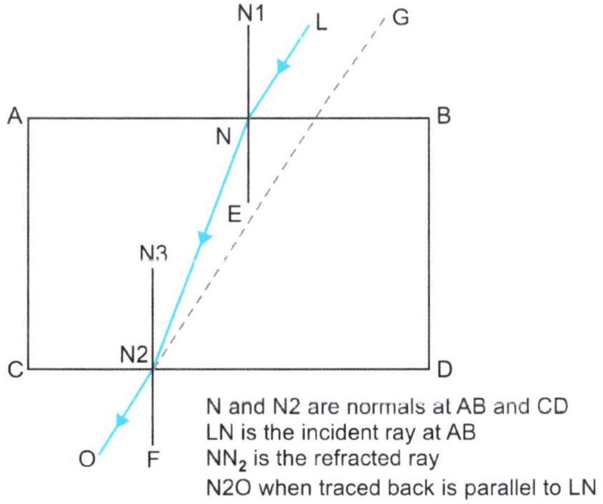

Fig. 2.20: Refraction through a plane sheet of glass ABCD

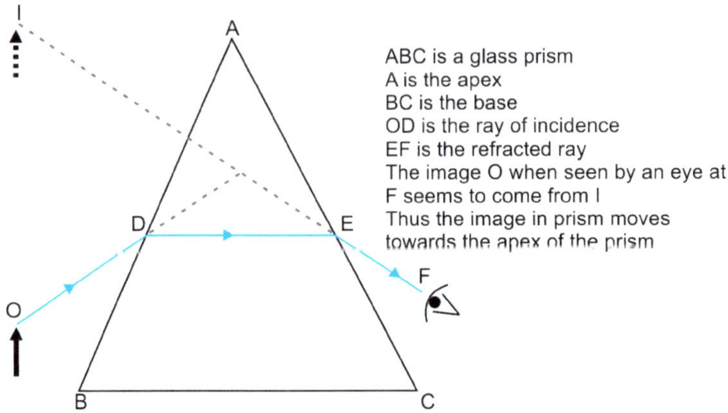

Fig. 2.21: Refraction through a prism

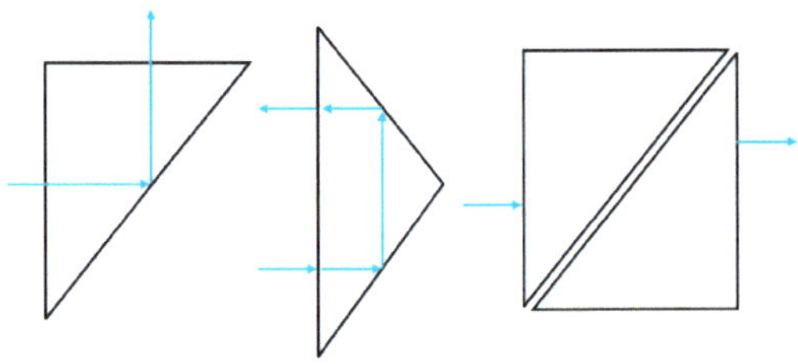

Fig. 2.22: Use of prism to deviate the rays

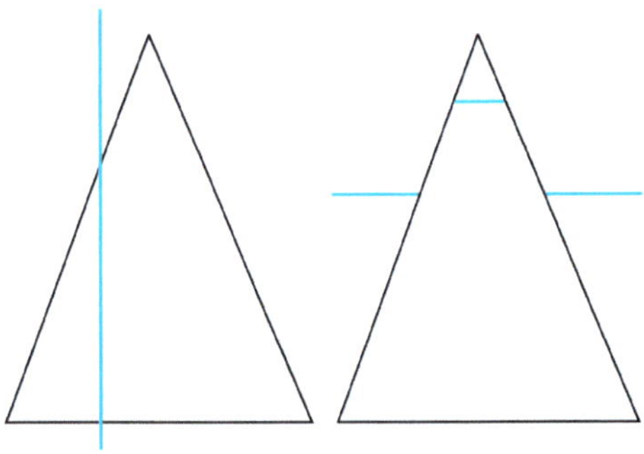

Fig. 2.23: Showing the image moves towards the apex only

If two prisms of equal refracting angle are placed base to apex, they act as a plate of glass. In ophthalmology prisms of small refractive angles are **used to measure angle of deviation of squint**. **Prisms do not improve vision** but move the image. This property is utilized to treat diplopia in paralytic squint. Prisms are widely used in various optical instruments to rotate the ray of light in place of plane mirrors.

If they are rotated in opposite direction, they behave like a single prism of increased power unless the apexes are in the direction which the total strength becomes sum of the power of two prism.

Power of prisms used in ophthalmology is measured in prism diopter.

How to Identify a Prism

It is not difficult to identify a large prism. It can be identified by looking at it. Difficulty arises when a prism is incorporated in a spectacle. To find out a prism in a spectacle glass, hold the glass near the eye and look at a vertical line. If the two ends of the line outside and the line inside the lens are in one line, there is no prism in the glass. If the line inside the lens is shifted towards one side, the lens has a prism. Now flip the lens, the line inside the lens will move towards the other side. Putting appropriate prism that will joint the three lines will be the power of prism (Fig. 2.24).

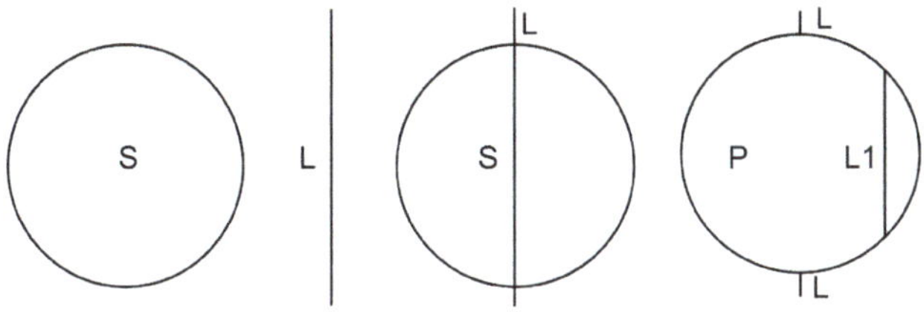

S is lens without prism
L is a linear object

When S is put in front of line L, there is no deviation in line L if there is no prism

P is a lens with prism, when put in front of line LL, the line shifts towards the apex as L1

Fig. 2.24: Identification of prism in spectacle lencs

LENSES

Lenses are transparent optical devices, which are bounded at least on one side by a curved surface which can be a part of a sphere or a cylinder.

They are three types of lenses:

1. Spherical
2. Cylindrical

   Both can either concave or convex.
3. A spherocylinder is partly spherical and partly cylindrical.

According to shape of the lens, the lenses are called **biconvex**, **planoconvex**, **concavoconvex**, **biconcave**, **planoconcave** and **convexoconcave**. The convex lenses are thin on the periphery and the concave lenses are thick at the periphery (Fig. 2.25).

Construction of Lenses

Convex lenses are considered to be a combination of prisms of equal strength placed base to base. The line between the two prisms is the principal axis (Figs 2.26 to 2.29).

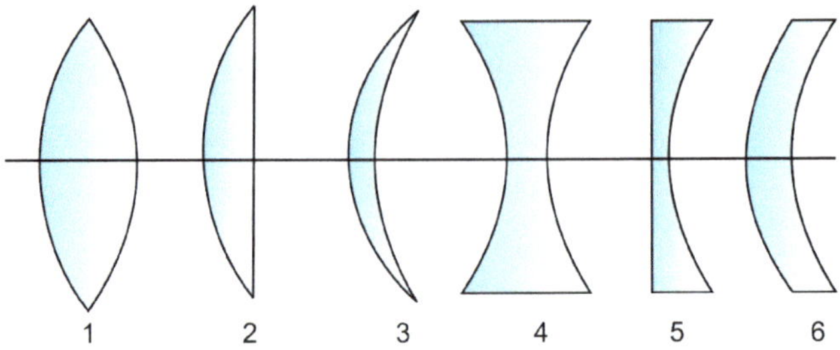

1 - Biconvex, 2 - Planoconvex, 3 - Concavoconvex, 4 - Biconcave, 5 - Planoconcave, 6 - Convexoconcave

Fig. 2.25: Types of lencs

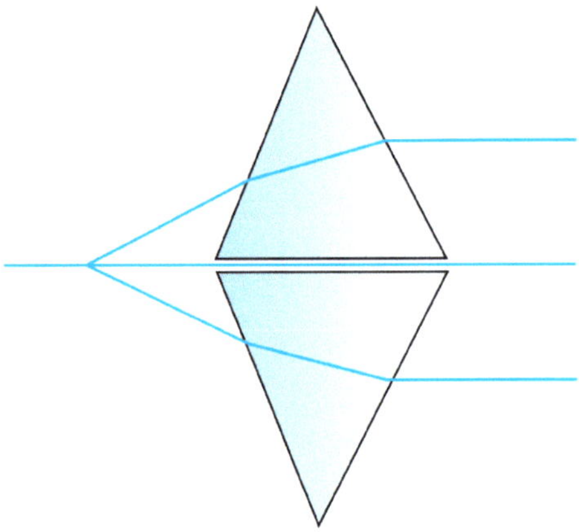

Fig. 2.26: Refraction through two similar prisms base against each other, behave like a convex lens

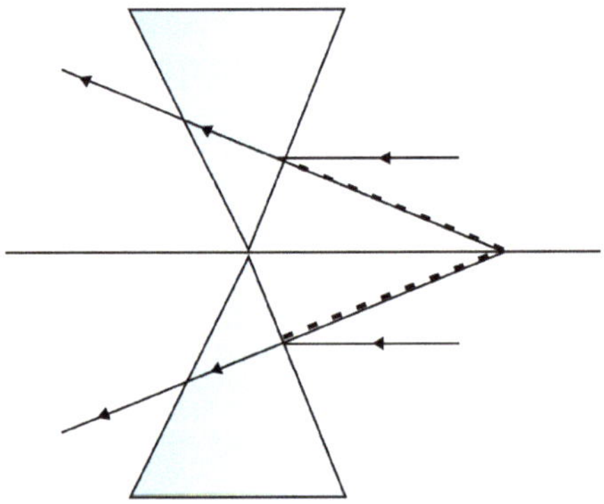

Fig. 2.27: Refraction through two prisms with apex against each other, behave like concave lens

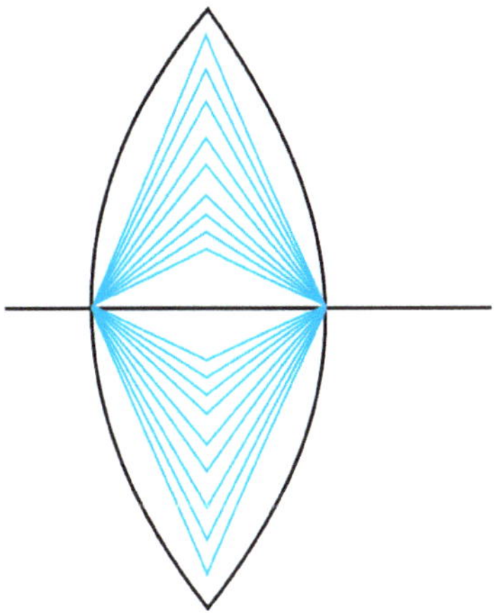

Fig. 2.28: Concept of formation of convex lenses by combination of prisms placed base to base

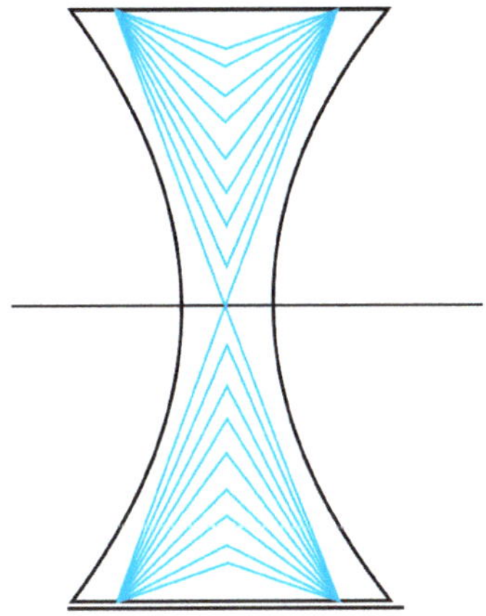

Fig. 2.29: Concept of formation of concave lenses by combination of prisms placed apex to apex

Similarly concave spherical lenses are considered to be made up of prisms of equal strength kept apex to apex. The line passing between the two apices is the principal axis.

The convex lenses bend the parallel rays to converge on the principal axis. The point where the parallel rays converge to meet the principal axis on the other side and is called **principal focus** and the distance between the principal focus and center of the lens is the **focal length** of the lens.

In concave lens the rays seem to diverge from the principal focus.

The convex lenses are called plus lenses and the convex lenses are called minus lenses.

The power of lens is calculated as reciprocal of focal length in meters and the unit of measurement is **diopter**. Thus, a lens of one diopter will have a focal length of one meter.

Diopter	Focal length
1/4 D	4 mt = 400 cm
1/2 D	2 mt = 200 cm
1 D	1 mt = 100 cm
2 D	1/2 mt = 50 cm
4 D	1/4 mt = 25 cm
10 D	1/10 mt = 10 cm

Optical center of lens is a point on the principal axis through which rays of light pass without deviation.

Construction of Image Formed by a Lens

Construction of an image formed by the rays passing through a lens requires minimum two rays (lines). One parallel to the principal axis and other through the optical center of the lens.

Image formed by the convex lens (Figs 2.30A and B to 2.34).

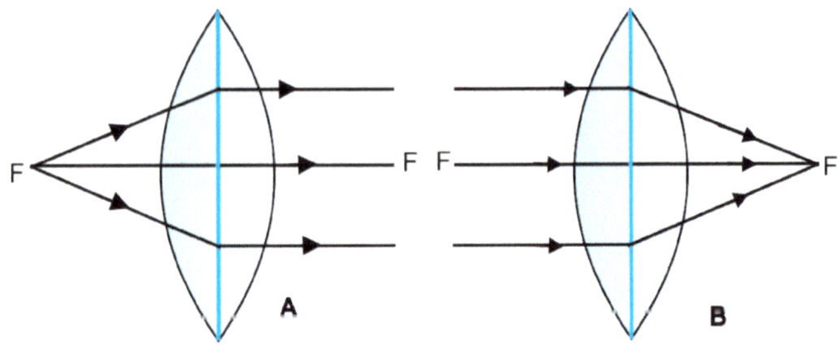

Figs 2.30A and B: Image formed by convex lens; (A) Object at focus, magnified image formed at infinithy; (B) Object at infinity, pinpoint real image at focus

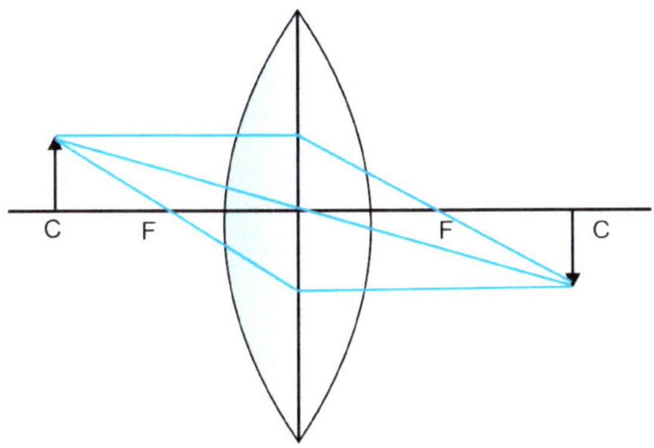

Fig. 2.31: Image formed by a convex lens when the object is situated in the center of the curvature

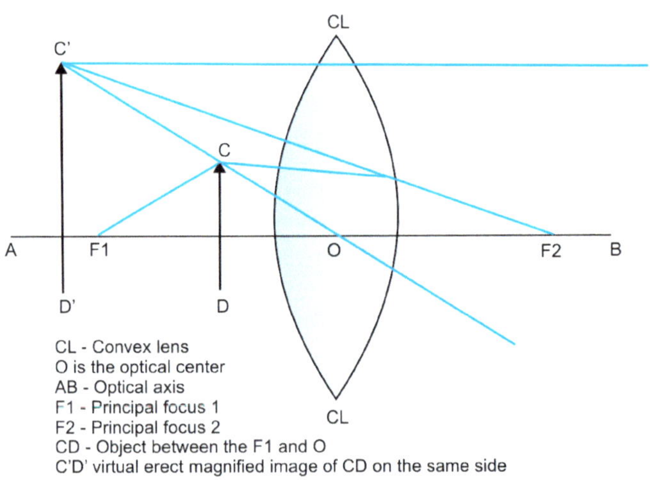

Fig. 2.32: Formation of image in a convex lens when object placed between the F1 and O

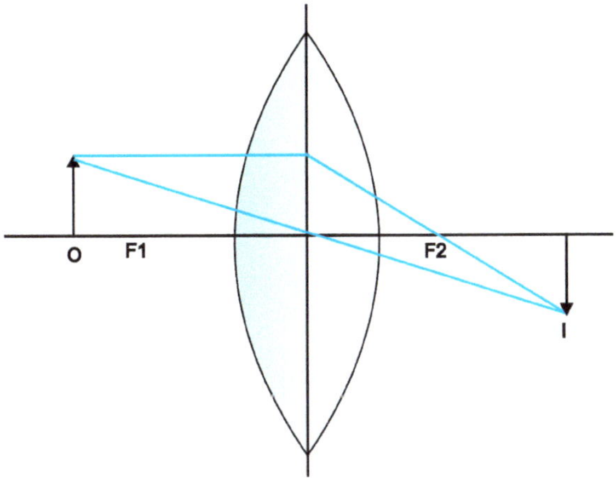

Fig. 2.33: Image formation by a convex lens when the object 'O' is beyond F1, the image 'I' is formed on the opposite side as real and inverted

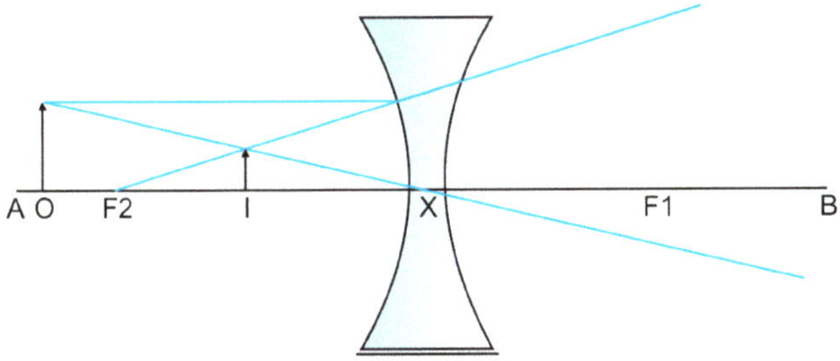

Fig. 2.34: Image formation by a concave lens, AB is the optical axis, X is the optical center, O is the object, I is image which is virtual, erect, small on the same side

Points to Remember Information of Image by Convex Lens

1. If the distance of the object is more than the focal length, the image will be formed on the other side, it will be real and inverted.
2. If the distance between the object is less than the focal length, the image will be virtual erect, magnified and formed on the same side of the object. This principle is used in simple magnified corneal loupe.
3. If the object is at the focus, the image will be formed at infinity and magnified.
4. If the object is at infinity, the image will be formed at focus. It will be real and pinpoint.

Image formed by a concave lens is always virtual, erect and smaller than the object, on the side of the object between the focus and the lens irrespective of distance of object from the lens.

Power of Combination of Two or more Lenses

The total power of multiple lens is the sum total of power of the lenses. This is true only when:

1. The center of the lenses are in the same line.
2. The distance between the lenses is very small.
3. The lenses are of small power (Fig. 2.35).

Cylindrical Lenses

These lenses can either be convex or concave. The convex cylindrical lenses are outer part of a solidcylinder. The concave cylindrical lenses are inner part of a hollow cylinder but parallel to the axis of the cylinder (Fig. 2.36).

A cylindrical lens has no power along the axis of the cylinder. The power is present at right angles to the axis. The rays passing through a cylindrical lens obey the rule of refraction of spherical lenses except that the **image formed by a cylindrical lens is a line** and not a point as by a sphere.

When cylindrical lenses are added to spherical lens, the combination is called **spherocylinder**. The cylindrical power is added to spherical power algebraically only at right angles to the axis of the cylinder.

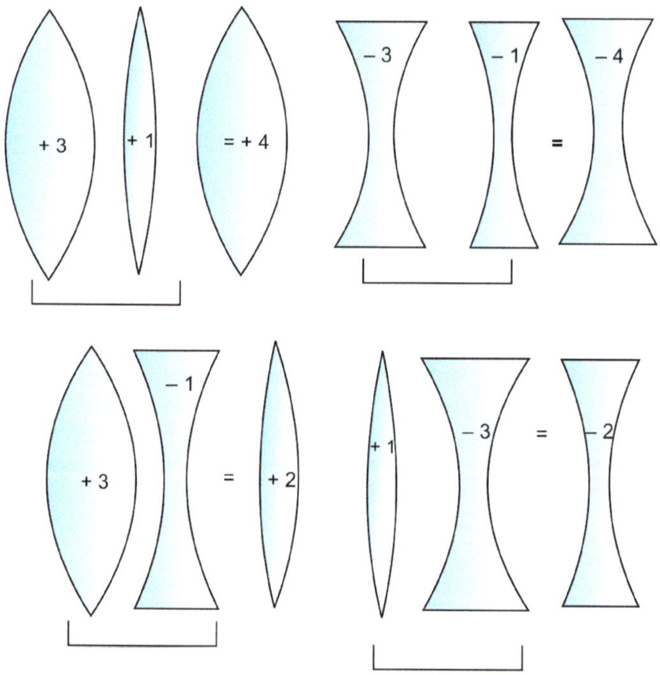

Fig. 2.35: Power of combination of spherical lenses is the algebric sum of lenses

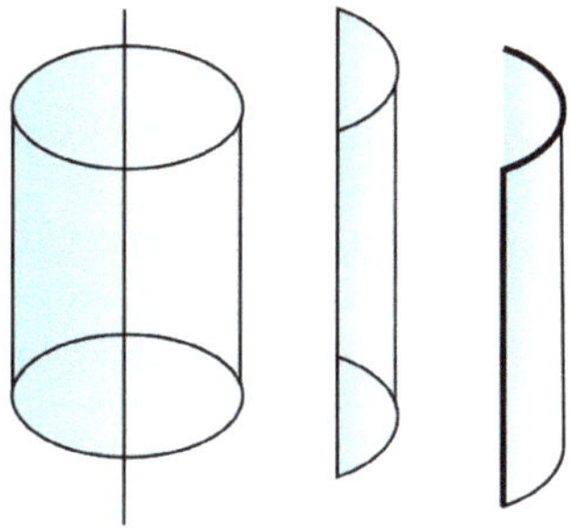

Figs 2.36A to C: Concept of cylindrical lenses

Identification of Lenses

Spherical

1. Convex
   i. The image moves against the movement of the lens.
   ii. The image is magnified.
   iii. If the lens is rotated, there is no distortion of the image.
   iv. The size of the image is equal in all meridia.
   v. The lens is thick in the center and thin on the periphery.
2. Concave
   i. The object moves with the movement of the lens.
   ii. The image looks smaller.
   iii. There is no distortion on rotating the lens.
   iv. The size of the image is equal in all meridia.
   v. The lens is thin in the center and thick in the periphery.
3. Cylindrical
   Convex cylinder
   i. The image moves against the movement of the lens only in one axis.
   ii. There is no movement at right angles to the axis.
   iii. The image is elongated at right angles to the axis.
   iv. There is distortion on rotating the lens.

   Concave cylinder
   i. The image moves with the movement of the lens only in one axis.
   ii. There is no movement at right angles to this.
   iii. The image is shortened at right angles to the axis.
   iv. There is distortion on rotating the lens.

CLINICAL OPTICS

Refraction of a Normal Eye

For all practical purposes, the normal eye at rest is considered to act as a single strong convex lens of +60 D with a focal length of 24 mm. It is better to break this into two system of +43 and +17 D. The former is due to **cornea** and second is due to **lens**. Both the systems are situated on the same axis (**coaxial**) and have common optical center (**homocentric**).

This simplified system has:

1. One principal plane 2 mm behind the cornea.
2. A nodal point situated 5 mm behind the plane.
3. Anterior focal point 15 mm in front of the cornea.
4. Posterior focal point 24 mm behind the cornea.
5. Refractive power +60 D = 43 D + 17 D.

In such a system, parallel rays are brought to focus on the retina provided the accommodation is at rest and the condition is called **emmetropia** (patient will not require glasses for distance). The image formed at place other than retina results in **ametropia**. (patient will require glasses for distant). If the image is formed in front of the retina, it is called **myopia** and when formed behind the retina it is hypermetropia.

The factors that cause abnormal position of retinal image are:

1. **Length of the globe**—Length of normal adult eye is 24 mm. A change of 1 mm produces ametropia of 3 D. If the eye is 23 mm long, it is 3 D hypermetropic. If the eye is 25 mm long, it is 3 D myopic.
2. **Corneal curvature**—The curvature of a normal cornea is 8 mm. If there is a change in corneal curvature, the image will not be formed on the retina. 1 mm increase will produce myopia of 6 D. Lessening of curvature by 1mm will produce **hypermetropia of 6 D**. Uneven curvature will produce **astigmatism**.
3. **Lenticular curvature**—An increase in lenticular curvature causes myopia, a decrease in lenticular curvature will cause hypermetropia.
4. **Refractive index of lens**—An increased refractive index causes myopia. A decreased refractive index cause hypermetropia.
5. **Accommodation–**
   i. When accommodation is at rest, the image is formed on the retina in emmetropia.
   ii. When there is increased accommodation, the image moves forward.

ABNORMAL REFRACTION

When all parallel rays of light are not focused on the retina with accommodation at rest, the condition is called error of refraction or **ametropia**. All the parallel rays are focused on the retina with accommodation at rest, the eye does not have any error of refraction and the eye is called **emmetropic** (Fig. 2.37).

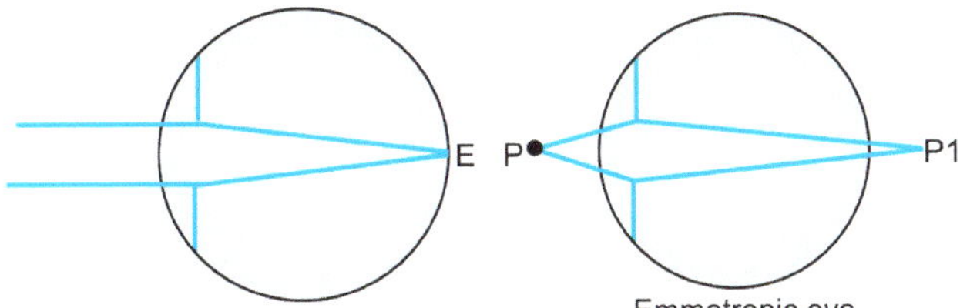

Fig. 2.37: Emmetropic eye

Types of Ametropia

1. Myopia
2. Hypermetropia
3. Astigmatism

Myopia

Myopia is defined as a condition where parallel rays are brought to focus in front of the retina, when accommodation is at rest but divergent rays from near point are focuszed on the retina. The myopia becomes worse by accommodation (Fig. 2.38).

Myopia is the **commonest** type of error of refraction in both the sexes. It is more common in **children**. It has a tendency to increase in first few years of onset. There after it stops increasing. It is easily corrected but have some serious complications like retinal detachment. Myopia has strong **genetic link**. If only one parent has myopia chances are that 10% of the children will have myopia. This percentage increases to 20% if both the parents have myopia. The brothers and sisters of a myopic child may have myopia of various grades. However, it is not uncommon to see myopia in children without family history. It is also common to have only one child in the family to have myopia.

Myopia **generally involves both eyes** but myopic power in both eyes are rarely equal. However, rate of increase of power is almost equal in two eyes. Children who develop myopia between 5 years to 10 years have more tendency to progress. The progress may be –1.0 D to 3.0 D every year up to 18 to 20 years. Patients who develop myopia in teens too have tendency to progress but the rate of progress is not more than 0.5 to 1.5 D per year till the patient reaches 20 years of age. **Wearing of glasses have no influence on progress of myopia**. Rarely myopia may be present in one eye and the child is not aware of it unless both eyes are tested separately. An adult with unilateral myopia may not complain of difficulty in near vision after forty years (presbyopia) because he uses myopic eye for near vision and normal eye for distant vision. Myopic children are more likely to present with esotropia (one eye is turned towards the nose).

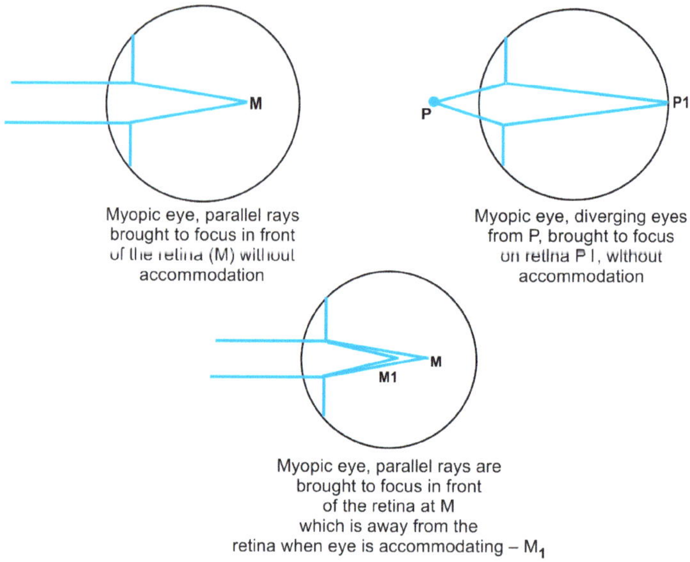

Fig. 2.38: Myopia, its relation to accommodation

Causes of Myopia

The exact cause of myopia is not known. Some of the anatomical factors that produce myopia are listed below. Many a times more than one factor may be the cause.

1. **Increased axial length of the eyeball**—Axial length (from cornea to retina) of normal eye is 24 mm. Parallel rays are focused 24 mm behind the cornea with accommodation at rest. If the eyeball is longer than 24 mm, the rays will come to focus in front of the retina to form a sharp image and then diverge to reach the retina to form a diffuse image which reduces the vision. **One millimeter of increase** in axial length produces myopia of **3 diopter**. Thus an eye that is 25 mm long will be myope by –3 dioptre, 26 mm long eye will be –6 D myope.
   Increased axial length is the commonest cause of myopia.
2. **Increased corneal curvature**—Normal curvature of cornea is 8 mm. If the cornea becomes more curved, the rays are focused in front of the retina even with normal length. This happens in two conditions—**keratoconus** and **keratoglobus**.
3. **Increased refractive index of the lens**—The refractive index of clear lens is 1.33. If this increase, the image again shift forward. This is commonly seen in early stages of **nuclear cataract** and in **untreated diabetes**. A person who is already myope, becomes worse when he develops nuclear cataract. A hypermetropic improve vision when he develops nuclear cataract.

4. **Increased curvature of lens** – This **is rare** and seen in two rare conditions of **anterior lenticonus** and **posterior lenticonus**.
5. **Anterior displacement of lens** also shifts the retinal image forward. This is again rare.

Clinical Signs of Myopia

1. A child may be born with myopia. This is called **congenital myopia**. Fortunately this is **rare**. The error of refraction in congenital myopia is generally high, i.e. about –10 D when detected first it generally does not increase much, the child remains prone for serious complication like retinal detachment.
2. **Simple myopia**—This is the **commonest** type of myopia, generally seen in children of both the sexes between 5 years to 15 years. It progresses gradually. A child at six year of age may be –1 D myope, by 15 years his power may increase to –5 D, –6 D. Increase of power is less if myopia develops in teens, i.e. a myope using –1.0 D at 13 years may increase to –3.0 D or –4.0 D by 18 years.
   The commonest symptom that brings the child to ophthalmologist is inability to see writings on black board in the school. The parents may complain that the child sits too near the TV set to watch.
3. A myopia is said to be **progressive** if the increment in power is fast, say from –3.0 D to –10 D within 3 to 4 years but the child can read 6/6 with each eye with best correction.
4. A myopia is said to be **degenerative or pathological** if the vision does not improve to 6/6 with best correction due to degenerative changes in the retina. A pathological myopia need not have very high power always.

Signs of Myopia

Mild to moderate myopia **may not have any sign** that may be correlated to myopia.

The distant vision is always less than normal. Generally on first visit the child may have vision between 6/18 to 6/60. The uncorrected child squeezes the lids to produce pinhole effect that improves vision. The vision improves to almost 6/6 with pinhole.

The near vision is normal. The child may keep the book too close to the eye to read.

In high myopia the eyeballs are larger than in emmetropia. The cornea too is large and the anterior chamber deeper than normal. The pupil is also large.

The fundus in simple myopia is normal but in pathological myopia shows degenerative changes.

Treatment

1. **There is no medical treatment.** Improvement of diet, supplementation of vitamins and antioxidants, eye exercises are not effective in preventing progress, eliminating glasses or remove glasses.
2. The definitive treatment is optical that can be by:
   I. Optical devices
      a. Spectacles (Fig. 2.39)
      b. Contact lenses
         i. Hard
         ii. Semisoft
         iii. Soft
   II. Surgery
      a. On the cornea
         i. Radial keratotomy (RK)
         ii. Photorefractive keratoplasty (PRK)
         iii. LASIK
      b. On the lens
         i. Phakic IOL
         ii. Clear lens removal

The spectacles are the best and cheapest form of management. They are easy to handle.

The spectacles should be prescribed after refraction under homatropiae.

All children under 10 years should be refracted under atropine.

Children above 10 years up to 20 years are refracted under home tropine or cyclopentolate.

Refraction under cycloplegia removes **pseudomyopia** and unmasks associated astigmatism.

Pseudomyopia is not myopia. It is in fact hypermetropia. If the child accommodate to have clear vision, the accommodation overshoots the required amount, the image is formed in front of the retina and the eye behave like myopia and improves with minus lenses. This in turn worsens the hypermetropia and the child accommodates more till he reaches a stage

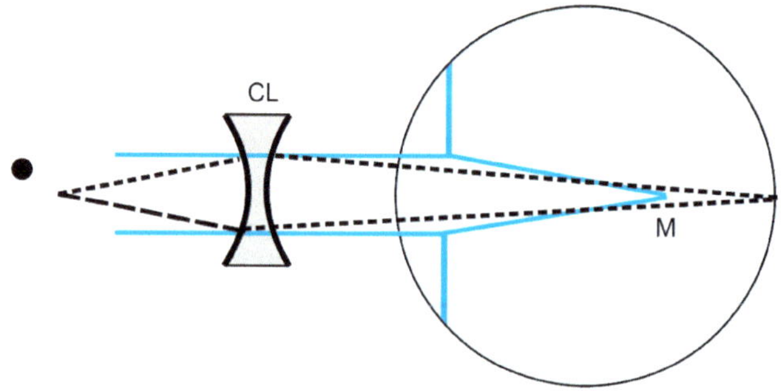

Fig. 2.39: Myopia corrected by concave lens, CL

where the vision does not improve and the child gets watering from the eyes and headache that is relieved by discarding the minus glasses.

HYPERMETROPIA (HYPEROPIA)

Hypermetropia is that condition of the eye where parallel rays from infinity are not brought to focus on the retina when accommodation is at rest. The image is formed behind the retina. Divergent rays arising from near point are focused farther away from the retina (Fig. 2.40).

Most of children at birth are hypermetropes due to short axial length of the new born eye (16–17 mm). The hypermetropia at birth ranges between 2 D to 3 D. As the child grows the axial length increases and at five years, it is almost 24 mm. Thus, the hypermetropia present at birth is neutralized by increased length of the eye.

If the eye fails to reach adult size by four to five years of age, the child will remain hypermetropic. If this hypermetropic is small, i.e. less than 2 D, it may be neutralized due to spurt in growth during puberty.

A person who has been emmetrope all through the adult life may become hypermetrope round about fifty years of age due to flattening of the lens and cornea and failure of accommodation.

Hypermetropia is also genetically determined disorder but the incidence is not so marked as in myopia. Hypermetropia too is a bilateral disorder and the power in two eyes are generally same. However, it may be unilateral as well or the power in two eyes may differ greatly putting the eye with higher power at a risk of convergent squint.

In contrast to myopia which becomes worse if the person accommodates, hypermetropia can be fully or partially corrected by accommodation (Fig. 2.40).

Cause (Etiology) of Hypermetropia

Like myopia, hypermetropia can also be divided into:

1. Axial
2. Curvature
3. Index
4. Displacement
5. Pathological

Axial Hypermetropia

This is the commonest type of hypermetropia. It is caused due to short length of the eyeball. 1 mm of shortening causes three dioptre of hypermetropia when accommodation is not at work. If axial length of an eye is 23 mm its will be +3.0 D hypermetrope and a 22 mm eye will be +6.0 D hypermetrope. This is generally associated with some degree of astigmatism.

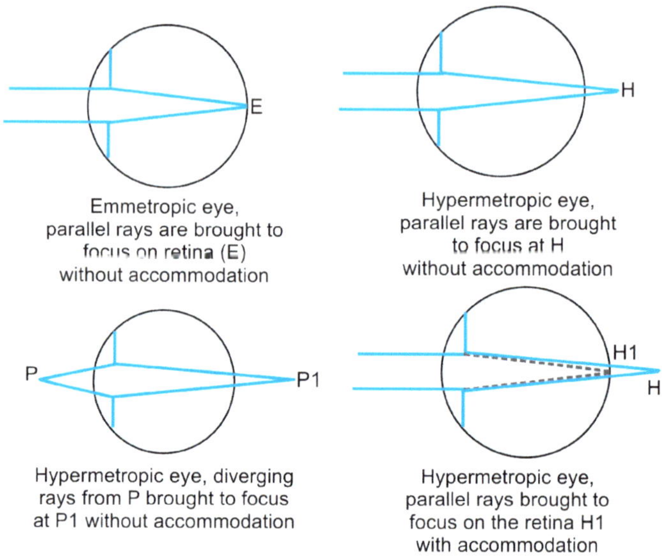

Fig. 2.40: Hypermetropia, its relation to accommodation and correction by convex lens

Curvature Hypermetropic

1 mm flattening of cornea results in hypermetropia of +6 D. Thus soft eyes, eyes with smaller cornea have curvature hypermetropia. A flat lens too causes hypermetropia and this is the cause of hypermetropia developing after 50 years of age.

Index Hypermetropia

The refractive index of clear lens is 1.34. If this is reduced, the eye becomes hypermetropic as seen in dehydration and hypoglycemic (less sugar in blood).

Displaced Lens

If the lens is displaced backwards, its focal length also shifts back, thus making the eye hypermetropic.

Accommodation in Hypermetropia

It has been discused earlier that if the power of a convex lens is increased, its focal length decreases. The same thing happen when the eye accommodates. The normal eye with a lens of +17 D focuses at 24 mm but by accommodation the lens becomes +20 or +22 D, hence the image moves forward.

The normal ciliary body has some tone physiologically. This can correct hypermetropia by +1 D. The hypermetropia corrected by ciliary tone is called **latent hypermetropia**. The remaining part is called **manifest**

hypermetropia. The manifest hypermetropia is divided into **facultative hypermetropia** and **absolute hypermetropia**.

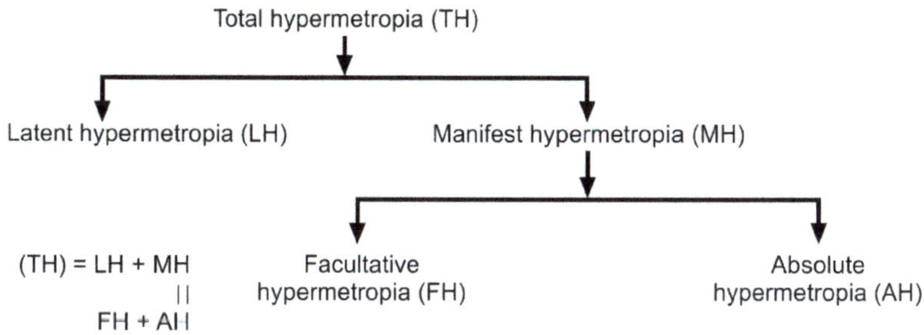

Example

1. A patient has diminished distant vision, with +2 D, his vision improve to 6/6. This is absolute hypermetropia.
2. Keep on adding plus lenses till the vision remains 6/6 say by +4.5 D, the vision remains 6/6, so his facultative hypermetropia is 4.5 D – 2.0 D = 2.5 D and +4.5 D is the manifest hypermetropia.
3. Under complete cycloplegia, the patient requires +6.0 D to remain 6/6. This 6.00 is the total hypermetropia and +1.5 is the latent hypermetropia.

Symptoms of Hypermetropia

To begin with moderate hypermetropia has less symptoms of diminished distant vision than myopia of same extent, i.e. a myope of –1.5 D will always have diminished distant vision but a hypermetrope of +1.5 D may have 6/6 vision.

Thus a hypermetropic can be:

1. **Asymptomatic** (no complains) because moderate hypermetropia is corrected by accommodation.
2. **Asthenopia**—The vision is fully corrected by accommodation but constant use of accommodation produce nonvisual symptoms—watering, photophobia, headache and tiredness of the eyes. These symptoms are called asthenopia or **tired eyes**.
3. **Diminished distant vision**—This happens when hypermetropia is not corrected by accommodation.
4. **Defective near vision**—When all the accommodation is used to correct distant vision, the patient has no accommodation left for near. Generally diminished near vision occurs after 40 years of age in emmetropia. However, if a patient round about 30 to 35 years complains of diminished near vision, chances are that the patient is high hypermetropic and his near vision will be corrected by distant correction only.

5. **Sudden blurring of distant vision**—This happens in children and young adults who use too much of accommodation to have clear vision, resulting in **pseudomyopia**.
6. **Convergent squint**—One eye may be turned towards the nose (esotropia). This may be the only symptom for which child may be brought to an ophthalmologist.
7. **Recurrent stye**, chalazia, blepharitis are common in uncorrected hypermetropia.
8. **Amblyopia** may develop in some cases especially if the power is different in two eyes or one eye squints.

Treatment

As in case of myopia there is **no medical treatment**. There are no special diets or exercises that can give relief to hypermetropia.

The only treatment is **optical** that can be achieved by optical methods only. They are **spectacles**, **contact lenses** or **surgery** (Fig. 2.41).

Spectacles should be prescribed only after refraction under cycloplegia. All children under six years or children with esotropia should be refracted under atropine one percent.

Prescription of atropine requires some special features:

- Use only one percent ointment in children.
- Apply ointment in both eyes irrespective of vision or squint.
- Use smallest possible strip of ointment.
- Use atropine three times a day for three days.
- Ask the parents not to put atropine on the day of refraction.
- Warn the parents that:

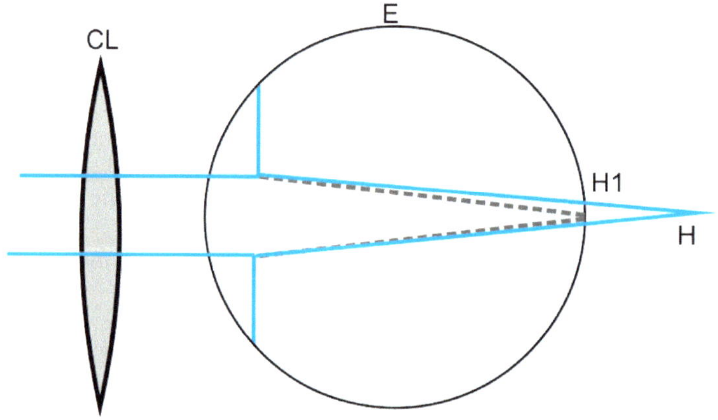

Fig. 2.41: Hypermetropia corrected by + lense. E is hypermetropic eye Parallel rays are brought to focus behind the retina at H. CL is a convex lens that brings the image H to retina at H1

i. The child will have diminished near as well as far vision.
ii. The child will have glare due to widely dilated pupil.
iii. The child will have a dryness of mouth and flushed (red) face.
iv. The child may have slight rise of temperature.
v. The effect of atropine will last for about a fortnight.
vi. There is no medicine to counter effect of atropine in eyes.

In persons above 10 years of age, may be refracted under homatropine two percent, cyclopentolate one percent or tropicamide 0.8 percent. These drugs are available only as drops. They are instilled three to four times a day at an interval of five minutes just before refraction.

The action of these drugs pass off in twenty four to thirty six hours.

There is no drug that can counteract mydriasis and cycloplegia caused by these drugs.

Sympathomimetics like phenylephrine have no role in refraction in hypermetropia.

While doing refraction utmost care should be given to amount and axis of astigmatism. For this purpose autorefractometer may give better result in noncooperative children.

Ideally hypermetropia should be corrected fully after the effect of cycloplegia has passed off, i.e. if atropine has been used, the glasses are prescribed after two weeks. In case of other drugs, the glasses are prescribed after 48 hours. This is called postmydriatic test (PMT).

A child may not accept full hypermetropic correction on the first instance. Such children are given glasses that have best vision for distance as well as near with greatest comfort.

The power of glasses is increased in small installment over next three to six months.

Pathological Hypermetropia

1. Where the parallel rays are being focused 24 mm behind the cornea but retina has moved forward. This happens in central serous retinopathy, retinal detachment, choroidal detachment or orbital tumors.
2. When the axial length of the eye is normal and retina is 24 mm behind the cornea but the rays are focuszed far behind the retina. This is seen when lens is absent from the pupillary area. This is called **aphakia**.

The commonest cause of pathological hypermetropia is absence of lens from the pupillary area. This is called aphakia.

The other causes of pathological hypermetropia are:

- Micro cornea (very small cornea)
- Soft eye
- Any growth pushing the sclera from behind
- Swelling of the macula (central serous retinopathy)

APHAKIA

Absence of crystalline lens fully or partially from the pupillary area is called aphakia.

It can be **congenital** (present at birth) or **acquired**.

True **congenital aphakia** that is present at birth is **very rare**. Here either the lens has not formed at all or has been absorbed before birth.

More common are condition where the lens is in place at birth but gradually gets dislocated. The dislocation is generally partial that is lens is absent partly from the pupillary area. Partial absence of lens from the pupil is called **subluxation**. The subluxated lens can be clear or hazy.

Commonest cause of **acquired aphakia** is **surgical removal** of lens to improve vision in cataract. This method is no more practiced and a better method of implanting an artificial intraocular lens (IOL) is done. The condition where an intraocular lens is put in the pupillary area is called **pseudophakia**. A well-performed pseudophakia behaves like emmetropic.

The dioptric power of an aphakic eye is different from other emmetropic or hypermetropic eye.

It will be recalled that an emmetropic eye has a dioptric power of +60 D and parallel rays are brought to focus on the retina which is 24 mm behind the cornea.

In aphakia the lens is removed that means the dioptric power is reduced by +17 (usual power of lens). Hence, the total power of an aphakic eye becomes +43 D and parallel rays are brought to focus, 31 mm behind the retina. **As there is no lens, there is no accommodation**. So the rays in no way can be brought to focus on the retina as happens in manifest hypermetropia.

Thus an aphakic eye not only has very **poor distant vision** but it has **no near vision**.

Signs of Aphakia

Generally there is a **scar** at the limbus. The anterior chamber **(AC) is deep**. The iris vibrates with movement (**tremulousness of iris**). Generally there is one or two holes in the iris (**iridectomy**). The pupil is **jet black** if the lens has been removed completely (Intracapsular cataract extraction = ICCI). If the lens is partly removed (Extracapsular cataract extraction), a white membrane (**after cataract**) is visible in the pupil. The third and fourth Purkinje images are also absent.

The vision is reduced to 1/60 to 2/60. There is no near vision.

The eye is absolutely hypermetropic. The hypermetropia varies between +10.0 D to +12.0 D with +1.0 to +2.0 Dyl at 180° (Fig. 2.42).

Management of Aphakia

The condition is corrected by prescribing +10 D to +11 D Dsp with +1.0 to +2.0 Dyl at 180°→ axis.

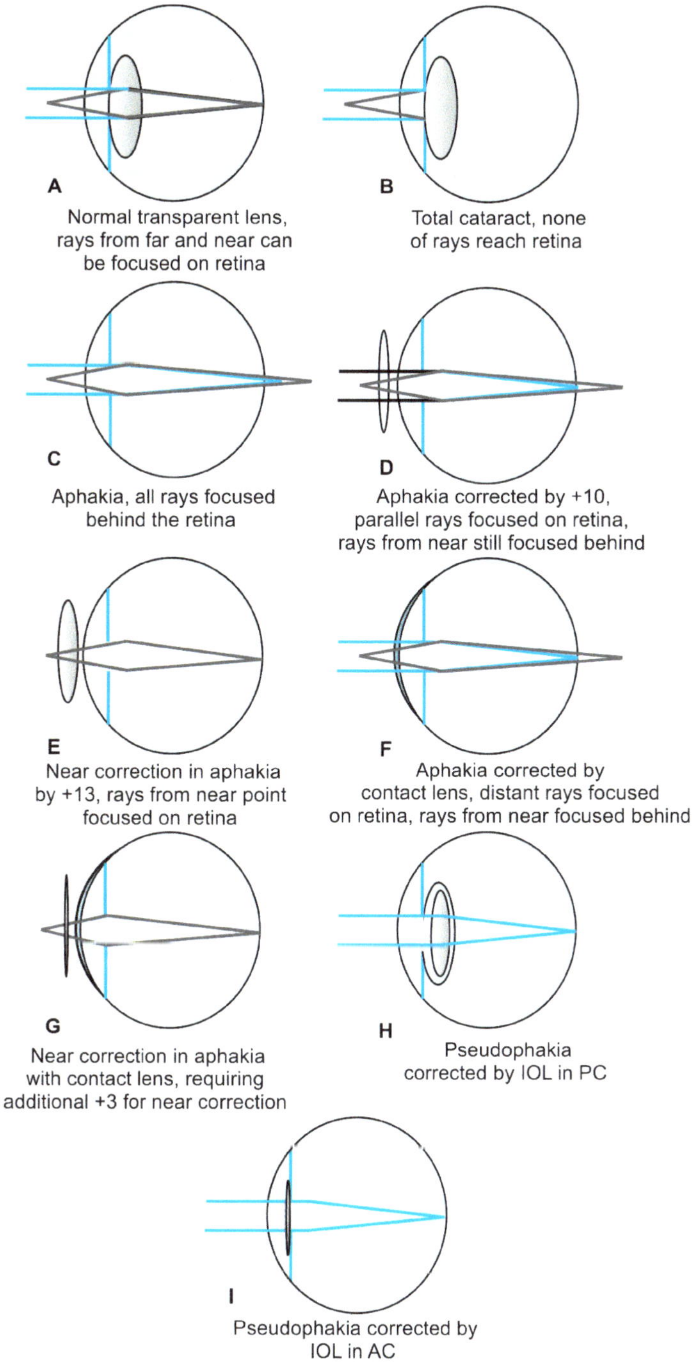

Fig. 2.42: Optics of aphakia and pseudophakia, their optical correction

A +10 D lens in the spectacle is as effective as a +17 D lens inside the eye.

As there is no accommodation, the eye requires additional +3.0 Dsph correction for near, which is added to distant correction. Thus a patient who requires +10 Dsp with +1 Dyl 180 → for distant will requre +13.0 Dsph with +1.00 Dcyl for near.

The other method to correct aphakia is by **contact lens.** A patient with contact lens will require +3.0 Dsp in spectacle for near vision in addition to contact lens. The best way to correct aphakia is by an **intraocular lens.**

The other acquired cause of aphakia is trauma. The injury can be blunt (by a rounded object) or penetrating (by a pointed object). Both can cause **traumatic cataract** which may get absorbed or may dislocate.

ASTIGMATISM

Astigmatism is that error of refraction where all parallel rays are not brought to focus at one plane with or without accommodation. In fact accommodation may worsen the astigmatism. In nonastigmatic eyes with error of refraction, the rays are brought to focus either in front of the retina producing myopia or behind the retina producing hypermetropia. In both the conditions, the image formed on the retina is not a point but a diffuse circle. In astigmatism the image formed is oval in shape (Fig. 2.43).

Mild degree of astigmatism is very common which does not cause any symptoms, hence do not require any treatment.

Astigmatism has been classified variously according to:

1. Cause (etiology)
2. Clinical finding
   i. Position of the axis
   ii. Position of image

The etiological classification depends upon the part of the optical system involved, i.e. cornea, lens or retina. Out of the above three, the cornea is the part responsible in most of the cases.

Corneal Astigmatism

The cornea has different curvature at different meridians. This difference may be as low as 0.5 Dcyl or as high as 5.0 Dcyl. The vertical meridian is more curved than horizontal. The meridian which is more curved is more myopic than the other. This change in curvature is due to pressure of the lids on the cornea. The lids squeeze the cornea in between them. Similarly swelling of the lid or a growth of the lid also changes the corneal curvature. The change in the curvature may be uniform, gradual and smooth. This is called **regular astigmatism**. Nonuniform change in curvature causes **irregular astigmatism**.

Lenticular Astigmatism

Incidence of lenticular astigmatism is very low. The lens can cause astigmatism in following ways:

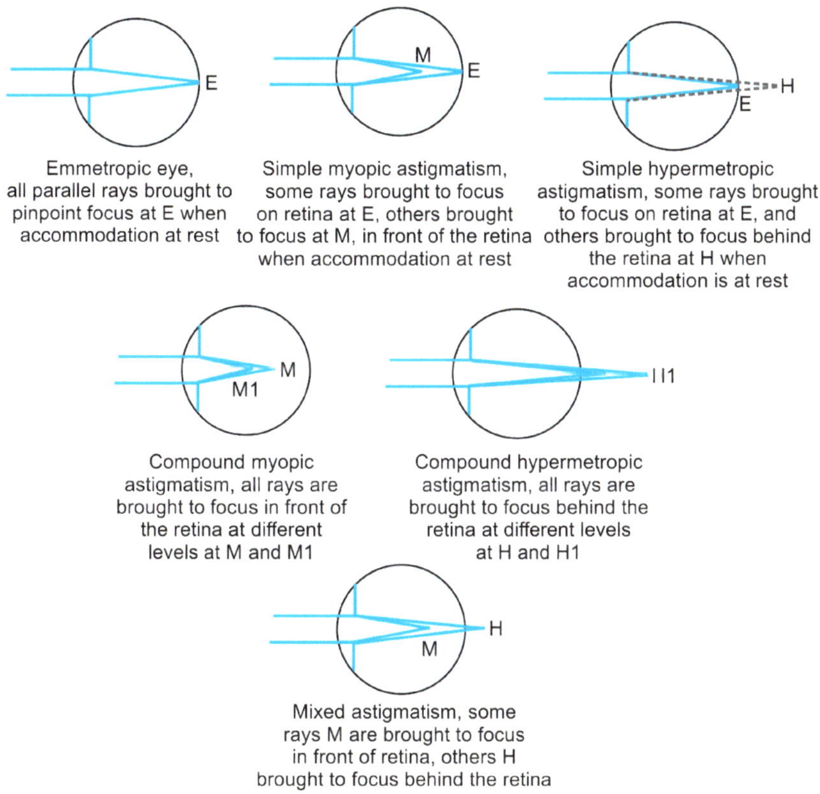

Fig. 2.43: Clinical type of astigmatism

1. The anterior or posterior surface is not smooth
   - **Anterior lenticonus**
   - **Posterior lenticonus**
2. The lens is tilted. **Subluxation of lens**
3. The refractive index of the lens is not uniform as in early stages of cataract.

Retinal Astigmatism

If the retina is not smooth, this may cause irregular image formation. It is also rare.

Clinical Types of Astigmatism

Clinically depending upon smoothness of the cornea the astigmatism can be

1. **Regular astigmatism:** In this type, the two main meridians are at 90° to each other and the power is same all along the meridian.

The regular astigmatism is further divided into following groups depending upon the curvature of the vertical meridian.

i. **Astigmatism with the rule**: This is corrected either by a concave cylinder at 180° or a convex cylinder at 90°. The meridia may vary slightly on either side by 20° but the angle between the two remains 90°.

ii. **Astigmatism against the rule**: This is corrected by convex cylinder at 180° or concave cylinder at 90° to each other. There may be slight variation in axis on each side of the principal axis.

iii. **Oblique astigmatism:** Here the principal axes are at right angle to each other. The axes are at 45° or 135°.

iv. **Bioblique astigmatism**: In this case the angles between the two axes are no more at right angles but have equal power all through the axis.

2. **Irregular astigmatism**

Here the two meridians are neither at right angles to each other nor the power is same all along a meridian.

According to position of image in relation to retina, the astigmatism can be classified as follows:

1. **Simple**
   - Myopic
   - Hypermetropic
2. **Compound**
   - Myopic
   - Hypermetropic
3. **Mixed**

Simple astigmatism is that astigmatism where image in one meridian is on the retina and the other is focused either (a) in front of the retina or (b) behind the retina. The former is called **simple myopic astigmatism** and the latter is called **simple hypermetropic astigmatism**. The simple myopic astigmatism is corrected by single myopic cylinder and simple hypermetropic astigmatism is corrected by single hypermetropic cylinder. Spheres are not required.

Compound astigmatism is that astigmatism where image is not focused on retina in any meridian. They are focused either (a) in front of retina or (b) behind the retina. They are called **compound myopic astigmatism** and **compound hypermetropic astigmatism** and require sphere and cylinder of the same sign to correct them, i.e. **minus sphere with minus cylinder** and **plus sphere with plus cylinder**.

Mixed astigmatism is that astigmatism where one meridian is focused in front of the retina (myopic) and the other is focused behind the retina (hypermetropic) and the condition is corrected by **sphere and cylinder of opposite sign**, i.e. plus sphere with minus cylinder or minus sphere with plus cylinder. The value of the cylinder in mixed astigmatism is always more than the value of the sphere. For example an eye with mixed astigmatism requires +1 Dsph with –2 Dcyl 180°→. He will also improve with –1 Dsph with +2 Dcyl at 90°↓.

Irregular Astigmatism

Irregular astigmatism is that astigmatism where dioptric value changes not only in two meridians but in the same meridian.

The common causes irregular astigmatism are:

- Pterygium
- Corneal opacity
- Keratoconus
- Growth at limbus
- Partial traumatic cataract

The vision can not be corrected by spectacles. Some improvement may be achieved by **contact lens**. Best results are obtained by **keratoplasty**.

Symptoms of Astigmatism

The symptoms of astigmatism depend upon severity and type of astigmatism. They are:

1. Visual
2. Asthenopia (feeling of tiredness of the eyes)
3. Muscle imbalance

Visual

Low degree of astigmatism are well tolerated in children and young adult they rarely experience diminished distant vision. It is high astigmatism that causes symptoms of:

a. Diminished distant vision.
b. Distortion of figures.
c. Difficulty in near work because accommodation that is required for near work worsens astigmatism. Thus neither rays coming from distance nor those coming from near are focused. If the patient is under 40 years of age, these symptoms are cured by proper astigmatic correction only.

Mixed astigmatism produces less symptoms than simple or compound astigmatism of same degree.

Signs

There are no **specific external signs** that may lead to diagnosis of astigmatism. Patient with high astigmatism may tilt the head to compensate for astigmatism.

Astigmatism is diagnosed by:

1. Retinoscopy under cycloplegia.
   Retinoscope may either be mirror retinoscope or self-illuminated streak retinoscope.
2. Autorefractometer
3. Keratometer (For corneal astigmatism)
4. Computerized keratoscopy

The glasses are best prescribed 48 hours after retinoscopy, when the accommodation has returned to precycloplegic level and pupils have returned to normal size.

Axis and extent of astigmatism is confirmed by—(Fig. 2.44):

1. Cross cylinder
2. Astigmatism dial
3. Astigmatic fan
4. Duochrome test
5. FRIEND test

Cross cylinder is a lens mounted in a frame with a handle. It consists of a sphere and a cylinder. The value of the cylinder is twice the value of the sphere and of opposite sign. The commonest combination is –0.25 Dsp with +0.50 Dcyl.

The axis of the cylinder is marked at 90° and 180°.

Astigmatic Fan

This consists of a horizontal line from the center of which radiating lines are drawn at an interval of 10°. All the lines are of same length, breadth, color and brightness. They are black lines on white background. A person with proper correction will see all of them as sharp lines at equal distance from each other.

One of the easiest methods is to examine the patient on Snellen's chart. If a patient is able to see all the letters on Snellen's E chart equally clear then his astigmatism correction is satisfactory.

Management

Mild degree of astigmatism without symptom need not be treated. Moderate to high astigmatism are treated by:

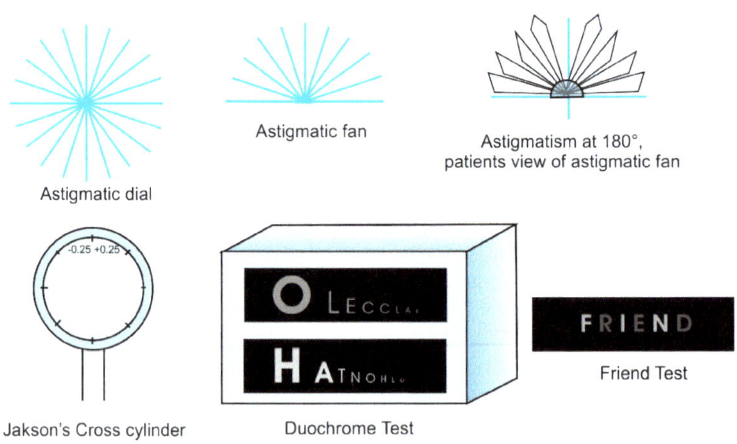

Fig. 2.44: Various methods used to correct astigmatism

1. **Spectacle**: While prescribing cylinder the value of cylinder must be the same as detected on refraction. It should neither be over corrected or under corrected.
2. **Contact lens**: Spherical contact lenses do not correct high astigmatism. In compound astigmatism they correct spherical power the cylindrical power may be left uncorrected or be neutralized by cylindrical power in spectacles. High astigmatism require special toric contact lenses. Irregular astigmatism is best treated by contact lenses.

Surgery

Many surgical procedures are available. They include photokerato refractive procedure and LASIK.

Presbyopia

Presbyopia is **not an error of refraction**. It is a **physiological condition** that develops round about 40 years of age, equally in both eyes in emmetropic eyes, in all races and both sexes those with poor health, uncorrected hypermetropia and habitual near worker develop presbyopia early.

Near work is usually done at about 30 cm in an emmetropic eye due to accommodation. As age increases power of accommodation diminishes. A patient can manage to see near things at 40 to 50 cm in bright light. After that he finds it difficult to do near work, this is called presbyopia.

The symptoms are:

- Inability to read small prints in usual light.
- Inability to thread needle.
- Running of letters and line.

The patient tries to overcome this by increasing the light and holding the book away as far as possible. Once this fails, he seeks help for correction of near vision.

The other causes of diminished near vision are:

- Uncorrected hypermetropia where all the accommodation is used for clear distant vision
- Use of parasympatholytic drugs locally, e.g. atropine, homatropine, cyclopentolate.
- Ingestion of parasympatholytic drugs.
- Internal ophthalmoplegia
- Aphakia and pseudophakia

Management of Presbyopia

1. Correction of distant vision.
2. Addition of plus lenses on distant correction according to age and profession of the patient.

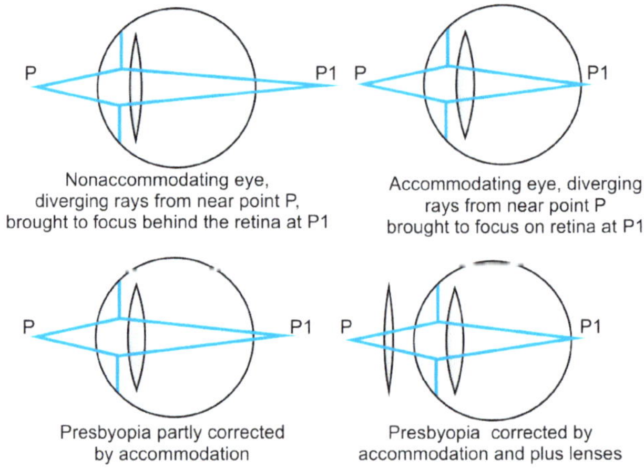

Fig. 2.45: Physiology of accommodation

The most commonly used formula for near vision addition

Age	*Addition*
40 years	+1 D
45 years	+1.5 D
50 years	+2 D
55 years	+2.5 D
60 years	+3.0 D

Example

1. An emmetropic at age of 40 years will require only +1 D for near correction.
2. A myope of –1 D at the age of 40 years will require—(–1) + (+1) = 0 D. He will be able to see the near object by removing his distant correction.
3. A myope of –2 D at 40 years of age will require—(–2) + (+1) = –1 D. He will be able to see near objects with –1 D.
4. A hypermetrope of +1 at the age of 40 years will require—(+1) + (+1) = +2 D Sph for near work.
5. A hypermetrope of +1 at 50 years will require—(+1) + (+2.0) = +3.0 D Sph.

Presbyopic Correction can be Given as (Fig. 2.45)

1. Unifocal for near only
2. Bifocal—Upper part for distance and lower part of near.
3. Trifocal—Upper part of distance vision, middle part for intermediate distance and lower part for near vision.
4. Progressive—Here the near correction gradually shifts towards above downwards.

CHAPTER

3

Symptomatology

Symptoms are the complains of the patient regarding the discomfort/disease that he or she is suffering from, i.e. pain, redness and diminished vision.

Signs are the features that the examiner finds in the person with complaints, i.e. type of diminished vision, redness, pupillary changes, etc. **Some of the symptoms are signs as well**, i.e. lowering of upper lid (ptosis), inability to close the eye (lagophthalmos) and deviation of one eye (squint). Some of the symptoms lead to diagnosis, i.e. normal distant vision with poor near vision after 40 years of age is presbyopia. Diminished night vision of short duration in a child is most probably due to vitamin A deficiency, which is preventable and curable condition. In contrast to this gradual diminished night vision in an adult is retinitis pigmentosa which can neither be prevented nor treated.

As far as symptoms are concerned, they can be broadly divided into the two groups:

1. Ocular
2. Nonocular (not directly related to eyes)

   The ocular symptoms are far more common than nonocular.

   The ocular symptoms can be **visual** (related to vision), **nonvisual**, or may have both at the same time.

The common visual symptoms are:

1. Diminished distant vision
2. Diminished near vision
3. Diminished vision in bright light
4. Diminished night vision (night blindness)
5. Diminished color vision (color blindness)
6. Colored haloes (rainbow round a light)
7. Diplopia (seeing everything double)
8. Diminished field of vision (scotoma)
9. Frequent change of glasses
10. Black spots in front of the eye

Less common visual symptoms are:

1. Polypopia (one object looks more than two)
2. Metamorphopsia (shape of the object looks distorted)
3. Glare (dislike for light)
4. Photophobia (intolerance to light)
5. Blepharospasm
6. Photopsia (flashes of light)
7. Chromatopsia (changes in color of the object)

It is common for one person to have more than one symptom in the same eye or may have different symptoms in two eyes, i.e. diminished distant vision in one eye and diminished near vision in the eye.

The causes of visual symptoms are:

1. Errors of refraction (patient needs glasses for distant vision)
2. Diminished accommodation (patient needs glasses for near work)
3. Opacities in media (cataract, corneal opacity)
4. Diseases of retina, choroid and macula.
5. Diseases of optic path—From optic nerve to visual cortex.
6. Disturbance of ocular motility (squint)
7. Amblyopia

Amblyopia is diminished, painless vision of long standing. The commonest age of onset is six years or earlier. **The common causes** are unilateral uncorrected error of refraction and difference in power of glasses in two eyes, opacities in media (corneal opacity, cataract), squint. It is not treatable after eight years of age. The child may not be aware of the condition unless there is obvious visible sign like squint, glare, corneal opacity.

DIMINISHED DISTANT VISION

Diminished distant vision is the commonest visual symptom. It could be associated with nonvisual symptoms like redness, pain, watering in the eyes. It could be **gradual** or **sudden**. It could be **painless** or **painful**. It can be **unilateral** (in one eye) or **bilateral** (both eyes). It may be **equal** or **unequal** between the two eyes.

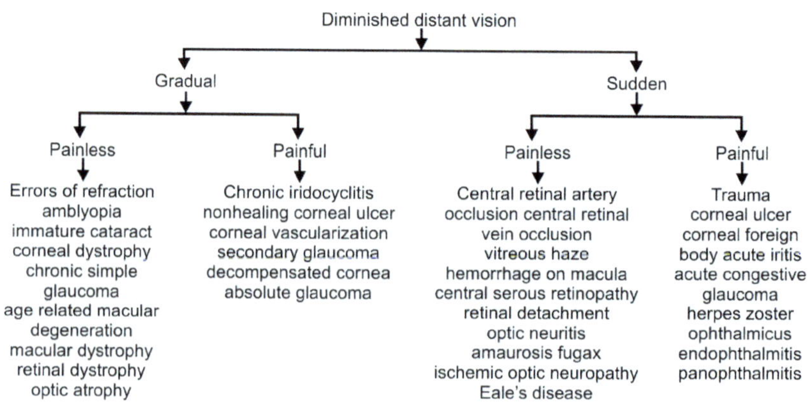

The causes of gradual painless diminished distant vision are:

1. Errors of refraction—Myopia, hypermetropia, astigmatism
2. Gradually developing opacities in the ocular media—Corneal dystrophy, corneal degeneration, treated cornea ulcer—various grades of immature cataract.

> The ocular media are—Cornea, aqueous, lens and vitreous.

Causes of sudden, painless loss of vision in both eyes

- Methylalcohol poisoning
- Quinine toxicity
- Malinger
- Transient ischemic attack

Amaurosis fugax is an unilateral, sudden, painless loss of vision that lasts for few minutes and then the vision returns to normal. Repeated attacks are common. This is due to diminished blood supply to the central retinal artery for short period. It is commonly seen in aged persons with raised blood pressure and diabetes.

Cortical blindness is sudden loss of vision in both eyes. It is painless. The loss of vision is profound but the patient does not realize that he has diminished vision. The eyes are normal in all respect. The commonest cause is injury to the back of the head. Other causes are absence of blood supply to visual cortex, infection and tumors. Some recovery is expected in majority of cases.

Methylalcohol poisoning is sudden bilateral loss of vision following drinking spurious alcohol where wood spirit or other toxic substances are added to usual drinking alcohol. Most of the persons drinking spurious alcohol die within few days. Those that survive are left blind with vision ranging from no perception of light to counting finger at three to four meters.

Causes of sudden painless loss of vision in one eye:

1. Central retinal artery obstruction
2. Central retinal vein occlusion
3. Vitreous hemorrhage
4. Central serous retinopathy
5. Optic neuritis
6. Acute ischemic optic neuropathy
7. Retinal detachment
8. Amaurosis fugax

DIMINISHED NEAR VISION

Generally an adult can read small letters kept at 30 cm (near point) without difficulty. As age advances the distance between the near point and the eyes increase. This is due to gradual decrease in accommodation. This condition is called presbyopia. It is not an error of refraction. This happens to everyone unless the patient is either myope or does not do near work.

Diminished near vision is commonly gradual in onset and involves both eyes equally and is corrected by adding plus lenses over distant correction.

Causes of gradual diminished near vision:
1. Presbyopia
2. Uncorrected high hypermetropia
3. Posterior polar cataract
4. Posterior capsular opacity
5. Macular degeneration
6. Bilateral large corneal opacities on the medial side.

Causes of sudden diminished near vision:
1. Instillation (putting medicine in the eye) of cycloplegic
2. Internal ophthalmoplegia (paralysis of iris and ciliary body)
3. Total ophthalmoplegia (paralysis of all the cranial nerves) serving the eye
4. Aphakia (absence of lens from pupillary area)
5. Pseudophakia (intraocular lens implant)
6. Over correction of myopia
7. Under correction of hypermetropia

Causes of diminished near as well as distant vision are:
1. Uncorrected aphakia and pseudophakia
2. Uncorrected hypermetropia, high myopia and high astigmatism
3. Advanced cataract
4. Macular degeneration
5. Corneal degenerations and dystrophies

DIMINISHED VISION IN BRIGHT LIGHT

The patient has good vision in dim light i.e. in the room. As soon as he steps out of room in bright light, or bright light from automobile fall on his eyes, his vision is reduced considerably. The commonest causes is **central nuclear cataract**. Other causes are **postpolar cataract, corneal opacity** and **macular degeneration**.

DIMINISHED NIGHT VISION

1. Vitamin A deficiency
2. Retinal dystrophy
3. Choroidal dystrophy

Vitamin A deficiency is generally seen in children. It generally develops over months and may be sudden in case of measles and diarrhea. The child has good vision in bright light (day light) but very poor vision in dim light. The child may not be able to move about even in his own house after sunset. He may not be able to locate his food kept in front of him. The condition is fully preventable by administering 2,00,000 IU of oral vitamin A to every child between six months to six years every six months. All children should also be immunized against measles because measles itself can cause vitamin A deficiency.

The next group of persons who develop night blindness are adults. The onset is gradual and equal in both eyes. The condition does not respond to vitamin A. The field is restricted. It may be seen in many members of the same family. These patients suffer from **retinitis pigmentosa**. There is no known treatment.

DIMINISHED COLOR VISION

This is commonly called color blindness but it does not fit in blindness in true sense.

It is a common disorder among **males**. About **eight percent of male** population suffer from this disorder. Women rarely suffer from color blindness. It is a **genetic defect**. The persons are generally not aware of the defect and come to know about it when tested specially for the defect. It is present from birth and there is no known treatment.

COLORED HALOES ROUND LIGHTS

A patient may complain of seeing **rainbows round artificial light**. It may be in one eye or both eyes. The commonest cause is **early stage of narrow angle glaucoma** where this may pass off after few hours or may terminate in acute attack of glaucoma. Other common cause is peripheral cortical cataract. The third cause of corneal edema due to any other cause.

DIPLOPIA (DOUBLE VISION)

The patient complains that everything looks two when both the eyes are open but the second image disappears when he closes one eye (any). This is the commonest type of **diplopia** and is called **binocular diplopia**. The commonest cause of such diplopia is **paralysis of one or more than one extraocular muscles**. The image that disappears on closing one eye is called **false image**. The false image may be separated from the true image horizontally and remain in the same level or may be at a higher level than the other but straight or the false image may be tilted. The separation between two images change with position of head (Fig. 3.1).

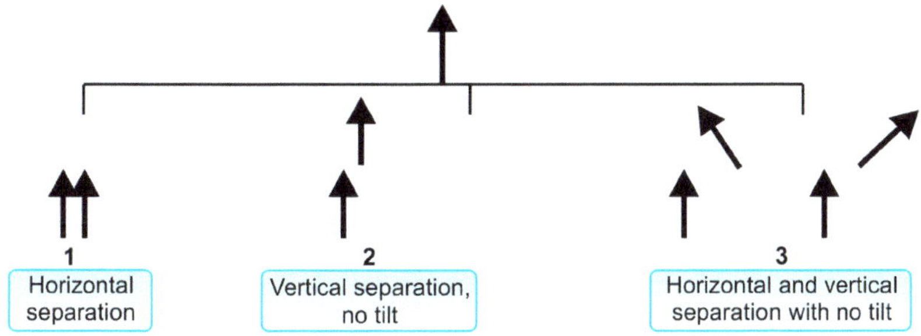

Fig. 3.1: Separation of images in diplopia

Uniocular diplopia is less common and the false image disappears only when an eye with pathology is closed. The common causes are **subluxated lens, iridodialysis, recent retinal detachment**. For example, if the right eye has subluxated lens that is causing diplopia, the diplopia will disappear only on closing the right eye and not the left eye. In contrast to this, if the right lateral rectus is paralysed, diplopia will disappear on closing any eye.

Causes of binocular diplopia are:

1. **Paralytic squint**—Paralysis of any of the extraocular muscles.
2. **Restrictive squint**—When any of the muscles is involved due to non-neurological cause:
   a. Fracture orbit
   b. Tumors of the orbit
   c. Thyroid disorder
   d. Myasthenia
3. **Anisometropia**—There is difference of more than 3 D power between two eyes.

DIMINISHED FIELD OF VISION (SEE CHAPTER PHYSIOLOGY)

Loss of field is called **scotoma**. It can be **central** or **peripheral**. The scotomas can be **unilateral** or **bilateral**, may not be of same grade. If the person is aware of the scotoma, it is called **positive scotoma**. If the patient is not aware of a scotoma, it is called **negative scotoma**. Positive scotomas generally develop suddenly.

> Lesions of retina and optic nerve cause unilateral loss of field of vision unless both the sides are involved simultaneously.

Causes of suddenly developing positive scotomas:

They are:

- Optic neuritis
- Ischemic optic neuropathy
- Central serous retinopathy
- Retinal detachment

Blind spot is an example of negative scotoma. It is present in every eye. It represents the **optic nerve head** which has no retinal element. It is situated on temporal side of the fixation point. The fixation point represents the macula. The blind spot is an oval area on the horizontal line. The horizontal line cuts the blind spot in two almost equal parts. The size of blind spot is 5.5° horizontally and 7.5° vertically.

The unilateral scotomas can be—(Fig. 3.2):

- Central (when involves macula)
- Centrocecal (when involved optic nerve head)
- Scattered (when retina, choroid are involved)
- Arcuate (when nerve fibers are involved)
- Hemianopia

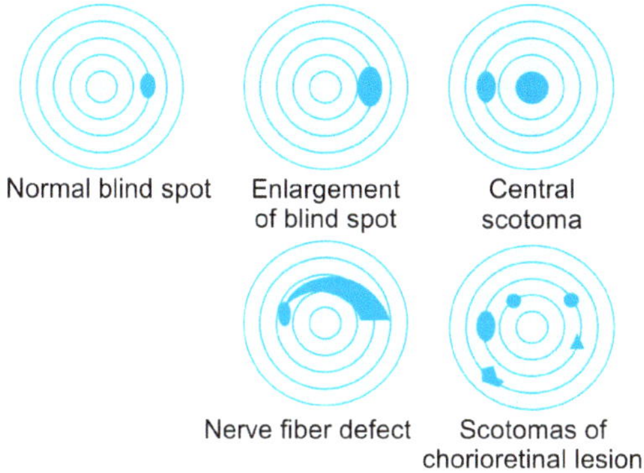

Fig. 3.2: Examples of central field changes

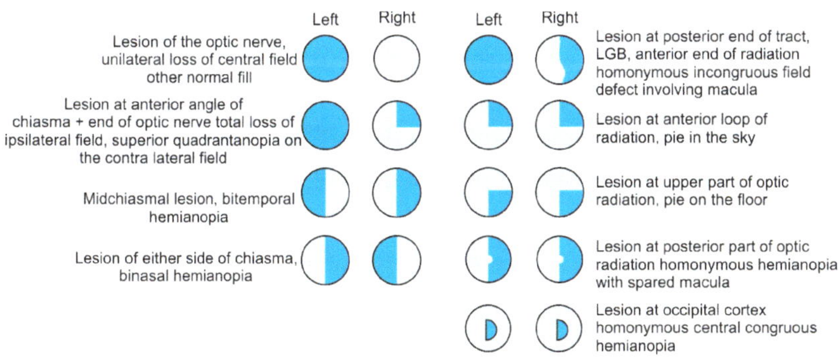

Fig. 3.3: Typical field changes at various levels of left visual path

- Enlargement of blind spot (papilledema, drusen of optic nerve)
- Peripheral constriction (retinitis pigmentosa)

Points to Note

1. Lesions of visual pathway from chiasma onwards causes bilateral field changes.
2. Lesions of chiasma cause heteronymous field changes, i.e. they are either temporal loss on each side or nasal loss on each side. The former is most common field change of involvement of chiasma and known as bitemporal hemianopia (Fig 3.3).
3. Lesions beyond chiasma cause homonymous field defect, i.e. there is loss of temporal field in one eye and nasal loss in the other eye.

A patient with central or centrocecal scotoma (Figs 3.4 to 3.6) may complain of seeing an area of less vision in the center of Snellen's chart. A person with bitemporal hemianopia (may not be able to read the letters correctly on the left side of the chart while looking through left eye and on the right side when looking through right eye. A person with peripheral constriction seems to see through a tunnel. Patients with constricted field and temporal hemianopia bump against persons on the road or furniture in the room.

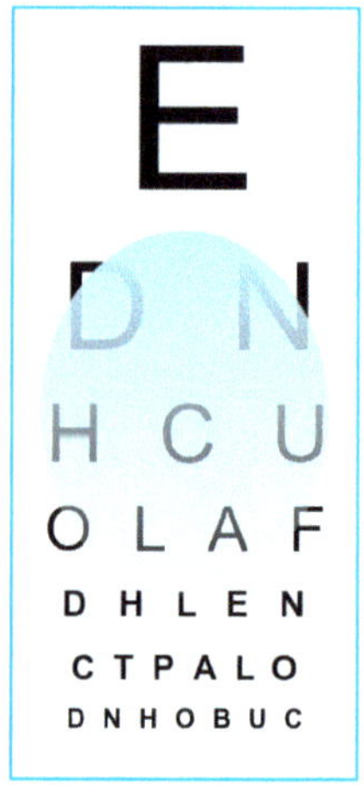

Fig. 3.4: Central scotoma as seen on Snellen's chart

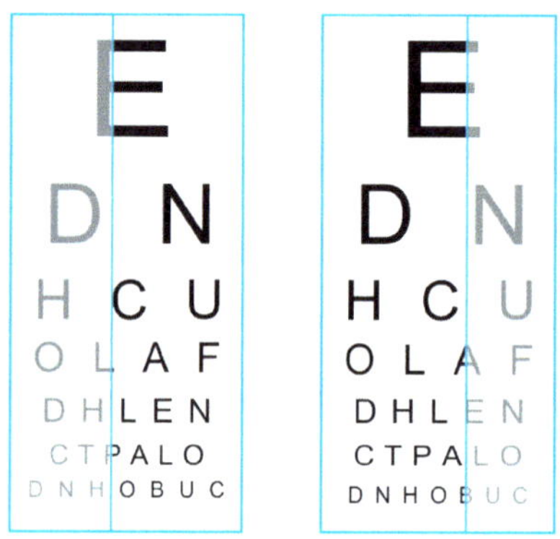

Fig. 3.5: Bitemporal hemianopia as seen on Snellen's chart

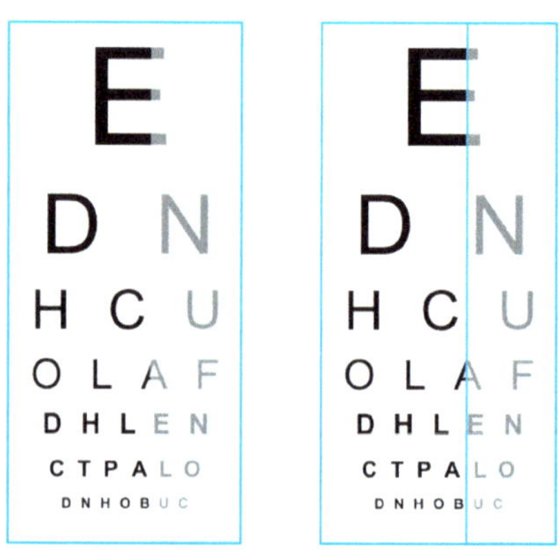

Fig. 3.6: Homonymous hemianopia as seen on Snellen's chart

FREQUENT CHANGE IN POWER OF GLASSES

1. Progressive myopia
2. Accommodative (facultative) hypermetropia shifting towards absolute hypermetropic
3. Central nuclear cataract
4. Diabetes
   i. Increased blood sugar (hyperglycemia) leads to myopia
   ii. Decreased blood sugar (hypoglycemia) leads to hypermetropia
5. Drugs taken orally
6. Drugs instilled locally:
   i. Miotics cause myopia
   ii. Cycloplegics cause hypermetropia

ASTHENOPIA

This is a vague feature of tiredness of the eye, which patient describe variously as pulling sensation, dull pain in eyes, watering, etc. This is caused by error of refraction and undiagnosed squint.

Less Common Visual Symptoms

1. Polyopia—Everything looks more than two. This is very common with distant lights like moon, street lights. The commonest cause is early lenticular changes.
2. Metamorphopsia—The object looks distorted. The straight lines look curved. Commonest cause is age related macular degeneration (Figs 3.7 and 3.8).
3. Glare—The patient does not like bright light.
   The common causes of glare are:
   a. Myopia
   b. Central nuclear cataract

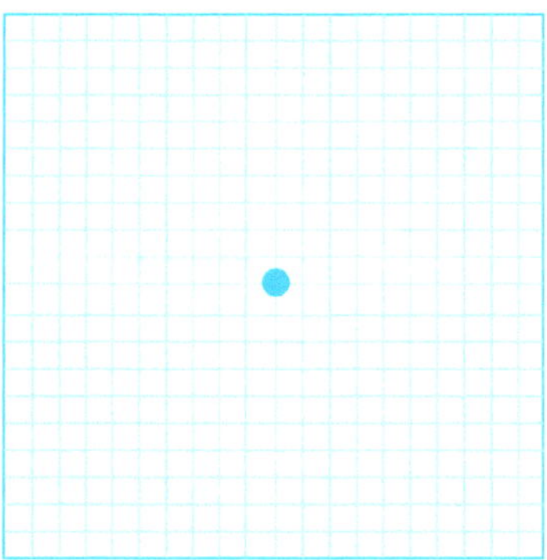

Fig. 3.7: Normal Amsler grid

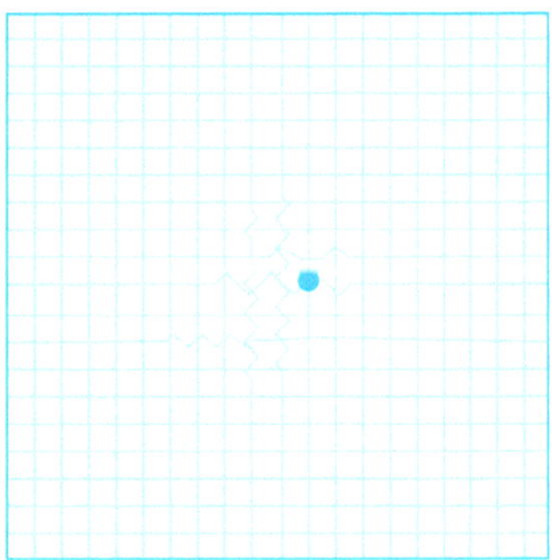

Fig. 3.8: Metamorphopsia

c. Instillation of mydriatic
d. Albinism

The symptoms are relieved by dark glasses.

4. Photophobia—This is intense intolerance to any light. This is generally associated with forceful closure of the lids and moving the face away from the source of light. Watering is very common in these eyes.
5. Blepharospasm—This is forceful closure of the eyes in presence of light. It is generally associated with photophobia and watering from the eyes. The symptoms are abolished for short time by instillation of local anesthetic agent. The symptoms are more marked in children.

   The common causes of blepharospasm are:
   a. Congenital glaucoma
   b. Phlyctenular keratoconjunctivitis
   c. Acute iritis
   d. Ultraviolet exposure of cornea
   e. Corneal foreign body, abrasion ulcer
6. Photopsia—The patient complains of seeing flashes of light even when the eyes are closed. This is a serious symptom and is most commonly seen in beginning of **retinal detachment**.
7. Chromatopsia—The patient complains that the light colored objects have colored tinge. The white wall may look to have faint blue color, or a pink color. This happens following removal of mature cataract. In jaundice the white color changes towards yellow. It should be remembered that there is no condition where black will look white or red or will look green.

Nonvisualocular symptoms can be unilateral or bilateral. They are:

1. Redness of the eye
2. Watering from the eye
3. Discharge from the eye
4. Pain in the eye
5. Drooping of the upper lid (ptosis)
6. Inability to close the lids (lagophthalmos)
7. Deviation of the eye (squint)
8. Swinging of the eyeball (nystagmus)
9. Whiteness on the black of the eye
   - Corneal opacity
   - Cataract
10. Bulging of the eye (proptosis)
11. Sinking of the eye in the orbit (enophthalmos)

REDNESS OF THE EYE

Redness of the eye is very common nonvisual symptom that may be present in one eye or both eyes may be involved. Redness of the eye can be free of pain without any visual loss or may be painful with visual loss. It may be associated with discharge.

The causes of redness of the eyes are:

1. Injury—Subconjunctival hemorrhage (Figs 3.9 to 3.11)
2. Acute infective conjunctivitis (Fig. 3.12)
   i. Viral conjunctivitis
   ii. Bacterial conjunctivitis
3. Allergic conjunctivitis
4. Acute iridocyclitis
5. Acute congestive glaucoma
6. Episcleritis and scleritis
7. Phlycten (Fig. 3.13)
8. Pterygium

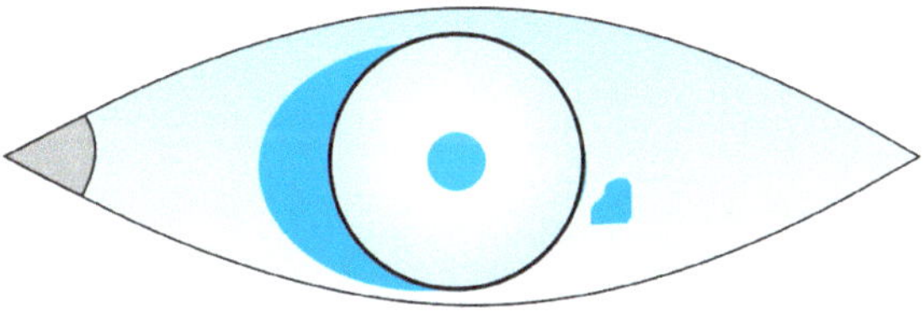

Fig. 3.9: Localized subconjunctival hemorrhage, periphery visible

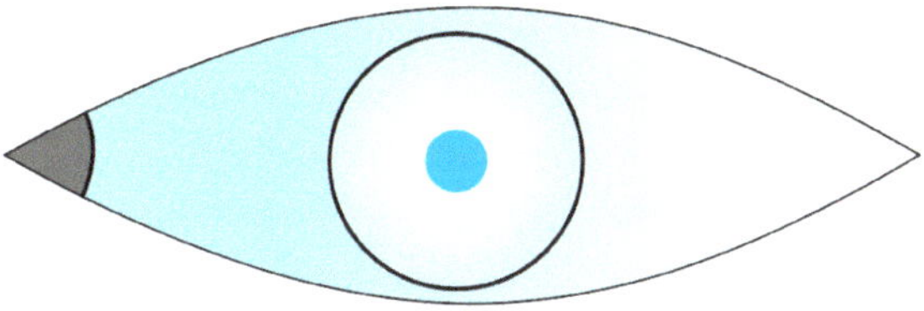

Fig. 3.10: Generalized subconjunctival hemorrhage, periphery not visible, may be due to head injury

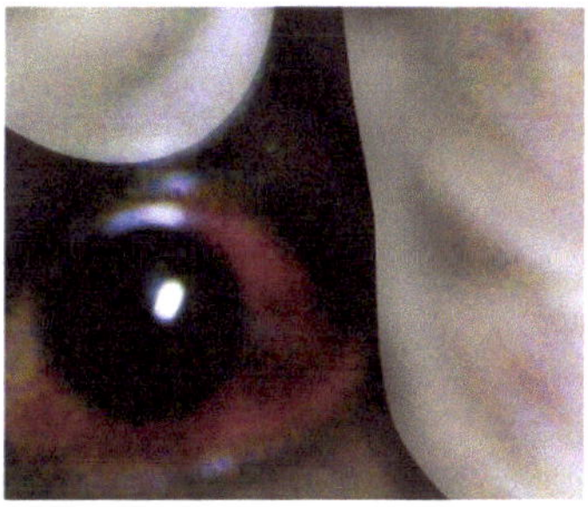

Fig. 3.11: Subconjunctival hemorrhage due to trauma

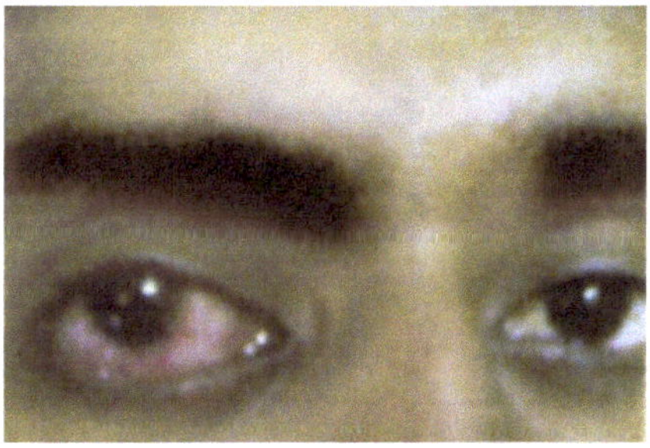

Fig. 3.12: Acute infective conjunctivitis

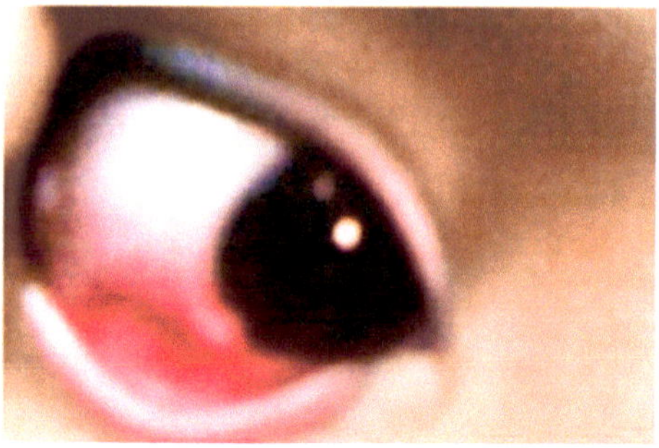

Fig. 3.13: Limbal phlycten

The congestion can be diffuse as in acute conjunctivitis or localized. The diffuse congestion generally starts on the periphery and spread towards the cornea.

The causes of localized conjunctival congestion are:

1. On the bulbar conjunctiva
   i. Small subconjunctival hemorrhage
   ii. Pterygium
   iii. Phlycten (Fig. 3.14)

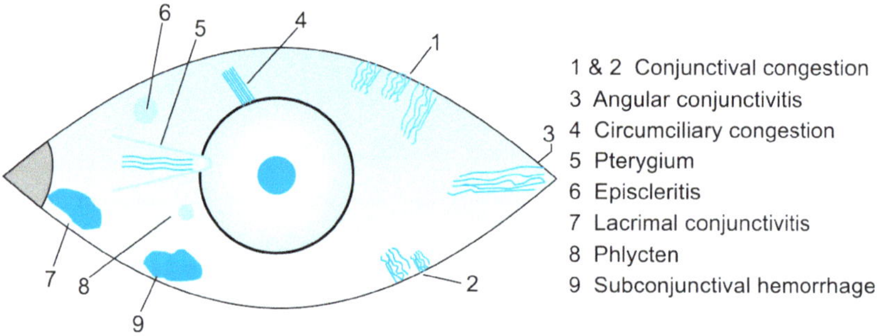

Fig. 3.14: Diagram showing localized conjunctival congestion

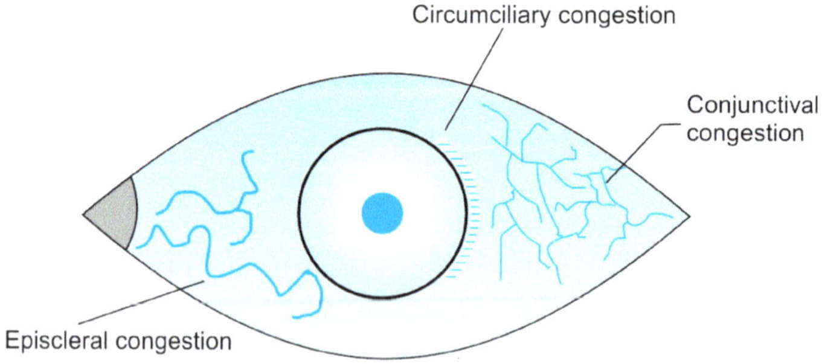

Fig. 3.15: Diagram showing three types of conjunctival congestion

iv. Episcleritis
v. Scleritis
vi. Angular conjunctivitis
vii. At the limbus
    i. Multiple phlyctens
    ii. Spring catarrh
2. Round the cornea (circumcorneal circumciliary) (Fig. 3.15)
    i. Corneal ulcer
    ii. Acute iritis
    iii. Acute congestive glaucoma

Watering from the Eyes

Normal eyes are always wet but the tears do not flow. A person is not aware of this wetness. When the person becomes aware of wetness, he complains of watering.

There are two types of watering from the eyes:
1. **Active watering**—This is called **lacrimation**. This is excess production of tears with normal drainage.
2. **Passive watering** is called **epiphora**. This is overflow of tears in presence of normal tear product.

In few cases both may be present.

Causes of Lacrimation

1. Injury to the outer eye—conjunctiva, cornea
2. Corneal foreign body
3. Keratitis, corneal ulcer
4. Phlyctenular keratoconjunctivitis
5. Acute anterior uveitis
6. Panuveitis
7. Acute congestive primary glaucoma
8. Acute congestive secondary glaucoma
9. Acute viral conjunctivitis
10. Acute allergic conjunctivitis
11. Reflex lacrimation due to irritation of nasal mucosa, throat, sinuses

Causes of Epiphora

1. Congenital nasolacrimal duct block (congenital dacryocystitis)
2. Ectropion of the lower lid
3. Absent or small lower puncta
4. Sac has been removed

Discharge from the Eyes

Discharge from the eyes denote disease of conjunctiva in the form of either infection (conjunctivitis) or allergy. The discharge consists of tear, mucus and microorganisms.

The discharge can be:
- Watery: Viral conjunctivitis
- Mucopurulent: Mild bacterial conjunctivitis
- Purulent: Severe bacterial conjunctivitis (gonococcal conjunctivitis)
- Roapy: Allergic conjunctivitis (spring catarrh)

Due to excess of mucopurulent discharge, the lids get stuck together when the patient sleeps.

Pain in the Eyes

The patient may complain of pain:
a. In the eyeball
b. Round the eyeball, i.e. in the lid, over the sac.

Causes of Pain in the Eyes

1. Injury
2. Iridocyclitis
3. Acute glaucoma
4. Corneal ulcer

Causes of Pain in the Lid

1. Stye
2. Infected chalazion
3. Lid abscess

Causes of Pain Over the Sac

- Acute dacryocystitis

Drooping of the Upper Eye Lid

The normal upper eye lid covers the upper 2 mm of the cornea. If it covers more than 2 mm, it is called drooping of upper lid (ptosis).

The causes of drooping of the upper lid can be:
1. Swelling of the upper lid (Fig. 3.16)
2. Growth in the upper lid (Fig. 3.17)
3. Small or absent eyeball (Fig. 3.18)
4. Congenital (Fig. 3.19)
5. Neurological
6. Myogenic (Fig. 3.20)
7. Myasthenia (Fig. 3.21)
8. Senile (Fig. 3.22)

The first three are called **pseudoptosis** while the last three are called **true ptosis**.

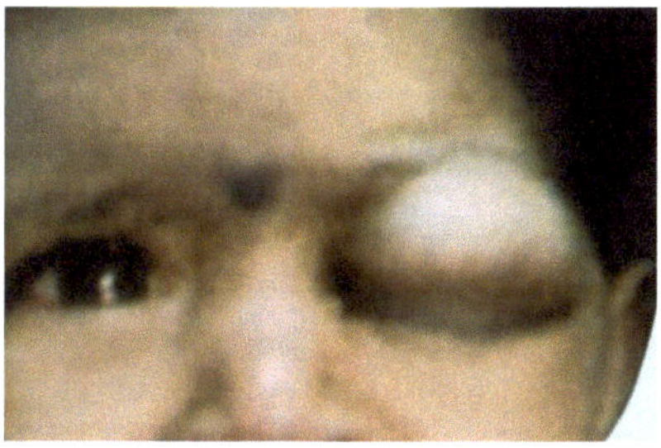

Fig. 3.16: Pseudoptosis due to swelling of the upper lid

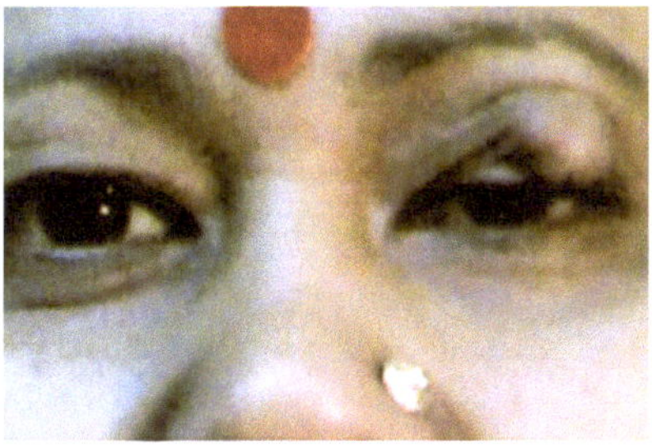

Fig. 3.17: Pseudoptosis due to growth in the left upper lid

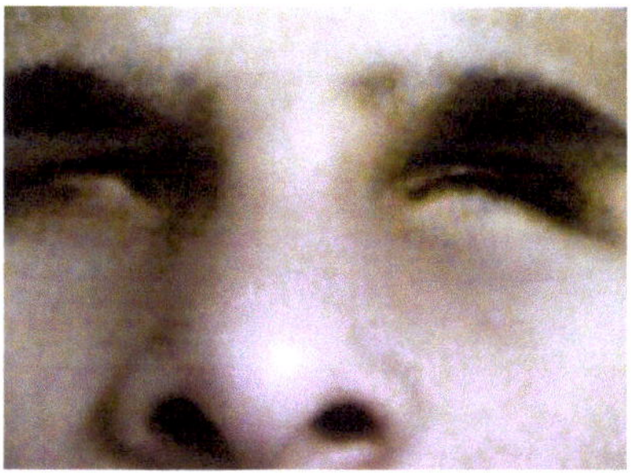

Fig. 3.18: Pseudoptosis due to small eyeball

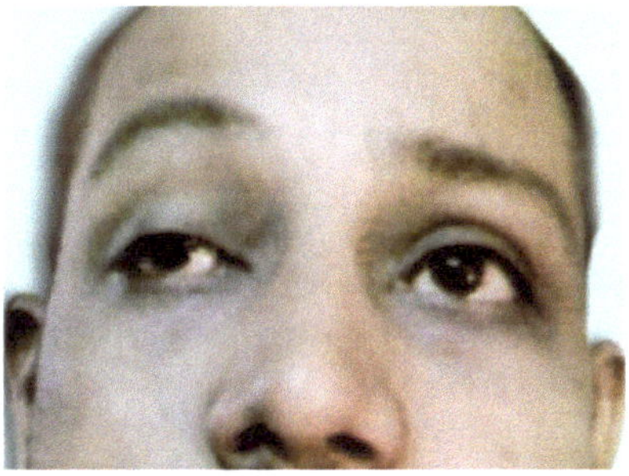

Fig. 3.19: Unilateral congenital ptosis

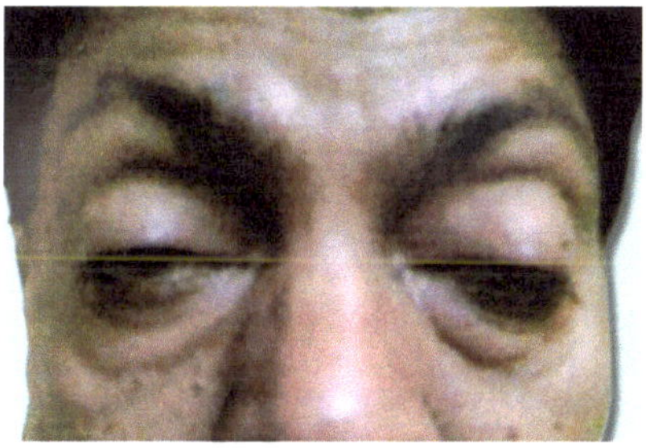

Fig. 3.20: Bilateral myogenic ptosis

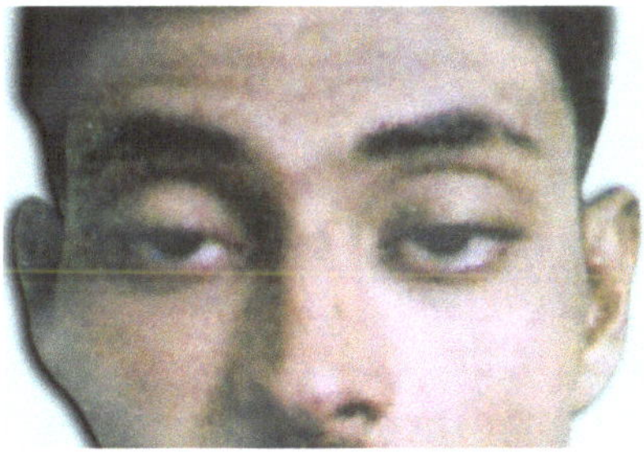

Fig. 3.21: Ptosis due to myasthenia

Inability to Close the Lids

A person should be able to close the lids voluntarily (at will, whenever he likes). Inability to close the lids is called **lagophthalmos**.

Lagophthalmos can be:

a. Neurological, i.e. paralysis of orbicularis (7th nerve palsy = facial palsy)
b. Mechanical—The large eyeball or protruding eyeball prevents the lids to close. This is brought about by **exophthalmos** or **large ciliary staphyloma.**

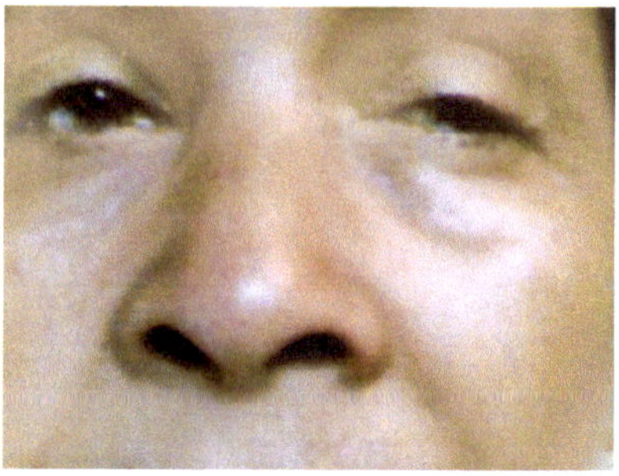

Fig. 3.22: Senile ptosis

Deviation of the Eyeball

Normally the two eyes are straight when looking at a distant object and the distance of the cornea from the canthi are equal in both the eyes and the image of the light held at 33 cm in front of the eye is at the center of the cornea. The two eyes are parallel to each eye when moving horizontally or vertically. While looking at a near object (converging), they are not parallel but the distance between the cornea and the medial canthus is the same in the two eyes (Fig. 3.23).

Any deviation of one eye in relation to the other eye when both eyes are looking at a distant object is called **squint**.

Squint can be present at birth, may develop in childhood or develop in adults.

There are two types of squint

1. Paralytic
2. Nonparalytic (concomitant)

Paralytic Squint

1. The main symptom of paralytic squint is **diplopia** (seeing everything double) which disappears on covering any of the eye. The cause of squint is paralysis of one or more than one extraocular muscles.
2. The next symptom is deviation of the eye. The eye is deviated away from the paralysed muscle, i.e. if the lateral rectus is paralyzed, the eye is deviated towards the nose.
3. The patient with paralytic squint complains that he can not move the squinting eye equally on all direction.
4. The patient may say that if he keeps his head turned on one particular side, his diplopia becomes less. Sometimes the person is not aware of this changed position of the head but the onlookers may point out the abnormal head position.
5. The symptoms of paralytic squint are of sudden onset.
6. The squint due to paralysis of extraocular muscles do not change sides (They do not alternate).

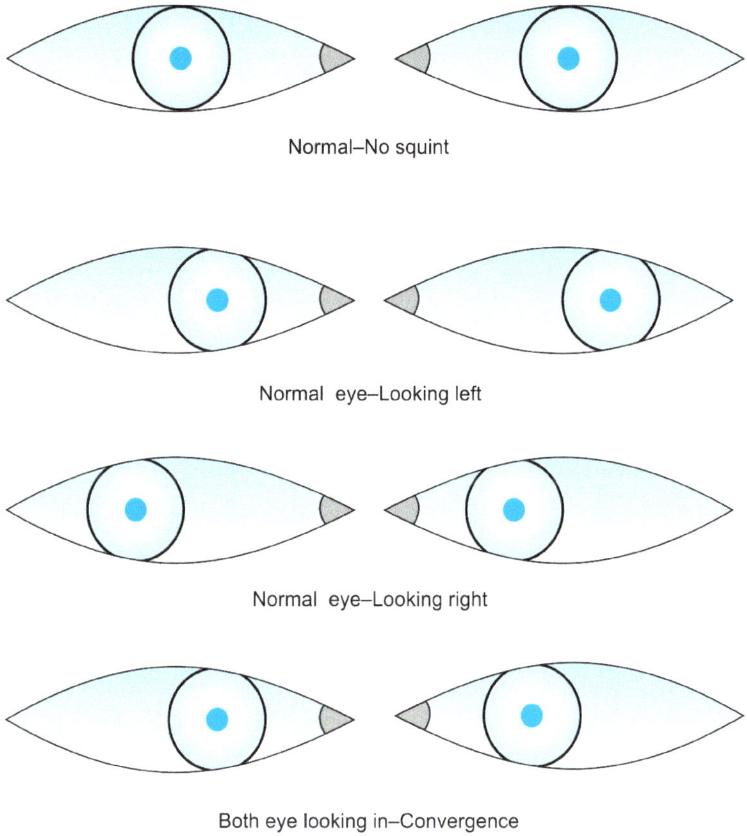

Fig. 3.23: Normal positions of the eye in various directions

Symptoms of Nonparalytic Squint

1. The patient may have a squint but the patient may not be aware of it unless pointed out.
2. The movements are maintained in both the eyes and are equal in both the eyes.
3. The squint may be limited to one eye only. This is called **unilateral squint** or may **alternate** between two eyes. This is called **binocular squint** or **alternate squint**.
4. There is no diplopia in nonparalytic squint.
5. There is no abnormal head posture.
6. The patient may have a gross loss of vision in the squinting eye.

Nonparalytic squint can be **latent squint** or **manifest squint**. The former is known as **phoria** about which the patient is not aware. Concomitant squint is that squint which is visible to the patient and the onlooker and one referred to as tropias. As per direction of the eye it can be **esotropia**, i.e. the eye deviates in, **exotropia** when the eye deviates out, **hypertropia**

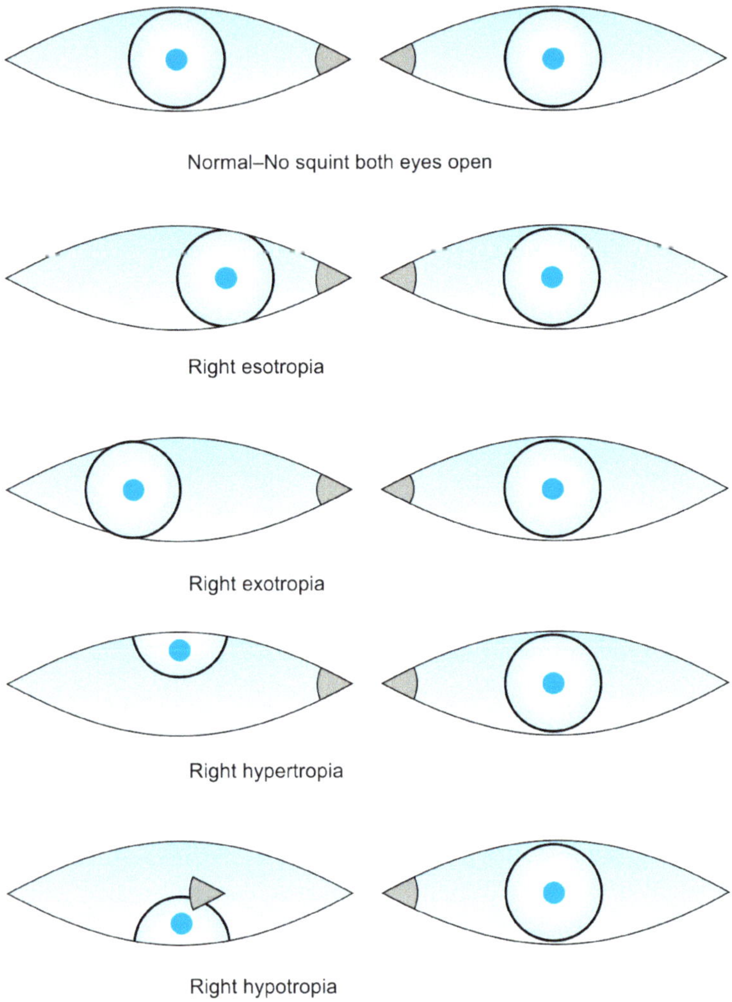

Fig. 3.24: Various types of tropia

when the eye deviates up and hypotropia when the eye deviates down. One eye may deviate always and the other eye remain straight, this is called **unilateral tropia** while both eyes squint equally and in the same direction when the fusion is broken, is called **alternative tropia** or binocular tropia. There is no diplopia in tropia. The movements are normal in all directions (Fig. 3.24).

Swinging of the Eyeball (Nystagmus)

Generally the patient is not aware of to and fro movement of the eye (oscillation). This is called **nystagmus** but the observers may notice it. Most of the time the oscillation are equal in two eyes. Horizontal oscillation are very common. Less common are vertical movements. Circular movements are least common.

Whitening of the Black Portion of the Eye

The portion of the eye that looks black (dark) is the **iris**. In the center of this large black portion is a central darker portion. This is **pupil**. The iris is not capable of turning white. The whiteness that the patient refers to is either in the cornea (**corneal opacity**) or in the lens (**cataract**) that is seen through the pupil.

A person becomes aware of corneal opacity when it is dense. Lighter opacities are not visible to untrained persons.

Persons become aware of lenticular opacity more often than corneal opacity.

Bulging of the Eye

There are two causes of bulging of the eyes:
1. Proptosis: In this generally a growth behind the eyeball pushes the eyeball forward.
2. Exophthalmos: This is seen in disease of **thyroid** gland due to a combination of many complex chemical changes.

Both the conditions can be unilateral or bilateral.

> Proptosis is more commonly unilateral while exophthalmos is generally bilateral.

The bulging of the eye is measured by an instrument called **exophthalmometer**.

Sinking of the Eyeball in the Orbit (Enophthalmos)

This is due to small eyeball (**microphthalmos**), soft eyeball (**phthisis**) or **fracture orbit**. This gives an appearance of ptosis as well.

Nonocular Symptoms

There are only two nonocular symptoms of ophthalmic interest. They are:
1. Headache
2. Vertigo

Out of the two, headache is more common.

It can be:
1. Migraineous (due to migraine)
2. Nonmigraineous

Vertigo is less common. It is generally accompanied by loss of hearing and nystagmus.

CHAPTER

4

Examination of the Eye

The examination of the eye consists of history of the disease and examination of the eye. The history taking should precede all other examinatins.

IMPORTANCE OF HISTORY TAKING IN OCULAR EXAMINATION

The patient is asked the purpose of his visit. These are the complaints of the person (symptoms). The symptoms may be **ocular**, **nonocular** or **both**. The person may have:

1. **Single symptom**, i.e. difficulty in near vision, diminished distant vision, squint. A patient may come with single symptom like squint. On close questioning and examination, he may have diminished vision in the squinting eye.
2. **Multiple symptoms** i.e. diminished near as well as distant vision, redness of eye with diminished vision, combination of redness, watering and diminished vision is very common.
3. Next step is to find out if the symptoms are unilateral (on one side only) or bilateral on both sides.
   When bilateral, find out if the symptoms in both sides started simultaneously (at the same time) or the other eye got involved after sometimes, may be days or weeks.
4. History of the disease many a times leads directly to diagnosis. Some of the common examples are:
   i. A school going child complains that he can not see the writings on the blackboard or the mother complains that the child moves near the TV set to see properly. Obviously this child has diminished distant vision which is most probably error of refraction. The commonest type of error of refraction at this age group with above symptoms is myopia.
   ii. A grandfather who was comfortable with near correction for years, finds that he can see near things better without glasses. Though the distant vision has diminished, is suffering from cataract.

iii. A child under five years, from slums is brought with complains of diminished night vision for few weeks. The mother may say that the child can not locate his food after sunset. This child is suffering from **vitamin A deficiency** and will improve with vitamin A injection.
iv. In contrast to this, an adult complains of diminished night vision for many months/years, the patient suffers from **retinitis pigmentosa** which will not improve with vitamin A injection.
v. A person over forty years complains that he has night blindness. On questioning, it is found that he finds difficulty in reading at night, he suffers from **presbyopia**. This is corrected by plus lenses.
vi. A person complains of diplopia of sudden origin, suffers from **paralytic squint**.

History of Past Illness

History of past illness may be or may not be related to the present illness. Some of the past illnesses/events can be related to present illness. The common examples are:

i. **Trauma**: A trauma in the past may result in many disorders later. The common are—Traumatic cataract, glaucoma, retinal detachment, corneal opacity.
ii. History suggestive of **anterior uveitis** may be related to complicated cataract, secondary glaucoma, cystoid macular edema.
iii. **Spring catarrh** treated by strong steroid for long time may lead to **steroid induced glaucoma**.

Past illness that are not related to present illness are mostly infective. Thus stye, chalazion, conjunctiritis, dacryocystitis, infective conjunctivitis in childhood can not be related to cataract, glaucoma or retinal detachment in old age.

History of Past Surgery

Amblyopia in patients may give history of **squint surgery** in childhood. A soft eye may have history of **glaucoma surgery**. **Retinal detachment** was very common following lens extraction.

History of Systemic Diseases

Specially diabetes, hypertension and thyroid diseases are associated with many ocular diseases.

Family History

Some of the diseases are seen in same family. Many members of the same family may suffer from the same disease.

Common examples are—Error of refraction, squint, early onset of cataract, glaucoma, retinitis pigmentosa, hereditary optic atrophy.

Examination of eye is broadly divided into following groups:

1. Recording of vision
2. External examination of the eye
3. Internal examination of the eye
4. Special investigation

Recording of Vision (Visual Acuity)

Recording of vision is one of the most important part of ocular examination. It should get priority over other tests.

Vision Consists of

i. Distant vision
ii. Near vision
iii. Color vision
iv. Field of vision

Recording of Distant Vision

There are various methods of recording distant vision.
There is a fixed order in which vision should be tested and recorded.

1. The right eye is tested first, this is followed by examination of the left eye. Then both eyes are tested together.
2. Vision is tested first without glasses.
3. This is followed by testing of vision with glasses.
4. The vision is recorded as:
   VA = Visual acuity
   RE denotes right eye and LE denotes left eye.
   BE means both eyes together.
   They are also written as OD, OS and OU respectively.

Testing of Distant Vision

Vision for distant is tested by various vision charts kept either at six meters or at three meters.They are:

1. Snellen's chart (Figs 4.1 and 4.2)
2. E chart (Fig. 4.3)
3. C chart (Fig. 4.4)
4. Log MAR chart (Fig. 4.5)
5. Pictorial charts
6. Dots

Out of the above **Snellen's charts** are most commonly used in literate persons. They are available in various languages. The E chart and C charts are used for illiterate persons. The pictorial charts and dots are not very accurate charts.

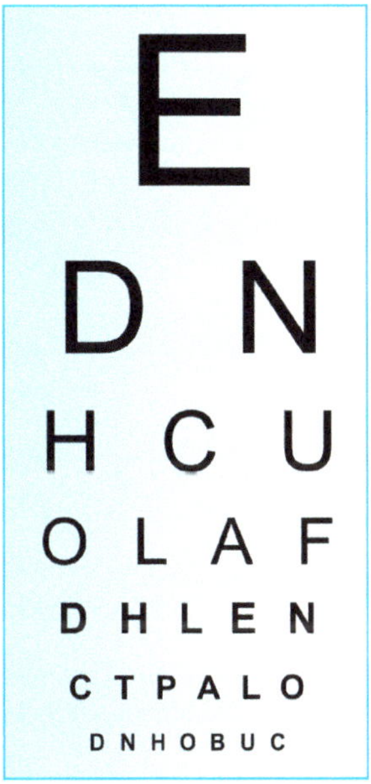

Fig. 4.1: Snellen's chart (alphabet)

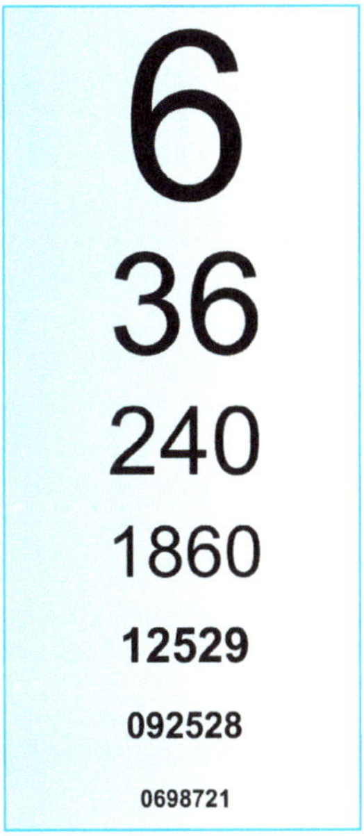

Fig. 4.2: Snellen's chart (number)

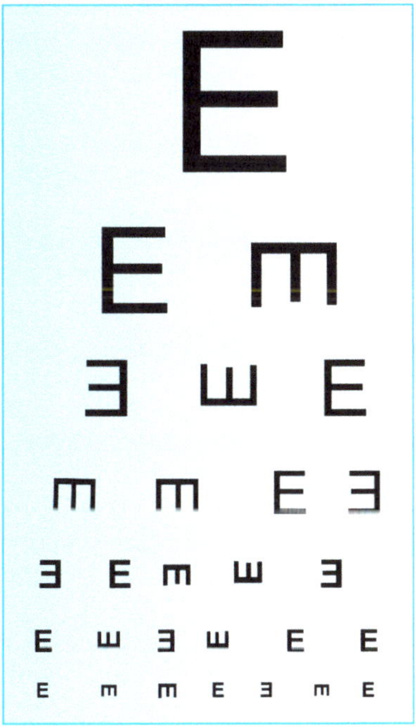

Fig. 4.3: E chart

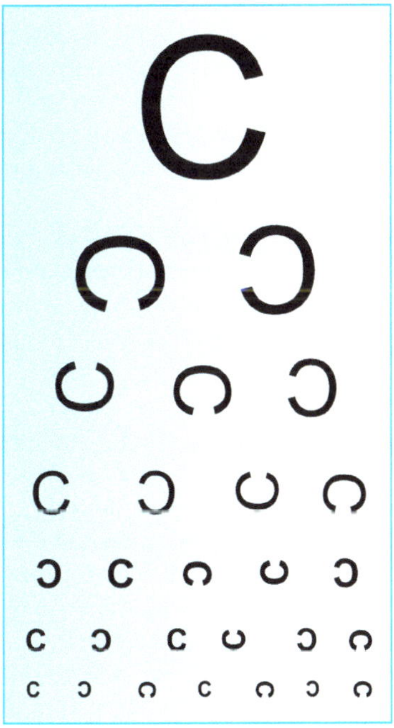

Fig. 4.4: C chart

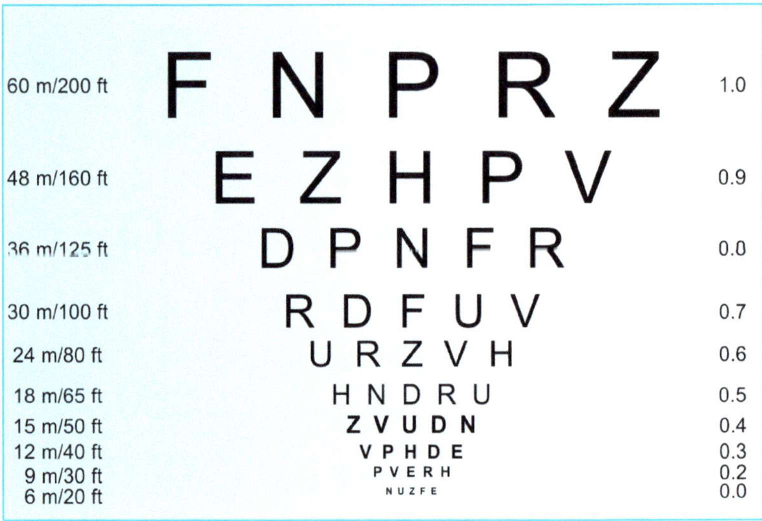

Fig. 4.5: Log MAR chart for distant to be used at four meters

Each Snellen's vision chart has seven lines of letters printed black on white background except. log MAR chart that has ten lines with equal number of letters i.e 5 letter in each line. The top most letter in other charts has only one letter. The second line has two letters. The numbers of letters in each successive line increases and the seventh line has seven letters. Letters in each line are of same size. The vision charts can be illuminated from outside or they may be illuminated from inside in a vision drum.

The vision charts are used at a distance of 6 meters or 20 feet. If the space available is less than 6 meters than there are two alternatives:

1. Reduce the size of the chart by half without changing the ratio of size between the two lines and keep at three meter.
2. Use a plane mirror at three meters and a large chart with letters reversed (Figs 4.6 and 4.7).

Chart that has letters which look the same when reflected through a plane mirror at three meters Fig. 4.6. The reversed chart is kept little behind, up above the head of the patient. If a self-illuminated vision drum is used, it should be seen that the illumination is uniform all over the chart.

To record vision

The patient sits at a distance of 6 meters from a regular large chart, or three meters from a 50% reduced chart or plane mirror. Log MAR chart is used at 4 meters (Fig. 4.5).

One eye is tested at a time. It is a convention that the right eye is tested first and the left eye later. While testing one eye, the other eye is fully covered without pressure on the globe. This can be done by:

1. Palm of the patient or examiner (Fig. 4.8A)
2. Occluder

i. In the trial frame (Fig. 4.8B)
ii. Hand held (Fig. 4.8C)

Figs 4.9A and B show incorrect method of closing one eye

Figure 4.10 shows various types of commonly used trial frames. Once the vision has been recorded in each eye, vision in both eyes together is tested thereafter.

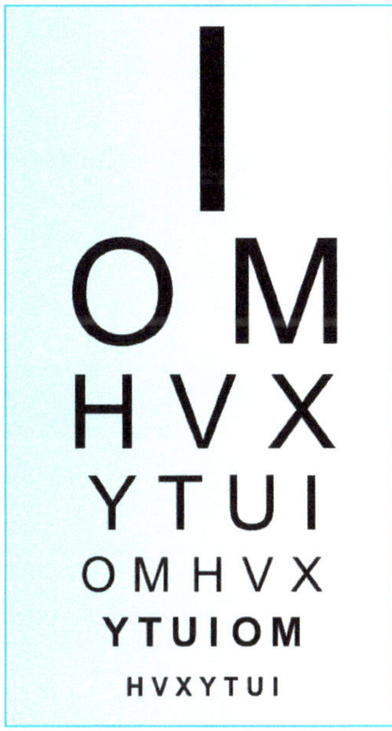

Fig. 4.6: Reversible Snellen's chart, the letters look similar in the chart as well as in the mirror used at three meters

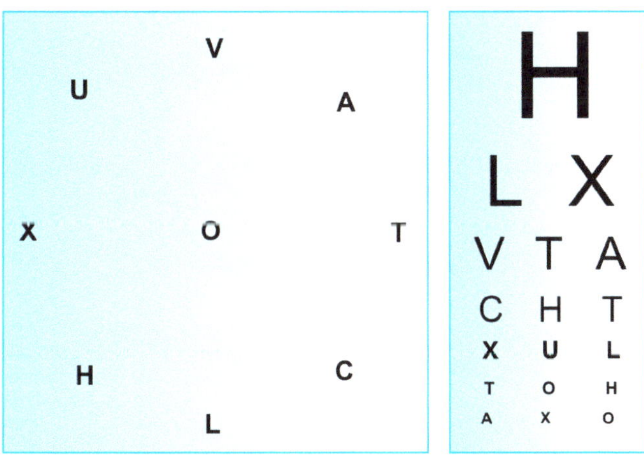

Fig. 4.7: Snellen's test for young children and retarded (STYCAR)

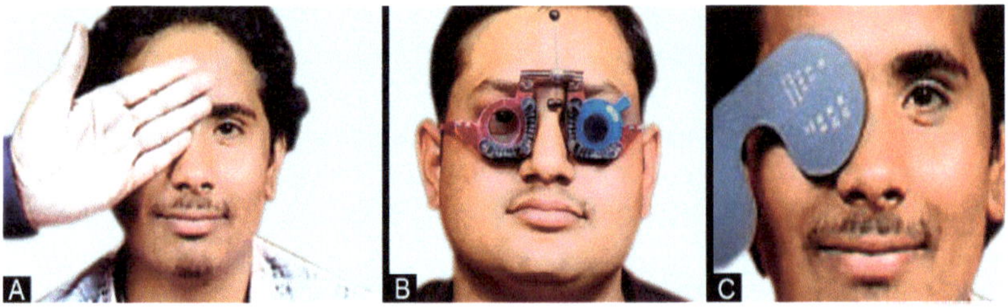

Figs 4.8A to C: Correct method of closing one eye for recording vision

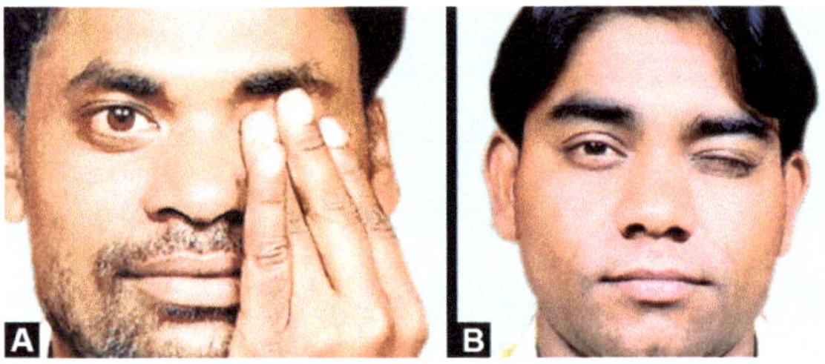

Figs 4.9A to B: Incorrect method of closing one eye for recording vision

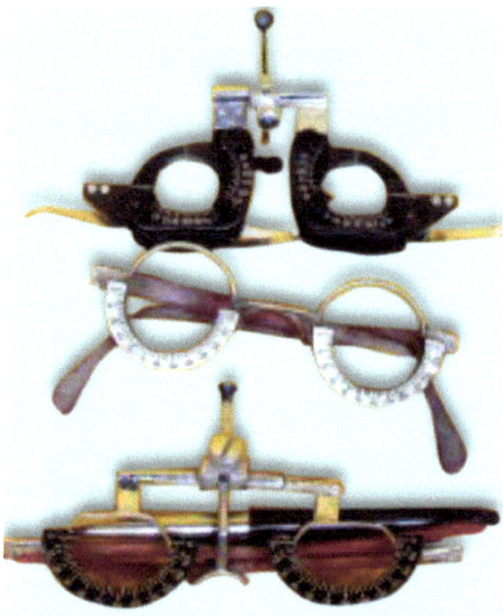

Fig. 4.10: Commonly used types of trial frames

> Vision in both eyes together is better than in one eye provided the other eye is fixing.

To record vision, the patient is asked to read the chart from above downwards. In usual vision chart, there are seven lines. If the patient can read all the letters in seventh line, it is called as 6/6 or 20/20. If the patient can read six lines, it is 6/9, 5th line is 6/12.

Line read	Vision
Seven	6/6 or 20/20
Six	6/9
Five	6/12 or 20/40
Four	6/18
Three	6/24 or 20/80
Two	6/36
One	6/60 200/200

> Vision 6/6 is normal vision. It means that the person can read the seventh line at a distance of six meters and the top letter at 60 meters.

If the patient is unable to read the top letter, he is moved towards the chart by one meters at a time and asked to read the top letter. If he can read the top letter at 5 meters, his vision is 5/60, at 4 meters it is 4/60, at three meters it is 3/60 and 1/60 at 1 meters.

If the patient can not read the top letter at one meter, he is asked to count the fingers of the examiner at one meter, half-meter and close to face and noted as CF 1 meter, CF 1/2 meter and CF close to face.

If the patient fails to count the fingers close to his face, he is asked if he can see the moving palm of the examiner. If he can do so, it is written as HM.

If patient fails to see examiners palm, light from a torch is thrown in the eye from front and the patient is asked if he can see the light. If he can see the light it is noted as perception of light or PL.

Then the torch is moved to left, right, above and below the eye and the patient is asked to tell the direction from which the light is coming. This is called projection of light and noted as Pr light.

Causes of Loss of Perception of Light

1. **Causes in the eyeball** (globe)
   i. Anophthalmos
   ii. Absence of total eyeball (enucleated eye)
   iii. Absence of internal structure of eye (eviscerated eye)
2. **Causes in the retina**
   i. Total retinal detachment of long standing
   ii. Central retinal artery occlusion

3. **Causes in optic nerve**
   Optic atrophy:
   i. Primary
   ii. Secondary
   iii. Glaucomatous
   iv. Transsection of optic nerve
4. **Causes of visual cortex**—Cortical blindness

Causes of Faulty Projection of Light (PrL)

1. Large retinal detachment
2. Absolute glaucoma
3. Advanced retinal dystrophy
4. Bitemporal hemianopia

Points to remember

1. Any amount of corneal opacity, lenticular opacity, high error of refraction or large macular lesion will not cause loss of perception of light so long the optic nerve is functioning.
2. Perception of light once lost can not be regained by any treatment.
3. Once it has been confirmed that there is no perception of light, there is no need to test projection of light.
4. It is not possible to have projection of light in absence of perception of light.

Once vision has been recorded, the next step is to find out if the person uses glasses, if so find out the purpose of it.

1. Is it for distance only?
2. Is it for near only? Generally these patients are above forty years without any power for distance vision.
3. Does the spectacle have power both for distance as well as near. These patients are generally past forty years of age.

If the pair of glasses has different powers for distance and near, find out if the person is using—(Fig. 4.11).

1. Bifocal glasses
2. Trifocal
3. Progressive

The next step is to find out the type and power of the glasses in each eye.

Procedure to Find Out Power of Spectacle Lens (Flow chart 4.1)

1. Hold the spectacle by the frame between thumb and index finger (Do not touch the lens).
2. Bring the spectacle near the eye (examiner) with side bars away from the eye.
3. Examine one lens at a time.

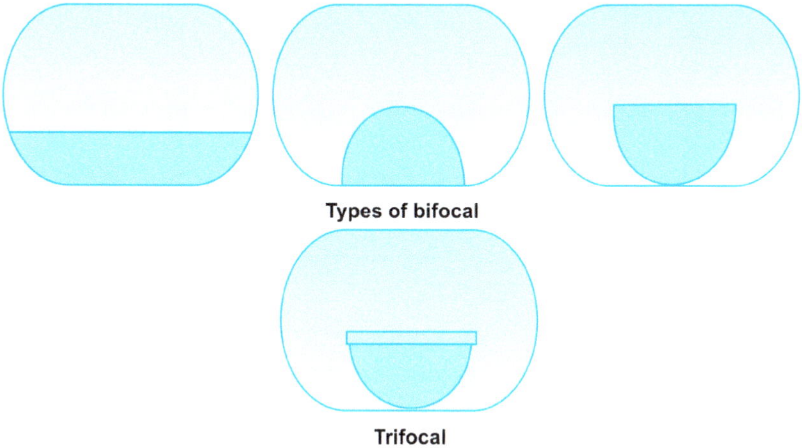

Fig. 4.11: Type of reading glasses

Flow chart 4.1: Procedure to find out power of spectacle lens

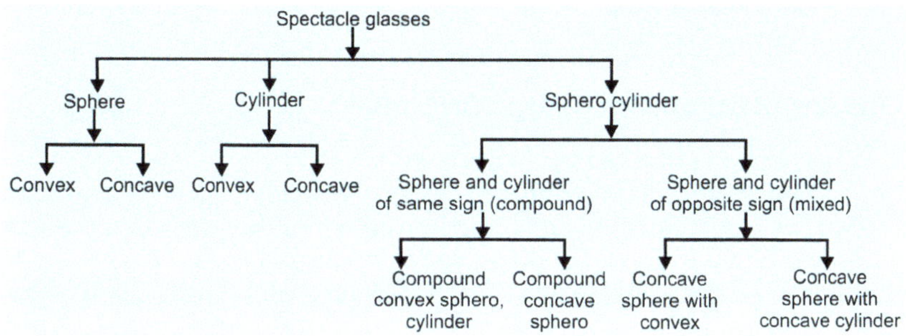

4. Look at a distant object.
5. Holding the spectacle away from the eye and seeing a near object is wrong.
6. Move the lens from side to side, up and down and rotate.
7. **Note:**
   i. The movement of the object, i.e. with or against
   ii. Size of the object enlarged, same or reduced
   iii. Look for distortion on rotation.
8. If there is no movement of the object, no change in size and no distortio,n the glass under examination is **plain glass** (without power).
   A lens is an optical device in which at least one surface is curved. The spherical lenses are part of a sphere and have equal power all over (in all meridians and axes). The cylindrical lenses are part of a cylinder. They have an axis. There is no power along the axis. The power is at right angle to the axis. According to shape, lenses can be—(Figs 4.12A to F)

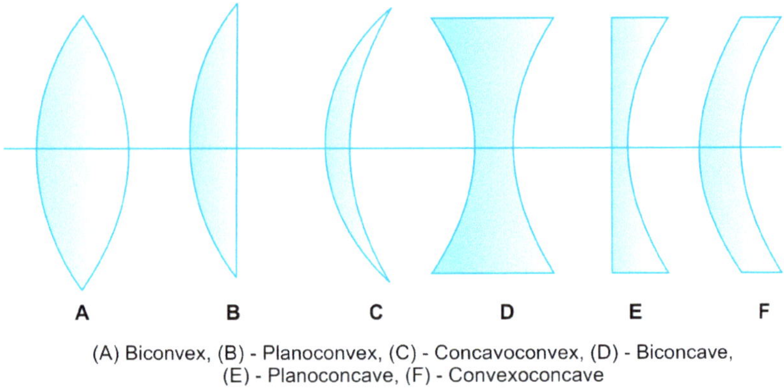

Figs 4.12A to F: Type of lenses; A. Biconvex B. Planoconvex C. concavoconvex D. Biconcave E. Planoconcave F. convexoconve

- Planoconcave
- Planoconvex
- Bi convex
- Convexoconcave
- Convexoconcave

Characteristics of Various Types of Lens

1. Plus (convex) sphere Figs 4.13 and 4.14
   i. The object looks magnified (larger) when seen through convex lens.
   ii. The object moves against the movement of the lens, i.e. if the lens is shifted to right, the image moves to the left.
   iii. The shape of the image does not change on rotating the lens (no distortion).
   iv. The lens is thin on the periphery and thick in center.

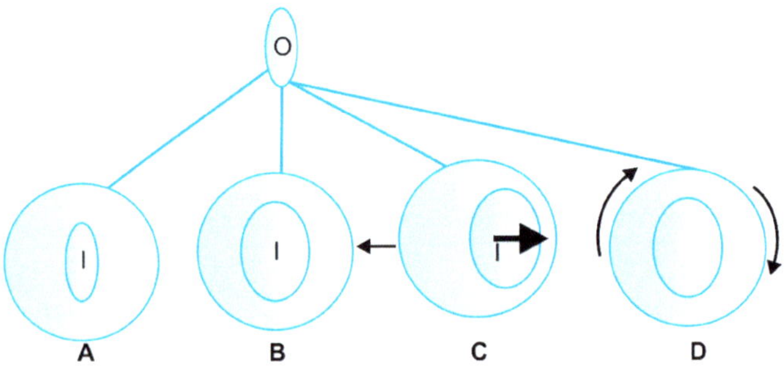

Figs 4.13A to D: Characteristics of convex lenses: change in size of object O when seen through; A. Plain glass, no change in size of the image I; B. Seen through convex lens, image I is enlarged movement of the image on movement of the lens; C. Image 'I' moves against the movement of the convex lens; D. No change in shape of image 'I' on rotating the convex lens

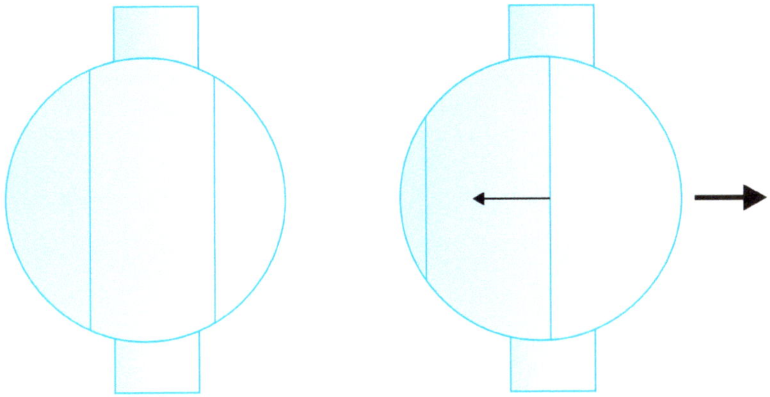

Fig. 4.14A: Movement of the image in a plus sphere

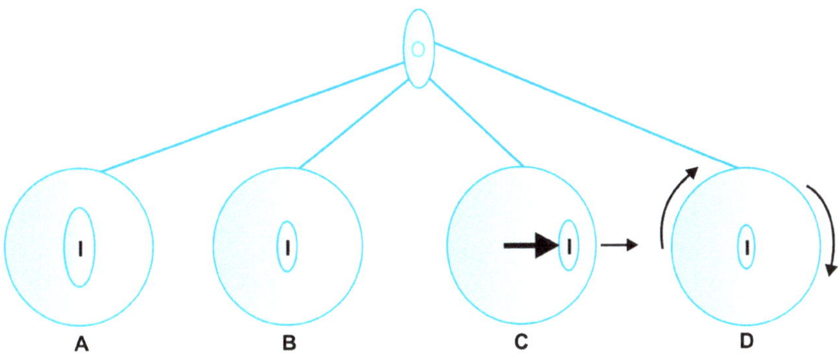

Figs 4.15A to D Characteristics of concave lenses, Change in size of object O when seen through; A. Plain glass, no change in size of the image I; B. Seen through convex lens, image I is diminished in size, movement of the image on movement of the lens; C Image 'I' moves with the movement of the concave lens; D. No chang in shape of image 'I' on rotating the concave lens

2. Minus (concave) sphere (Figs 4.15A to D and 4.16):
    i. Object looks **smaller** when seen through concave lens.
    ii. The object moves **with movement of the** concave lens.
    iii. The shape of the object does not change with rotation of lens (no distortion).
    iv. The lens is thick on the periphery and thus in the center.
3. Plus (convex) cylinder (Figs 4.17A to C)
    i. The object elongated in one direction (at right angles to the axis).
    ii. The object is widened at right angles to the axis.
    iii. If the axis is rotated by 90°, the image is shortened along the axis.
    iv. There is distortion of the image when the lens is rotated.

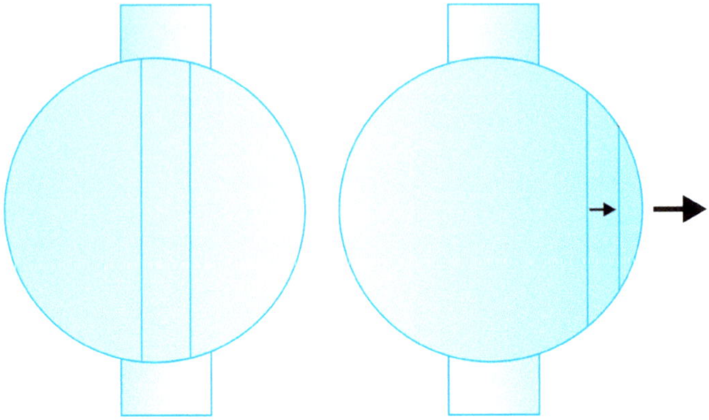

Fig. 4.16: Movement of the image in a minus sphere

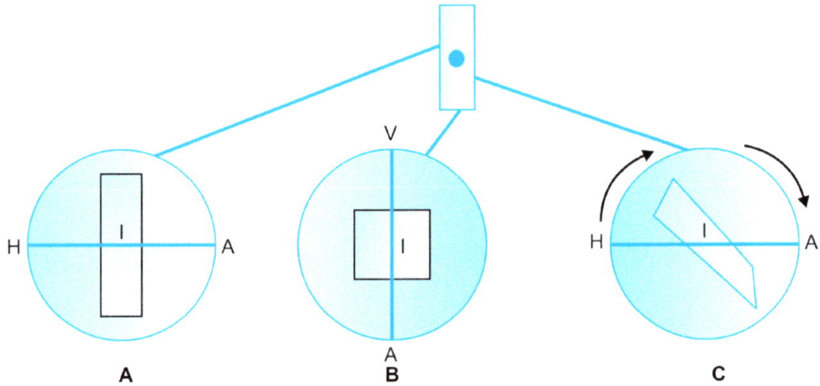

Figs 4.17A to C: Characteristics of plus cylinder; Object O seen through cylinder; A. The image 'I' looks longer at right angle to horizontal axis HA; B. The image 'I' looks short and broad at vertical axis VA; C. The Image 'I' looks distorted when the cylinder is rotated

4. Minus (concave) cylinder (Fig. 4.18A to C)
   i. The object is shortened at one meridian (at right angles to the axis).
   ii. The object is narrowed at right angles to the axis.
   iii. If the axis is rotated by 90°, the image is elongated (narrowed) along the axis of the cylinder.
   iv. There is distortion of image when the lens is rotated.

A Comparison of plus and minus sphere in made in table 4.1.

Uses of Lenses

The lenses are used in spectacles or in optical instruments.

Use of plus spherical lenses in spectacles:

   i. Hypermetropia
   ii. Presbyopia
   iii. Aphakia

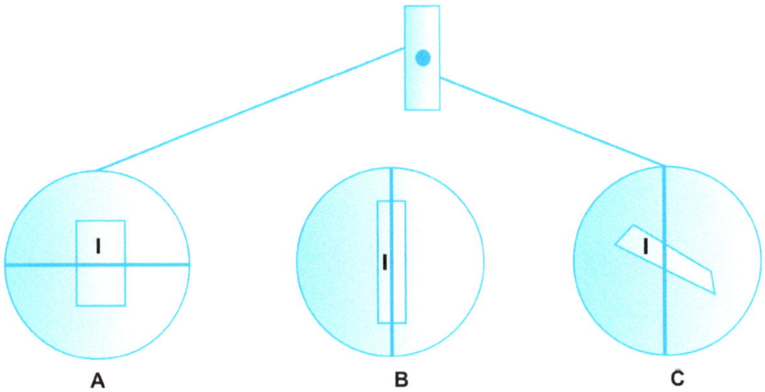

Figs 4.18A to C Characteristics of minus cylinder: Object O seen through cylinder; A. The image 'I' looks shorter and wider at right angles to the axis of the cylinder, B. looks longer and narrower along the axis of the cylinder, C. Smaller, narrower and distorted when rotated

Table 4.1: Comparison between plus and minus sphere

Features	Plus lens	Minus lens
Movement of image	Against	With
Size of the image	Large	Small
Distortion on rotation of lens	NIL	NIL
Thickness of lens	Thickest at the center	Thinnest at the center
Edge of the lens	Thin	Thick

Optical instruments
1. Corneal loupe (+40 D) (Fig. 4.19)
2. Condensing lens (+15 D, +20 D, +30 D, +60 D)

Uses of minus spherical lenses in spectacles: Myopia
In optical instruments: Hruby lens

Uses of Plus Cylinder

1. Simple hypermetropic astigmatism—Only plus cylinder is used. No sphere is required.
2. Compound hypermetropic astigmatism—Both plus cylinder and plus sphere are used.
3. Mixed astigmatism
   A plus cylinder with a minus sphere is used.

Uses of Minus Cylinder

1. Simple myopic astigmatism
   Only minus cylinder is used. No sphere is required.

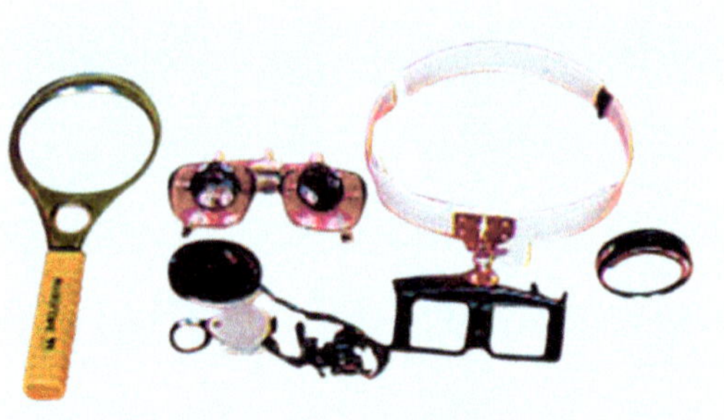

Fig. 4.19: Various types of loupes

2. Compound myopic astigmatism
   Both minus cylinder and minus spheres are used.
3. Mixed astigmatism
   A minus cylinder with a plus sphere is used.

> Note: In mixed astigmatism, the value of the cylinder is always more than the value of the sphere.

Examination of Near Vision

Near vision is tested in normally illuminated light with light falling upon the reading material.

Before near vision is tested, it is mandatory that distant vision in each eyes is tested separately.

1. Near correction is addition of convex lenses to distant correction.
2. An uniocular myope may use his myopic eye for near vision and the other eye for distant vision and need not require near correction.

The near vision is tested on various types of near vision charts. Commonly used charts are Snellen's near vision chart and Jaeger's chart (Figs 4.20 and 4.21). The illiterates are tested on near vision of E chart, C charts and dots.

The patient is asked to read the smallest print at 30 cm or his usual working distance, one eye at time and then both eyes together. The smallest letter is designated as N 5 or J 1 and the largest is N 48.

While testing near vision, find out:

1. His distant correction.
2. The distance at which he does his near work.
3. Has he instilled any cycloplegic in the eye.
4. Has he taken any oral medicine that cause cycloplegia.

How to Find out Power of Spectacle Lenses (Neutralizing)

1. Hold the spectacle as shown in photograph (Figs 4.22 and 4.23).
   Hold the spectacle by the frame between thumb and index finger near the eye with side bars away and look at it distant object (Fig. 4.22).

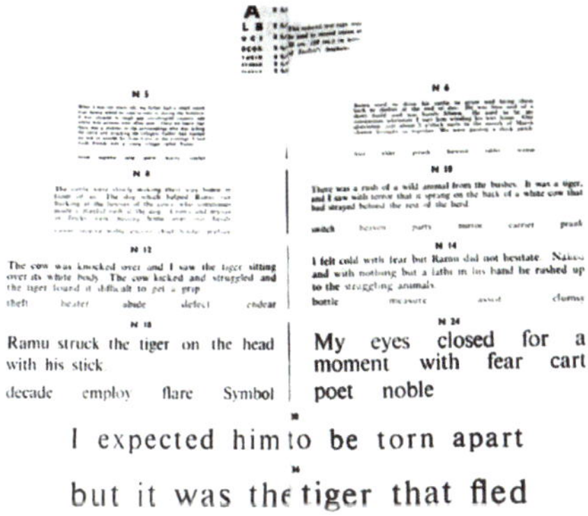

Fig. 4.20: Near vision chart

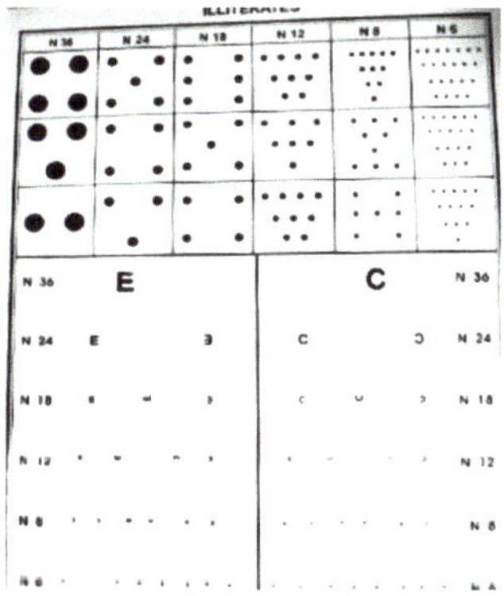

Fig. 4.21: Near vision charting for illitrate

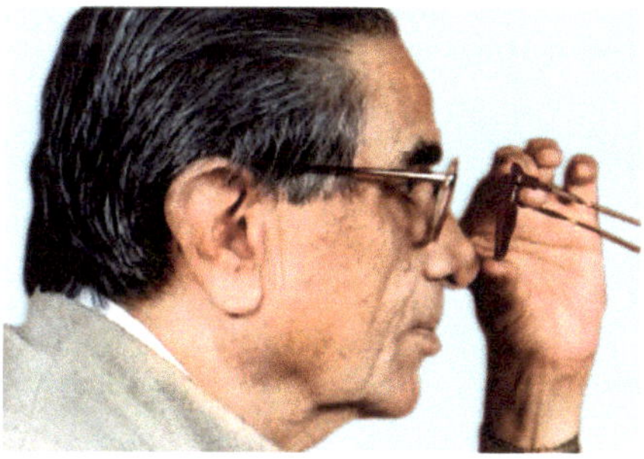

Fig. 4.22: Correct method of holding a spectacle to finding out its type

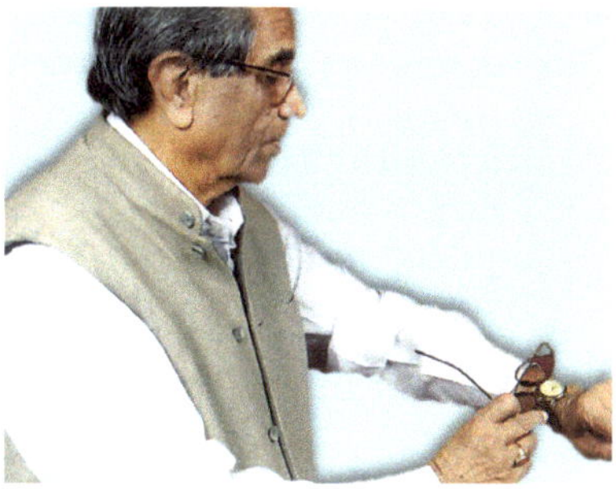

Fig. 4.23: Wrong method of holding a spectacle to find out its type

2. It is not advisable to hold the spectacle by the lens, keeping the side bar towards the observer, holding the spectacle away and seeing a near object (Fig. 4.23).
3. Find out if the type of the lens, i.e. concave or convex by observing movement of image.
4. Find out if:
   i. The lens is sphere only
   ii. Cylinder only
   iii. Spherocylinder
5. Find out if the movement is:
   i. Only in one direction—Simple astigmatism
   ii. Are the movements in two meridians different but in the same direction—Compound astigmatism
   iii. Are the movements in two meridians are opposite—Mixed astigmatism

There are two methods to neutralize a lens:

1. By putting lens of opposite sign over the lens till all the movements are abolished
2. By lensometer

Neutralizing by Lenses

i. Find out whether the lens is concave, convex or mixed.
ii. Find out whether it is a sphere only/cylinder only or a spherocylinder.
iii. Start putting spherical lenses of opposite sign:
  If the image move with, add plus lenses.
  If the image moves against, add minus lenses.

The neutralizing lens should be kept very near the spectacle lens.

In case of a sphere, the sphere will be neutralized by a sphere of opposite sign.

In case of spherocylinder, the spherical part will be neutralized by sphere. Additional cylinder will be required to neutralize cylindrical part. Only cylinder will be neutralized by cylinder of opposite sign.

For example—To neutralize a plus one cylinder at 180°, a minus one cylinder at 180° will neutralize the cylinder. It a minus one sphere is used it will neutralized the plus cylinder at 180° but add – 1.00 D at 90°.

The lensometer is an optical device that finds out:

- Power of sphere
- Power of cylinder
- Axis of cylinder
- Presbiopic addition
- Optical center of the glass
- Presence of prism

There are two types of lensometers:

1. Optical
2. Computerized

The computerized lensometer give a printout of the measurement.

The power of a lens is measured in dioptre (diopter). It is a unit measurement of converging/diverging power of a lens. It is reciprocal of focal length of the lens in meters (meters). A lens of one diopter will have a focal length of one meter (Table 4.2).

Higher is the power of the lens, shorter is the focal length. The following table give focal lengths of various diopters.

Table 4.2: Relation between dioter and focal length

Diopter	Focal length
1	100 cm = 1 m
2	50 cm = 1/2 m
3	33 cm = 1/3 m
4	25 cm = 1/4 m
5	20 cm = 1/5 m
10	10 cm = 1/10 m

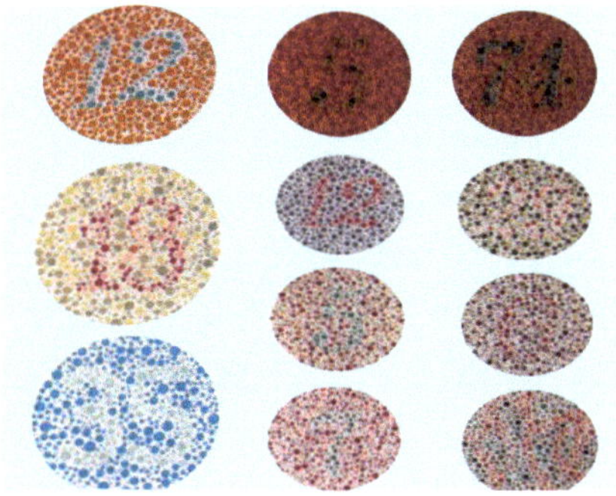

Fig. 4.24: Various types of color vision charts

Examination of Color Vision (Fig. 4.24)

About eight percent of male population have defective color vision. **Though defective color vision is generally called color blindness, it is not blindness.**

There are many devices by which color vision is tested. Most widely used device is **Ishihara plates** (chart). They are generally available in book form. Each page has one plate that shows a number made up of multiple dots in primary colors. The background is made up of dots of confusing color. Each plate has a number which is referred to an index provided at the end of the book.

> The color defects are present at birth and inherited. They do not progress. There is no treatment for color defect.

The second type of color defect develops in disease of macula and optic nerve. They are associated with diminished vision.

Examination of Field of Vision

When an eye looks at an object, it is not only the object that is visible but objects situated within a large area round the point of fixation are also visible. The area seen round the point of fixation is field of vision for the eye at that time. **The normal peripheral field of an eye is not circular** (Fig. 4.25). It is maximum at the temporal side and deficit at superinasal and interonasal. When both the eyes are open, the total amount of area visible is added. **The central field is circular** and extend all-round the fixation point 30° (Fig. 4.26).

The defects in the field of vision are called **scotomas**. They are nonseeing areas in the field.

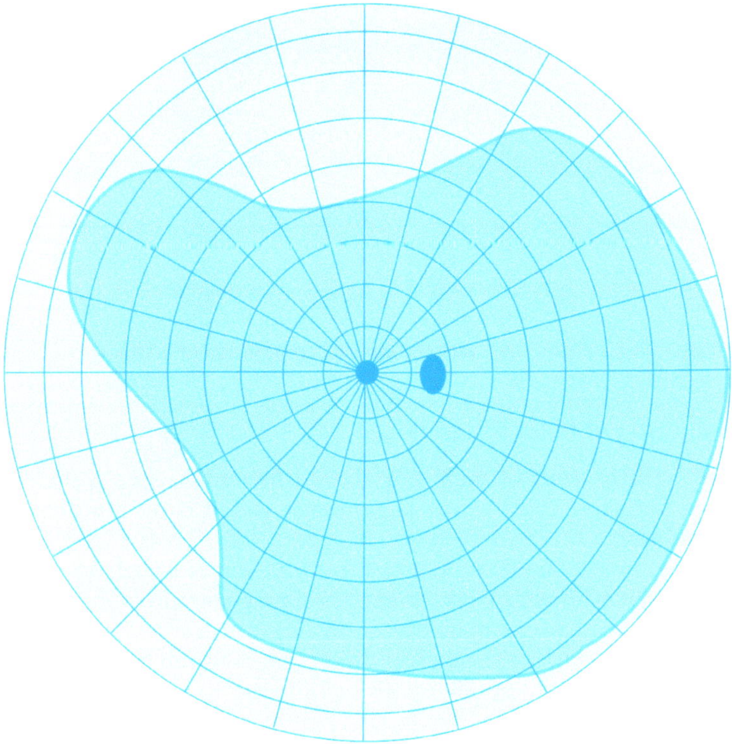

Fig. 4.25: Perimetry chart for peripheral field (right eye)

The presence of scotoma gives the following information:

i. Location of the lesion in the visual path
ii. Size of the lesion

The field changes can be:

i. Unilateral (only on one side) (Fig. 4.27)
ii. Bilateral (field changes on both sides)

Unilateral field changes are seen in lesions of retina, macula and optic nerve.

Bilateral field changes are seen in lesions of chiasma, optic tract, optic radiation and visual cortex (Fig. 4.28).

The bilateral field changes can be:

i. On the same side, i.e. right side of fields or left side of fields.
ii. One eye has field defect on right side and the other on the left side.

The fields have been divided into two types:

i. Central—30° all-round the point of fixation (4.26).
ii. Peripheral—Beyond 30° all-round (Fig. 4.25).

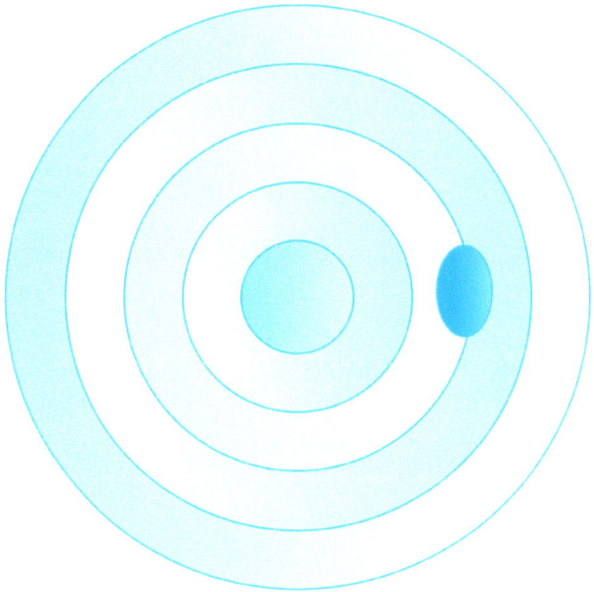

Fig. 4.26: Normal central field

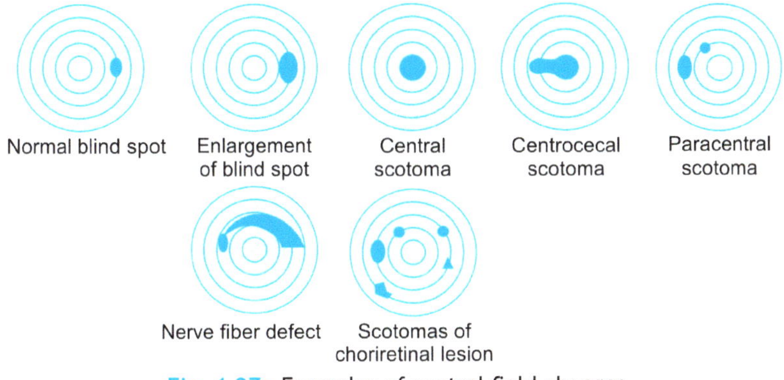

Fig. 4.27: Examples of central field changes

The central field changes can be tested:

i. 10° round the point of fixation by.
   Amsler grid held at reading distance (Fig. 4.29).
ii. 30° round the point of fixation by.
   Bjerrum screen at 1 meter or 2 meters

Peripheral field changes are charted by

1. conformation method –
2. Lister's perimeter
3. Goldmann perimeter
4. Automated perimeters

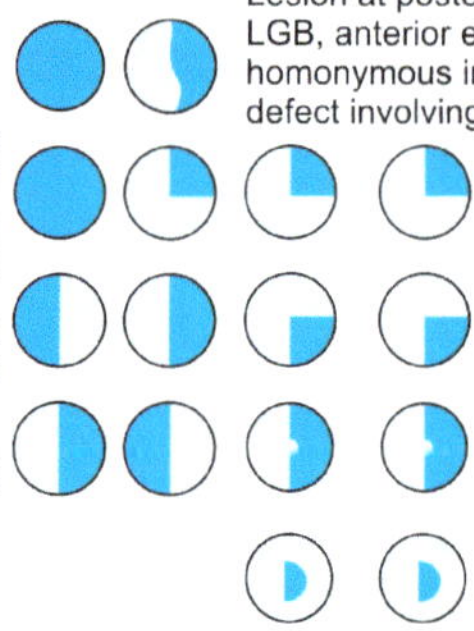

Fig. 4.28: Examples of bilateral field changes

The central field defects are—(Fig. 4.27)

i. Enlargement of blind spot
ii. Seidel scotoma
iii. Arcuate scotoma
   a. Single
   b. Double
iv. Roenne's step
v. Tubular field

Type of field defect (Fig. 4.27)	Probable cause
1. Enlargement of blind spot	Papilledema Opaque nerve fiber near the disc Early glaucoma
2. Seidel scotoma	Early stage of glaucoma
3. Arcuate scotoma	Moderately advanced glaucoma
4. Roenne's step	Advanced glaucoma
5. Tubular field	Retinitis pigmentosa Very advanced glaucoma

Automated perimeters are the best equipments to chart central as well as peripheral field. They can detect early changes. They have mostly replaced other methods. They are very costly and require special skill to interpret them.

External Examination of the Eyes

External examination of the eyes consist of:

1. Examination in diffuse light
2. Examination in focal (sharp and bright)
3. Examination by special instruments
4. Special investigation

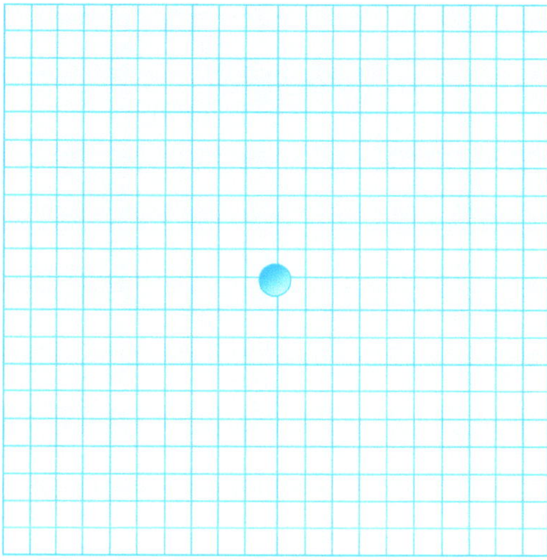

Fig. 4.29: Amsler grid

Examination in Diffuse Light

This is done under usual light of the room. The patient is made to sit comfortably about one meter from the examiner. The examination should be preceded by history taking (See page 130).

Examination of Eye with Subnormal Vision

1. Find out if the loss of vision is sudden or gradual.
2. Sudden loss of vision are mostly unilateral and do not improve with glasses.
3. Sudden painful loss is due to trauma, infection, inflammation or painful glaucoma. They also do not improve with glasses.
4. Record distant vision without glasses and with glasses.
5. Find out the purpose of the glasses.
6. Find out the power of the glasses.
7. If the vision is subnormal without glasses, put a **pinhole** in front of the eye, keep the other eye closed and ask the patient to read the same letter on Snellen's chart.
8. If there is improvement of vision, patient has error of refraction (he requires glasses for distance).
9. Do dynamic retinoscopy, i.e. without cycloplegia. This can be done with **retinoscope**, **streak retinoscope** or **autorefractometer**.
10. If in doubt about the power of the cylinder, do a **static retinoscopy**, i.e. under cycloplegia. Commonly used cycloplegics are atropine for children under 10 years of age. **Homatropine**, **cyclopentolate**, **tropicamide** for patients between 10 years to 40 years. Phenylephirne 10% for persons over 40 years. This drug is not cycloplegia this is only mydriatic.

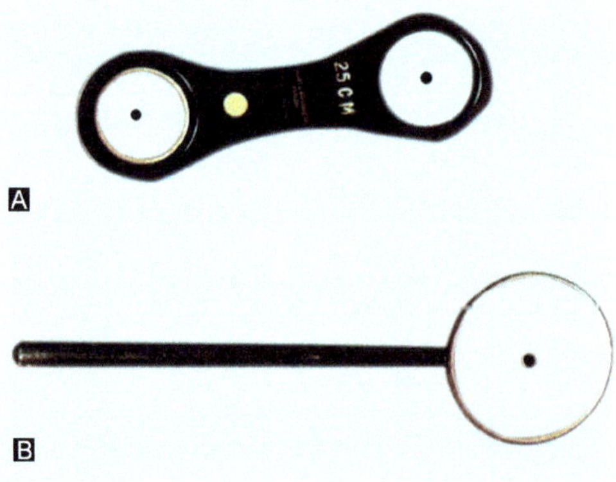

Figs 4.30A and B: A. Double retinoscope The white spot denotes plane mirror, the other is concave mirror B. Single plane mirror retinoscope

11. Find out the glass that gives best vision but do not prescribe these except following refraction without cycloplegic.
12. If the vision does not improve satisfactorily, examine the fundus to find out the cause.
13. Near vision correction is added to distant correction in presbyopic persons.

Method of Doing Retinoscopy

Commonly retinoscopy is done with **plane mirror retinoscope**. Concave mirror retinoscopy is used in hazy media and high errors of refraction (Figs 4.30A and B).

The patient sits at a distance of 1 meter from the examiner with a source of light behind slightly shifted to one side so that the face of the patient is in dark.

The light is thrown in the dilated pupil of the patient with a plane mirror. The pupillary area lights up as pink glow if there is no opacity in the media. If opacity is present, it stands out as black area.

Move the retinoscope from side to side, first horizontally and then vertically.

Note the movement of the pink glow.

1. If it moves with movement of the mirror, the eye is – emmetrope, hypermetrope or myopic less than 1 D.
2. If there is no movement, the eye is myope by 1 D.
3. If the image moves against, the eye is myopic, more than 1 D.
4. If the image moves with, put a +1.5 D in front of the eye, if the movement is stopped, the patient is emmetrope.
5. If the image moves with, add + lenses till all the movements are abolished.
6. If the image moves against with +1.5 D, the patient has myopia less than 1 D, gradually reduce the power towards the minus side till movements

are abolished. This is the myopic retinoscopy. The patient will require -1.5 D sphere more than this for distant correction. For example, the myopic refraction is -2.0 D sphere in all axes, the patient will require (-2) + (-1.5) = -3.5 D for distance. To this plus addition will be required as per age and profession of the patient in presbyopic age.

7. If the image moves with movement of the retinoscope after putting +1.5 D, the patient is hypermetropic. To find out the hypermetropic retinoscopy, keep adding plus sphere till all movements are abolished. The distant correction will be less by -1.5 D for distance. For example, if the retinoscopic finding is +2 Dsph in all axes, he will accept (+2) – (+1.5) = 0.5 Dsph for distance. To this plus lenses will be added as per age and profession of the patient in presbyopic age.
8. If there is a difference of power in two axes, the patient has astigmatism.

Difference of the power of two axes is the value of cylinder. The value of the cylinder does not change by adding plus or minus spheres.

OPHTHALMIC EXAMINATION

The ophthalmic examination is divided into two parts:

1. External examination of the eye
2. Internal examination of the eye

1. External examination is done under two heads:
   i. Examination under diffuse illumination
   ii. Examination under focal illumination by special instruments.
2. Internal examination requires special instruments.

Details of Examination Under Diffuse Illumination

Examination under diffuse illumination comprise of:

1. **Head posture**
   i. Position of chin
   ii. Turning of head to left or right side
   iii. Tilting of head
2. **Symmetry of face**
3. Position of eyebrow—(i) raised, (b) flat
4. Loss of eyebrow
5. Interpalpebral aperture (distance between upper and lower lid)
6. Deviation of eye–squint
7. Oscillation of the eye (abnormal movement of the eye = nystagmus)
8. Bulging of the eyeball (proptosis/exophthalmos)
9. Sunken eyeball

Head Posture

1. Position of the chin:
   a. It may be elevated. The causes are:
      i. Ptosis (drooping of the upper lid)
      ii. Paralysis of elevators (superior rectus and inferior oblique)

iii. High errors of refraction
iv. Loss of upper field of vision

b. Causes of depression of the chin are:
   i. Paralysis of depressors (inferior rectus and superior oblique)
   ii. Loss of lower field of vision

2. Turning of the head—The head may be turned towards right or left.
   a. The causes of turning of head towards right are paralysis of right lateral rectus or paralysis of left medial rectus.
   b. Causes of turning of head towards left are paralysis of left lateral rectus or right medial rectus.
3. Tilting of head is seen in paralysis of cyclovertical muscles, i.e. superior rectus, inferior rectus, superior oblique and inferior oblique in any eye.
4. Symmetry of the face (Fig. 4.31).
   For all practical purposes, the two sides of the face are symmetrical. The conditions when the symmetry is lost are:
   a. Congenital (present from birth)
   b. Trauma (injury to face)
   c. Facial palsy (paralysis of seventh nerve)
5. Position of the eyebrows (Fig. 4.32).
   The eyes brows are symmetrically arched in the lower part of the forehead.
   It may be raised in case of ptosis and pseudoptosis.
   It becomes flat in facial palsy.
6. Loss of eyebrow
   The eyebrows may become scanty (less) or may become absent in
   a. Old age
   b. Thermal burn
   c. Leprosy
   d. Hypothyroid
   e. Chemotherapy (Fig. 4.33)

Changes in Interpalpebral Aperture

The space between the two lids is called inter palpebral aperture. When the eyes are looking at a distant object (primary position), the upper lid covers the upper 2 mm of the cornea and the lower lid just touches the lower limbus.

It becomes narrow when the upper lid comes down as in **ptosis** (Figs 4.34A and B), **pseudoptosis** (Figs 4.35A and B), **phthisis bulbic** (soft eye), **microphthalms** (small eye) or when the eyeball has been removed. It becomes wide when the upper lid fails to cover the upper 2 mm of the cornea or the lower lid is retracted. The causes of **lid retraction** are:

- Lagophthalmos (inability to close the eye due to facial palsy) (Fig. 4.36).
- Proptosis (bulging of the eye due to tumor).
- Exophthalmos (bulging of the eye due to disorder of thyroid) (Fig. 4.37).

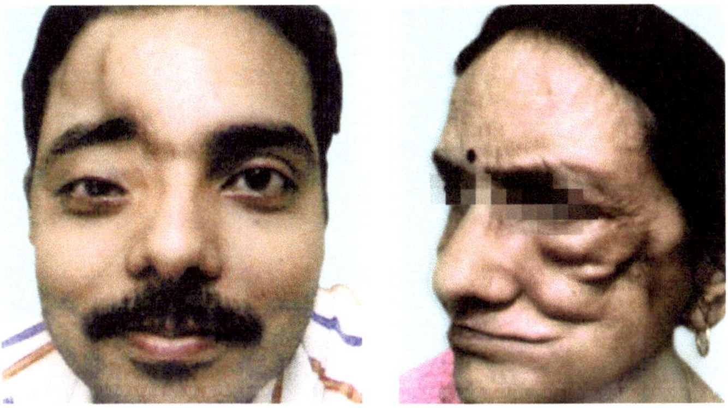

Fig. 4.31: Post-trumatic asymmetry of the face

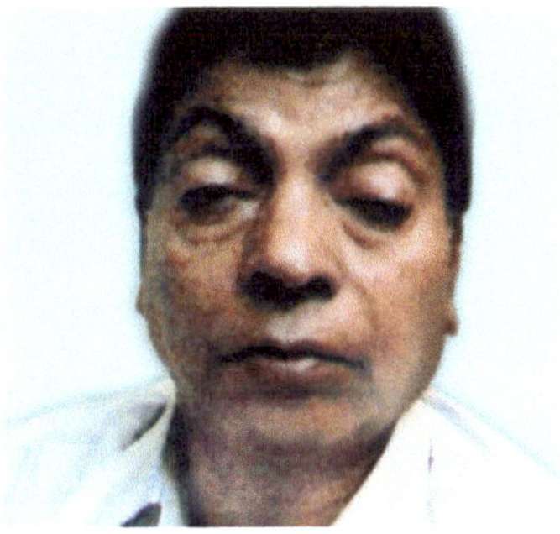

Fig. 4.32: Raised eyebrow in ptosis

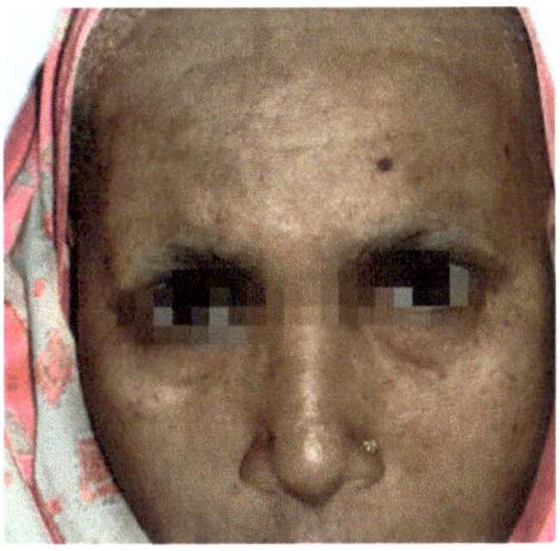

Fig. 4.33: Total loss of eyebrow following chemotherapy

Squint

Large degree of squint are very clearly visible, (Fig. 4.38). Small degree of squint requires careful observation.

Nystagmus—Normally the eyes do not oscillate in any direction but if it shows movement, it is called nystagmus. Most of the nystagmus are pathological (due to disease). It is generally associated with poor vision and squint or both. The cause may be in the eyes or in the brain.

Bulging of the eyeball

Abnormal bulging of the eyeball is of two types:

1. **Proptosis**—This is due to a growth behind the eyeball. This is generally unilateral (on one side only).
2. **Exophthalmos**—This is due to disease of the thyroid. This is generally bilateral. other signs and symptoms of thyroid diseases are generally present.

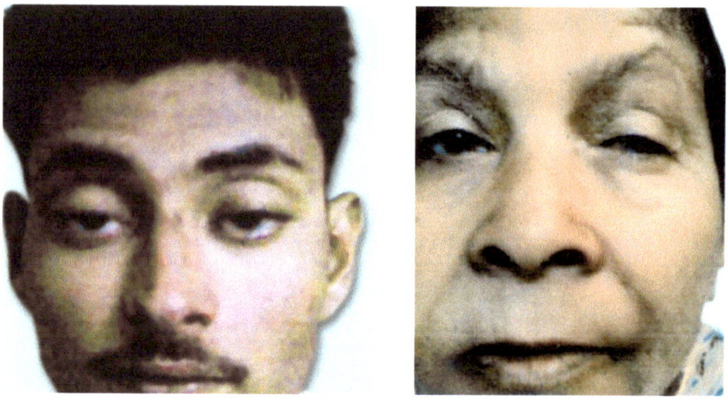

Figs 4.34A and B: Ptosis

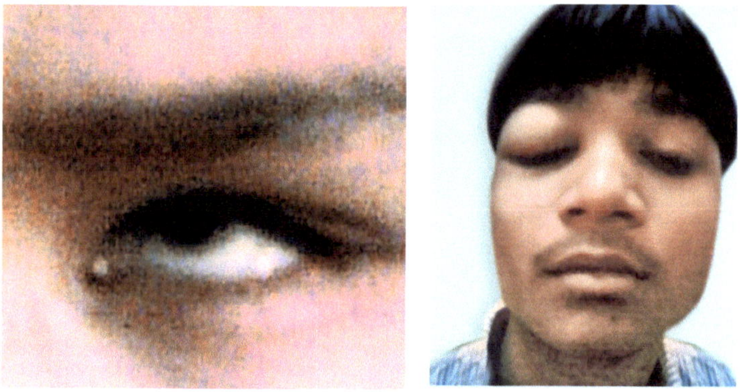

Figs. 4.35A and B: Pseudoptosis

The **bulging** can be very minimal or very large. The bulging eyes are always associated with wider palpebral fissure. There may be **lid retraction,** i.e. the upper part of the sclera is visible. If the bulge is large there may be **lagophthalmos** (inability to close the lids). Exophthalmos/proptosis is measured by an instrument called **exophthalmometer**.

Sunken Eyeball (Enophthalmos)

The interpalpebral fissure is narrow (Pseudoptosis). The cornea is flat and the eyeball is soft.

Examination Under Focal Illumination

This is done by a sharp bright light which can be handheld or in the form of a slit lamp. Handheld source of light may require a magnifier.

The handheld sources of light are:

1. Torch
2. Electric operated light

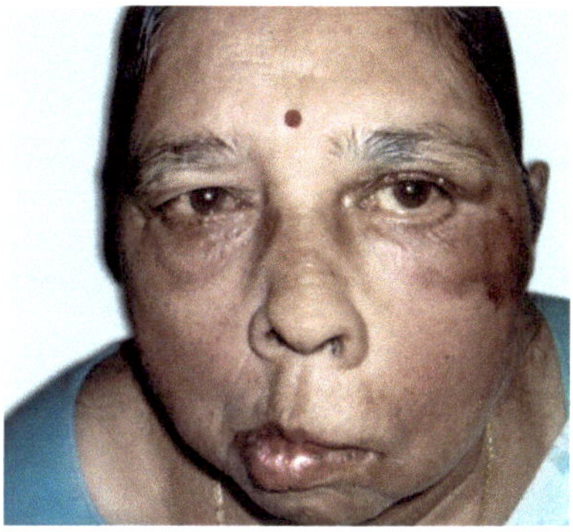

Fig. 4.36: Lagophthalmos

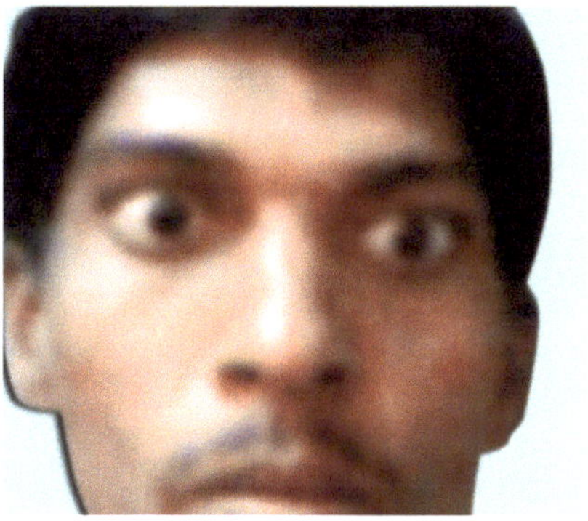

Fig. 4.37: Lid retraction in thyroid disease

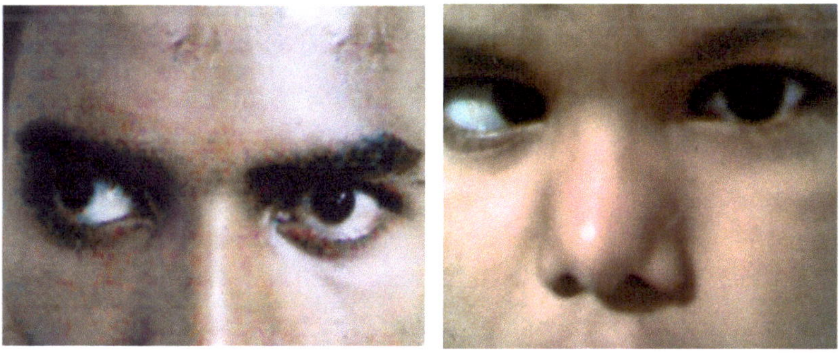

Fig. 4.38: Large degree of squint

The commonly used magnifiers are:

i. Corneal loupes (Photograph 4.4)
   a. Uniocular
   b. Binocular

ii. Telescopes (operating loupes)

None of the above appliances are self-illuminating. They require a separate source of light.

Slit lamp and operating microscope, both of them have source of illumination and magnifier in the same instrument.

Torch: A three-celled dry battery operated torch is most suitable. The width of the beam can easily be adjusted. A small pencil torch does not give good illumination and has a very small illuminated area.

Electric lights: These lights work on mains through a step down transformer. A rheostat in the transformer regulates brightness of the light. They generally have a condensing lens that changes wide beam to pin-point. The beam of light can be converted into a slit. A blue filter is also added to the light to see areas stained by fluorescein.

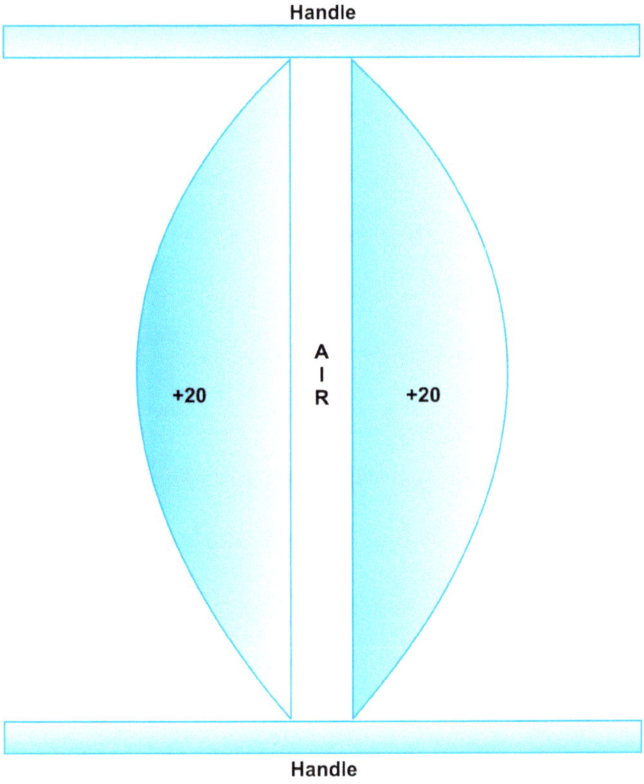

Fig. 4.39: Structure of uniocular corneal loupe

Corneal Loupes

There are two types of corneal loupes:
1. Uniocular corneal loupe
2. Binocular corneal loupe

The uniocular loupe is a handy, very cheap and good magnifier. It is basically a +40 D biconvex lens. In fact, it is a combination of two planoconvex lenses put together with their plane surfaces parallel and separated by a space of 2 mm, mounted in a plastic frame. The focal length of the combined lens is 2.5 cm and magnification is x10 (ten times). When the object is between the lens and its focal length, i.e. the object has to be at a distance of less than 2.5cm. The image formed by the loupe is enlarged erect, virtual and ten times magnified (Figs 4.39 and 4.40).

It requires a separate source of light (a torch or an electric light). Generally the loupe is held in left hand and torch in the right hand. The examiner has to move very close to the patient. The loupe is used to examine fine structures of the anterior chamber, iris, pupillary margin and lens. Structures beyond lens are not visible by a corneal loupe.

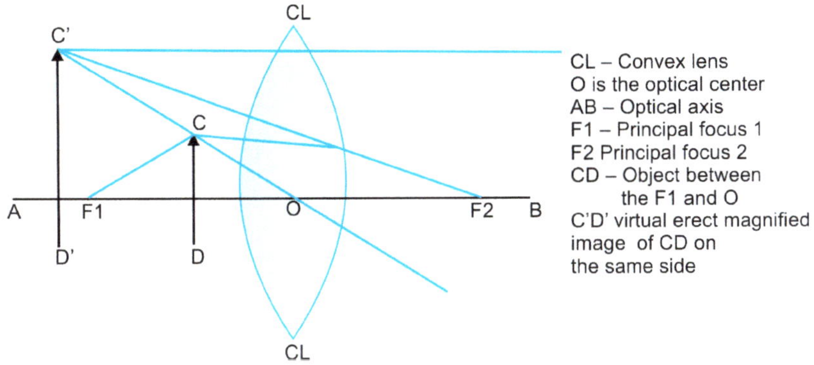

Fig. 4.40 Optics of corneal loupe

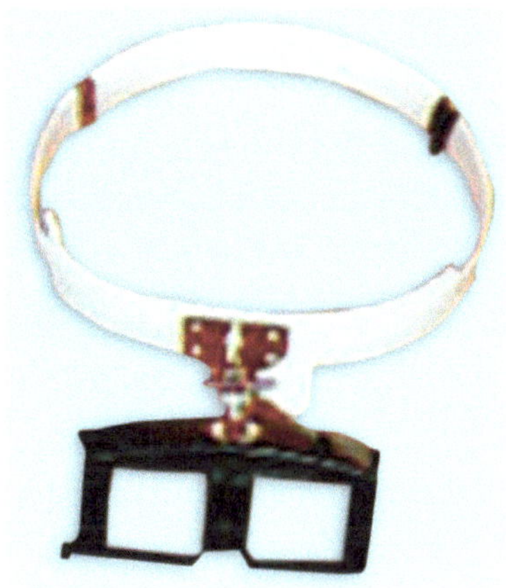

Fig. 4.41: Binocular loupe

The uniocular corneal loupe is a very useful instrument. It has some drawbacks too. They are:

1. The focal length is very small, i.e. 2.5 cm. To see an object clearly, the observer has to move very close to the patient.
2. The loupe is held in the left hand, the right hand holds a source of torch. Hence, both the hands of the examiner are engaged at the same time.

Binocular Loupe (Fig. 4.41)

Instead of one lens of uniocular loupe, the binocular loupe has two lenses. One for the right eye and the other for the left eye of the observer. The lenses are either mounted on a spectacle or a special frame that has a headband which can be worn round the forehead of the examiner.

The lenses used in binocular loupes are weaker than those used in uniocular loupe. Each lens is +6 D that has focal length of 17 cm. The magnification is only 1.5x.

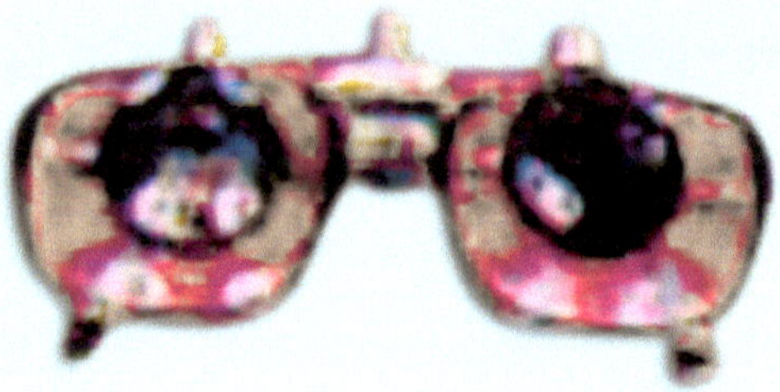

Fig. 4.42: Operating telescope

The advantages of binocular loupe is that one hand is always free. The examiner need not go very near the patients face. Being binocular it has some depth of focus.

The greatest disadvantage is poor magnification.

Operating Telescopes (Fig. 4.42)

These are in fact binoculars mounted on spectacle frames. The distant power of the observer can be incorporated in the spectacle frame. The binoculars have short farpoint and variable working distance. The distance between the two telescopes can be adjusted to suit the interpupillary distance of the examiner. The operating telescopes have magnification of 4x and 6x. More is the magnification, shorter is the working distance and smaller is the field. They also require a separate source of light. They can be used not only to examine the anterior segment of the eye but can be used during surgery of anterior segment where much magnification is not required.

Slit Lamp Biomicroscope (Fig. 4.43)

As the name suggests, the instrument is a microscope in which the source of light is in the form of a slit beam. The optical system of the microscope of slit lamp is horizontal in contrast to clinical microscope where the optical system is vertical and the illumination comes from behind the object. The object is almost transparent. In slit lamp, the light falls on the object from front.

The parts of the slit lamp can be broadly divided into two parts:

1. Optical
2. Mechanical

The optical part consists of –

1. Microscope
2. Illuminator

   i. The microscope is binocular. It has two eye pieces but a common objective. The distance between the two eye pieces is adjustable. The whole of the optical system can be moved towards or away from the eye of the observer. It can be moved sideways as well. The power of

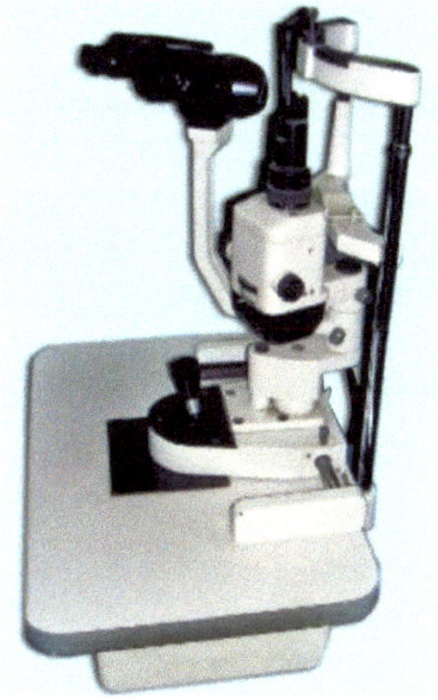

Fig. 4.43: Slit lamp biomicroscope

the eye pieces is also changeable. The magnification in a slit lamp varies between 5x to 50x. Commonly used magnification is 10x to 15x. As the microscope is binocular, it also has depth perception (stereoscopic vision).

ii. The illumination system consists of an electrically operated low-voltage bulb that works on mains through a rheostat. The rheostat adjusts the brightness of the light. The light passes through many lenses and prisms to be converted into a circular beam of light which can be converted into a slit by an adjusting screw. The length, width and position, i.e. vertical, horizontal or oblique, are adjustable by reducing the height and width, both at the same time. The bean can be converted into a point focus of 1 mm x 1 mm. Suitable colored filters can be interposed to change the color of the slit. The commonest filter used is a cobalt blue filter that is used to see the fluorescein staining of the cornea, applanation tonometry, contact lens fitting and tear film break up time.

The slit lamp microscope can examine only the anterior segment of the eye without special attachments.

The various attachments used are:

1. Plus lenses—El Bayadi, Volk, +60 D to +90 D
2. Minus lenses -55 D

With addition of these lenses, the central part of posterior segment, i.e. disc and macula can also be seen but not the periphery for which a three mirror gonioscope is required. Besides three mirror, one mirror gonioscopes are available to see the angle of the anterior chamber.

An applanation tonometer is a common attachment available with most of the slit lamps. In more advanced slit lamp, there are attachments to fit keratometer.

Cameras can be fitted to the eye pieces to obtain photograph of anterior segment.

The mechanical part of the slit lamp consists of:

1. Adjustable table
2. The base of the slit lamp. This can be moved in various direction.
3. Devices to adjust
   i. Height of the illumination system
   ii. Height and width of the beam
   iii. Angulations between the microscope and illumination
   iv. Chin rest
   v. Headband
   vi. Fixation light

The microscope can be moved from one eye to the other eye. It can be moved towards or away from the eye.

External examination of the eye:

EXAMINATION OF THE LIDS

Symptoms of Disorders of the Lids

1. Drooping of the lid
2. Widening of interpalpebral aperture
3. Inability to close the lids
4. Pain and tenderness in the lid
5. Growth on the lid

To examine the lid—Observe the position of chin—The chin is elevated in cases of ptosis.

Look for the position of the eyebrow.

- Raised eyebrow is seen in ptosis
- Flat eyebrow is seen in lagophthalmos

Examine the lid under the following heads:

1. Skin of the lid
2. Lid margin
3. Size of the interpalperbral aperture
   i. Height
   ii. Length

Skin of the lid is examined for evidence of:

1. Rashes—**Herpes zoster ophthalmicus** (Fig. 4.44). These rashes are limited to one side of the face only. They not only involve the lid of the skin but also the forehead and extend in the head. If there are rashes at the tip of the nose, there are chances that the cornea is also involved.

Other causes of rashes over the lid and skin are

1. Chickenpox, measles, herpes simplex.
2. Boils (Fig. 4.45)

Swelling of the skin—The skin may be minimally swollen or the swelling may obliterate the IPA due to pseudoptosis.

Causes of lid swelling are

1. Cellulitis lid (Fig. 4.46)
2. Allergy
3. Hemorrhage—Black eye (Fig. 4.47)
4. Insect bite
5. Tumors

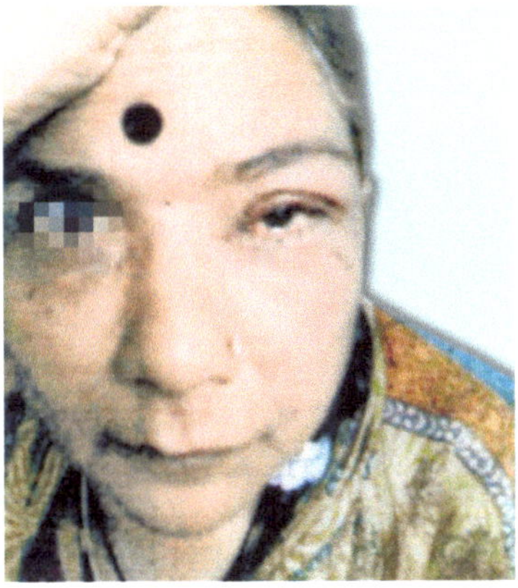

Fig. 4.44: Rashes of herpes zoster (left side)

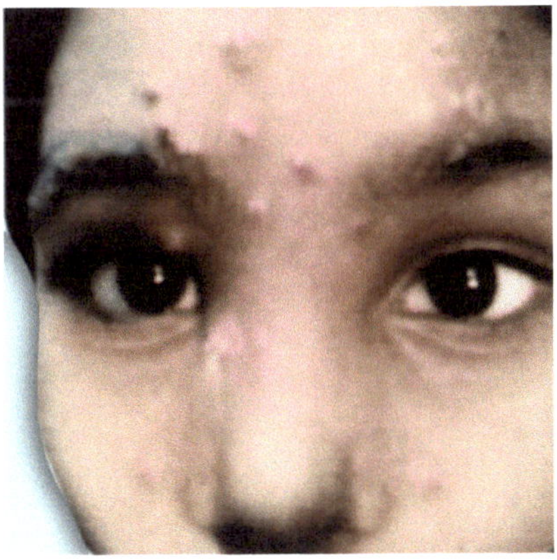

Fig. 4.45: Boils

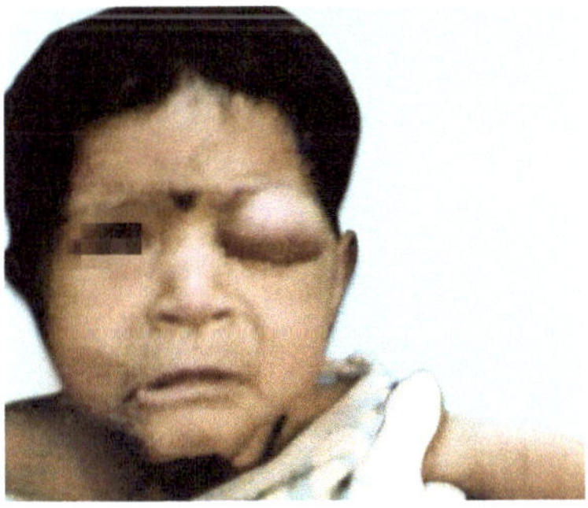

Fig. 4.46: Cellulitis lid

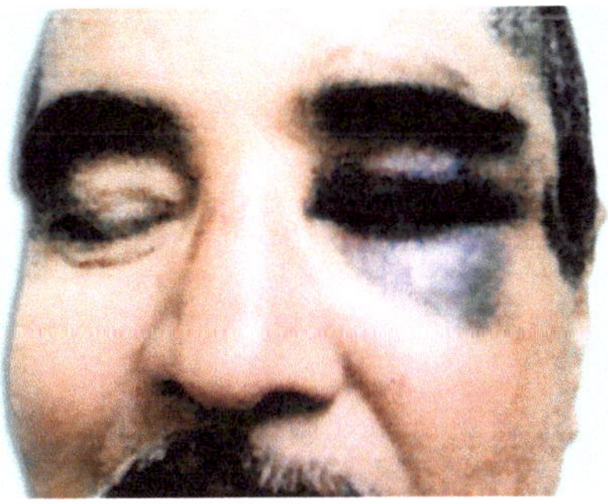

Fig. 4.47: Black eye

The lid margin is examined for:

1. Abnormal position of the lid margin
   i. Entropion
   ii. Ectropion

   Entropion is inturning of the lid margin.

   There are two types of entropion:

   a. **Spastic or senile**—This is seen in old age.
   b. Cicatricial—The common causes of cicatricial entropion are:
      - Trachoma
      - Leprosy
      - Chemical burn of the conjunctiva

   Ectropion is outturning of the lid margins. There are two types—

   a. **Senile**, seen in old age (Fig. 4.48)
   b. **Cicatricial** seen in scar on the lids.
2. Abnormality of the lid margin:
   i. **Coloboma of lid margin** can be **congenital** (present at birth) or **traumatic** due to injury either accidental or surgical. The colobomas may be present anywhere in any lids. The congenital coloboma of the upper lid is generally on the medial side while that of lower lid is at the lateral side of lower lid (Figs 4.49 and 4.50).

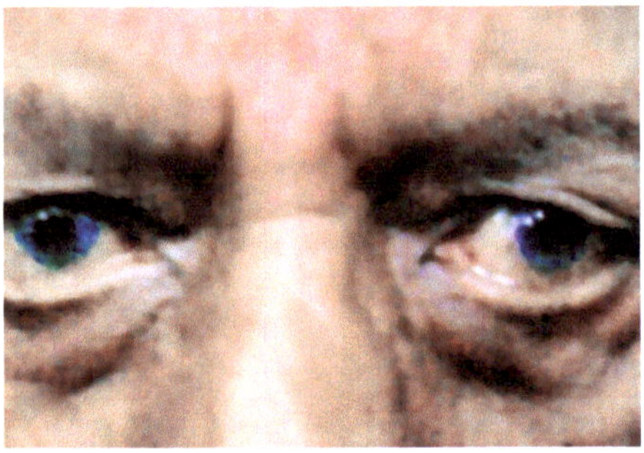

Fig. 4.48: Senile ectropion lower lid

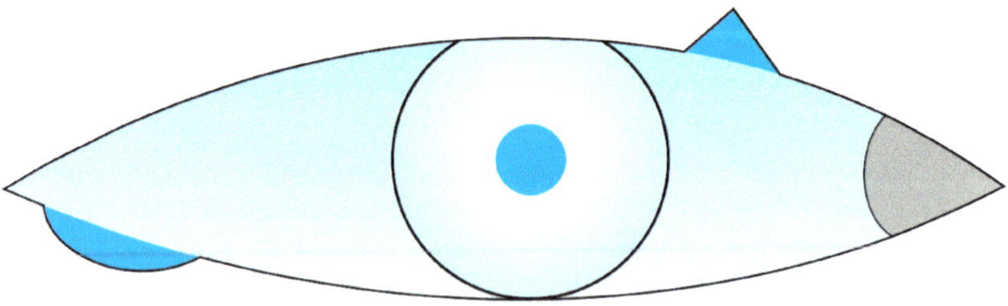

Fig. 4.49: Congenital coloboma—Upper and lower lid

ii. **Trichiasis**—This is very common disorder of the eye lashes. Normally the eye lashes point away from the cornea. In trichiasis, the lashes are turned towards the cornea. The number of lashes turned in vary from single to many (Fig. 4.51).
    The causes are—trachoma, leprosy, chronic ulcerative blepharitis, injury and idiopathic (when no cause can be detected)
iii. Madarosis—This means loss of lashes. Generally lashes fall of at regular interval and are replaced. When they do not grow after falling, a condition of madarosis sets in. In can involve any of the lids. All the lashes may be lost or there may be a patch from the lashes are missing. The common causes are **trachoma, leprosy** and **blepharitis**.

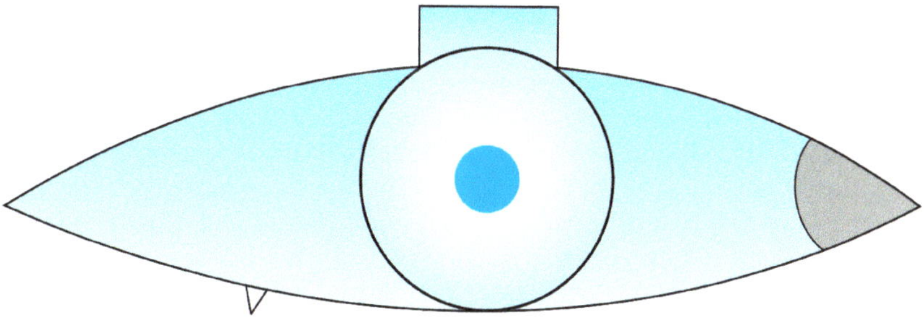

Fig. 4.50: Acquired total coloboma of the upper lid at the center and a notch coloboma of the lower lid

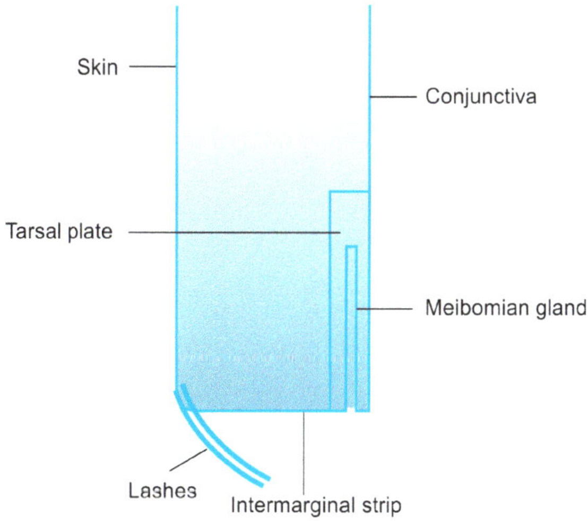

Fig. 4.51: Trichiasis

iv. Tylosis—Tylosis is uniform swelling of the lid margin. In normal lid, the inner margin is sharp and outer margin is rounded. In tylosis, whole of the lid margin is rounded and swollen. This is generally associated with madarosis. The commonest cause is **ulcerative blepharitis**.

Infection of Lid Margin

Infection of lid margin is called **blepharitis**. There are two types of blepharitis:

i. **Ulcerative blepharitis**—It is generally seen in both eyes. Upper lid is more commonly involved. There are scales at the base of the lashes. On removing the scale, there is little bleeding from the spot.
ii. **Squamous blepharitis** seen in both eyes. There are dry scales. There is no bleeding on removing them.
iii. **Stye**—This is acute infection of the root of the lashes. A small red painful swelling develops at the base of a single lash. The swelling is tender (pains on pressure). It is more common in children. If it develops in adults, they should be tested for diabetes. It may develop in any lid. More than one lid may be involved. There may be more than one stye in the same lid. Recurrence is very common. Preauricular lymph glands are generally enlarged (Fig. 4.52).
iv. **Chalazion**—Chalazion is chronic inflammation of tarsal gland. It is situated away from the lid margin. It develops slowly, is painless. There is no pain on pressure. The skin over the swelling moves over the swelling. which is spherical and diffuse. The number may vary between one to many. Any of the lids may be involved. Recurrence is common. (Fig. 4.53).

   The chalazion can gets infected, an infected chalazion is very painful. Recurrent chalazion in adult is a bad sign. It can be cancer.

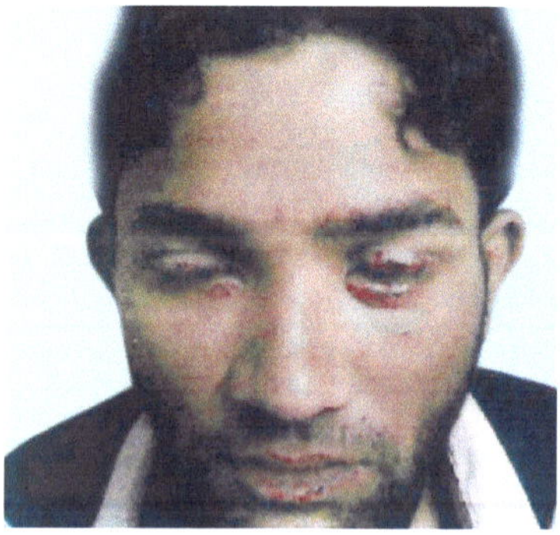

Fig. 4.52: Stye (both eyes, both lids)

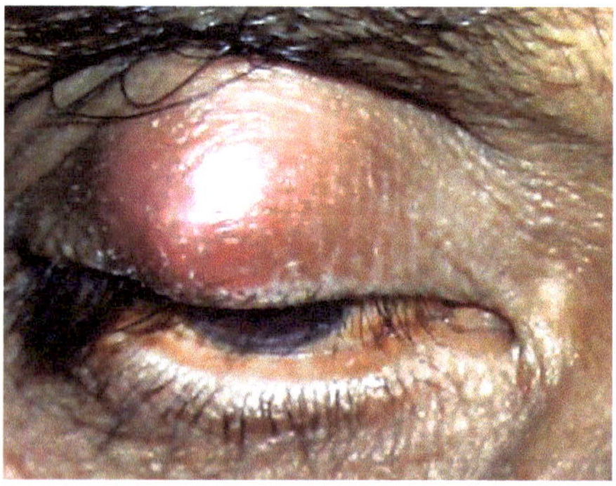

Fig. 4.53: Chalazion

Change in Interpalpebral Aperture

The space between the two lids is called interpalpebral aperture. It is about 30 mm long and 10 mm wide. It is widest in front of the cornea.

The upper lid covers upper 1/5 (2 mm) of the cornea and the lower lid just touches the lower edge of cornea.

The two ends of interpalpebral aperture are called canthi. The one towards the nose is called **medial canthus** while the one towards the ear is called **lateral canthus**.

The changes in interpalpebral aperture can be:

1. Reduced in height:
   i. Ptosis
   ii. Pseudoptosis
2. Increased in height:
   i. Lid retraction
   ii. Lagophthalmos
3. Decreased in height as well as length—Blepharophimosis

Ptosis

Drooping of upper lid is called ptosis. When upper lid covers more than 2 mm of the cornea, it is called ptosis (Fig. 4.54).

It can be:

- Congenital (present at birth)
- Acquired (after birth)

Congenital ptosis can be unilateral or bilateral. Acquired ptosis is generally unilateral.

Ptosis can be mild, moderate or severe (Fig. 4.54).

Signs of Ptosis

1. The patient keeps the chin elevated.
2. The eyebrows are raised.
3. The cornea is covered more than 2 mm.
4. If the lid covers the pupil, there is diminished vision.
5. Action of levator is diminished.

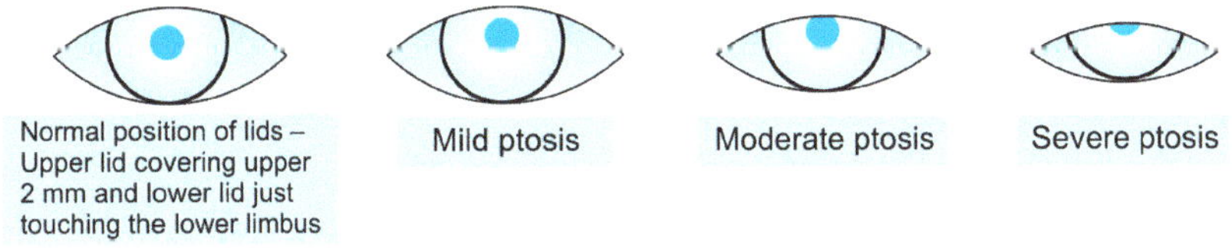

Fig. 4.54: Various grades of ptosis

Symptoms of Ptosis

1. Cosmetic—Changed look
2. Diplopia—In case of myasthenia only

Causes of Ptosis

1. Congenital
2. Acquired
   i. Neurologic - Paralysis of third nerve (Fig. 4.32)
   - Paralysis of sympathetic.
   ii. Myogenic - Myasthenia (Fig. 4.34A).
   - Trauma to levator
   iii. Mechanical - Tumors of the lid
   iv. Pseudoptosis
   In pseudoptosis the action of levator is normal.

Causes of Pseudoptosis

- Microphthalmos (small eye) (Fig. 4.35A).
- Phthisis (soft eye)
- Fracture of orbit
- Swelling of lids (Fig. 4.35A).

Lid Retraction

Normal lid covers upper 2 mm of cornea and lower lid just touches the lower border of cornea and no sclera (white of the eye) is visible. If sclera is visible above or below or both, it is called lid retraction (Fig. 4.37).

The commonest causes of lid retraction is thyroid disease of the eye.

LAGOPHTHALMOS

Inability to close the lids fully is called lagophthalmos. It is mostly unilateral and rarely bilateral.

It is commonly unilateral and acute. The commonest cause is Bell's palsy that is paralysis of seventh nerve. Other causes are injury to the seventh nerve, head injury and leprosy. Leprosy is commonest cause of bilateral lagophthalmos (Fig. 4.36).

The complaints of the patient with lagophthalmos are:
1. Inability to close the lids.
2. Watering from the eye.
3. Redness of the eye.
4. Deviation of the mouth.

Bell's Phenomenon

This is a protective mechanism of the eye. When the lids close, the eyeball rolls up under the lid. It is lost in third nerve palsy but retained in seventh nerve palsy.

Blepharospasm

This is forceful closure of both the lids on two sides. This is a reflex and involuntary. It is more marked in children. The causes are–corneal foreign body, corneal injury, keratitis and phlycten (Fig. 4.55).

Tumors of the Lid

Lids are common sites for tumors. The tumors can be **benign** (noncancer) or **malignant** (cancer).

The common benign tumors are—Hemangioma, neuroma and nevus. The malignant tumors are

- Rodent ulcer (Basal cell cancer)
- Epidermoid cancer
- Malignant melanoma

Examination of the Lacrimal Sac

Symptoms of Diseases of the Lacrimal Sac

1. Watering
2. Swelling over the sac

Examination of a Case of Watering from the Eyes

Normal eyes are always wet but tears do not fall out of the eyes. Tears can fall out of eyes in two conditions:

1. When there is excessive production of tears. This is called **lacrimation**.
2. When there is diminished drainage. This is called **epiphora**.

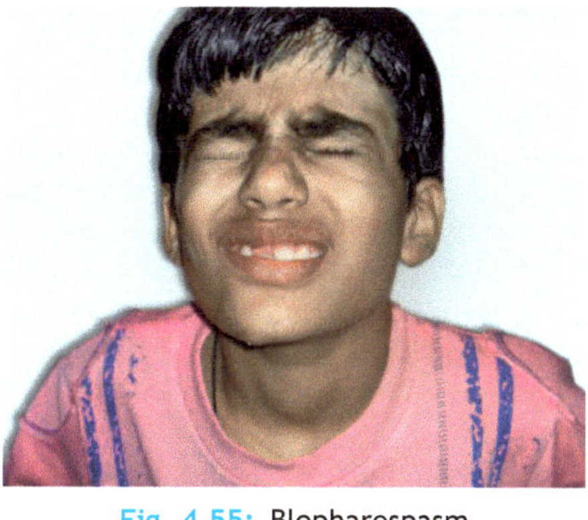

Fig. 4.55: Blepharospasm

Causes of Lacrimation

1. Anything that irritates the eyes
2. Acute conjunctivitis
3. Foreign body: lid or cornea
4. Corneal injury
5. Corneal ulcer
6. Keratitis
7. Acute iritis
8. Acute glaucoma

Causes of Epiphora

1. Lagophthalmos
2. Ectropion
3. Chronic dacryocystitis

Examination of a Case of Dacryocystitis

Dacryocystitis is inflammation of lacrimal sac. It can be congenital or acquired.

Congenital Dacryocystitis

This develops after 15 days of birth. It is generally unilateral. There is watering from the eye. There may be discharge from the eye. On pressure over the sac pus comes out from the puncta. **Congenital dacryocystitis** must be differentiated from **ophthalmia neonatorum**, which is acute infection of conjunctiva of new born, it starts with in first week of life is bilateral. Congenital dacryocystitis does not develop before 15 days.

Acquired dacryocystitis can be **acute** (sudden) or **chronic** (gradual). Acute dacryocystitis generally develop on chronic dacryocystitis.

The patient comes with redness, pain, swelling over the sac region. There is pain on pressure over the swelling. There is watering.

Chronic Dacryocystitis

1. Seen after 30 years of age.
2. More common in females.
3. Complains of watering from the eye.
   There may be a diffuse swelling over the sac. Pressure over sac causes pus discharges from the puncta. This is called regurgitation (Fig. 4.56).
4. Normally if a drop of chloromycetin is put in the conjunctiva. After few minutes the patient feels bitter taste in the throat. In case of chronic dacryocystitis, the drop does not reach throat.

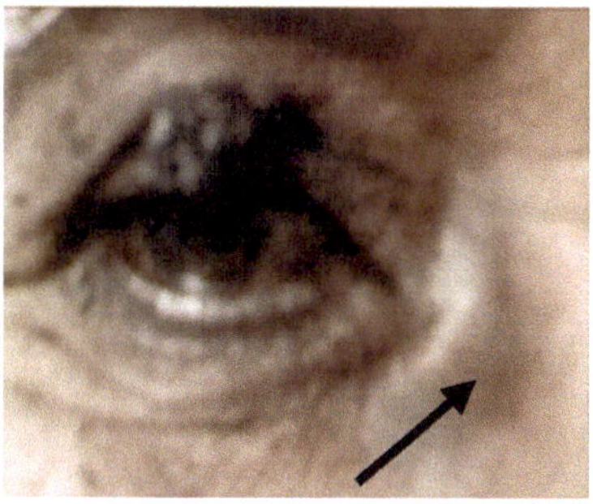

Fig. 4.56: Chronic dacyocrystitis

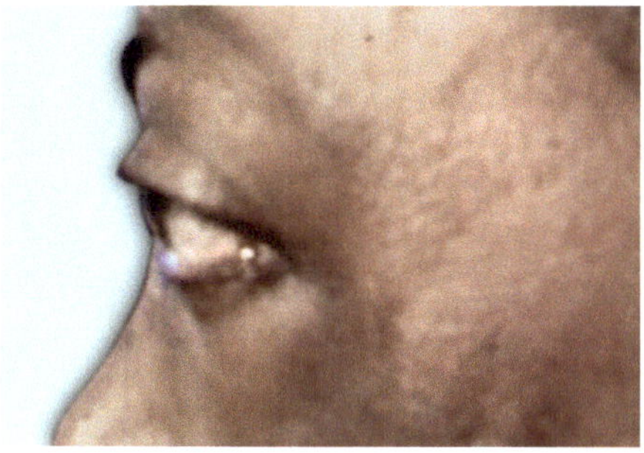

Fig. 4.57: Mild proptosis

5. If saline is injected in the lower canaliculus, it goes in the throat in persons without chronic dacryocystitis. This is called **syringing of sac**. In cases of chronic dacryocystitis, the saline does not reach throat but comes out of upper puncta. This is called negative syringing.

Examination of Orbit

The orbit is examined for:

1. Protrusion of the globe
   i. Proptosis
   ii. Exophthalmos
2. Retraction of globe—Enophthalmos

Proptosis (Fig. 4.57)

1. The eyeball bulges forward.
2. The bulge is measured by an instrument called **exophthalmometer** (Fig. 4.58) or clinically by standing behind the patient and observing the position of the globe in relation to the upper orbital rim. (Fig. 4.59).
3. The proptosis can be
   i. Congenital
   ii. Acquired

The **congenital proptosis** are generally bilateral due to congenital small orbits.

Acquired proptosis is mostly unilateral.

The cause of proptosis is generally a tumor behind the globe.

The tumor can be noncancer or cancer.

Exophthalmos

This is a type of protrusion of the globe due to disease of thyroid gland. Exophthalmos can be unilateral or bilateral.

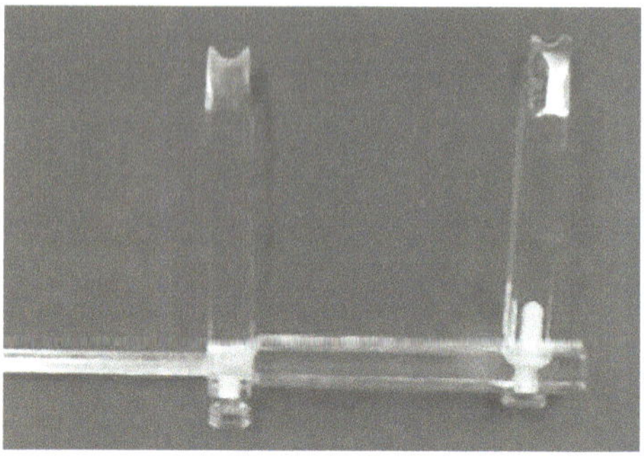

Fig. 4.58: Exophthalmometer

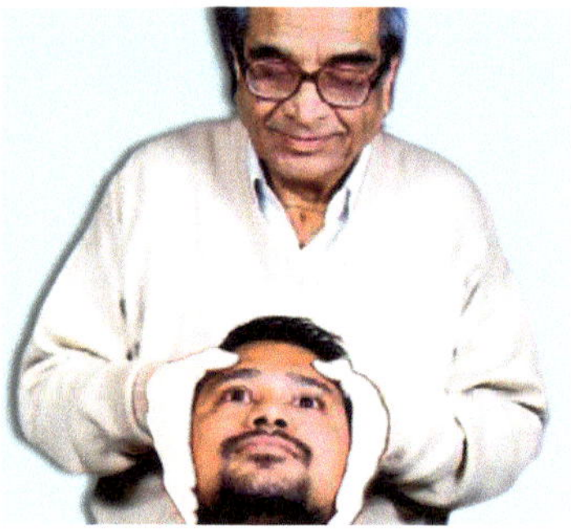

Fig. 4.59: Clinical examination of a case of proptosis

It may be associated with
- Lid retraction
- Restricted movements

Examination of Conjunctiva

Conjunctival diseases can be seen in all ages from newborn to very old age. The common symptoms are:
1. Watering from the eye (lacrimation)
2. Discharge from the eyes
3. Sticking of the lids
4. Redness of the eyes
5. Itching
6. Dryness of the eyes
7. White spots on the conjunctiva (xerosis—Bitot's spot)

Causes of Watering from the Eyes

1. Conjunctivitis
2. Deformity of the lids
3. Corneal ulcer
4. Keratitis
5. Injury to the cornea
6. Chronic dacryocystitis

Causes of Discharge from the Eyes

1. Infective conjunctivitis
   i. Watering—Viral infection
   ii. Thick discharge—Bacterial conjunctivitis
2. Allergic conjunctivitis
   i. Watering
   ii. Roapy discharge.

Redness of the Eye

Redness of the eyes can be
1. Conjunctival
2. Circumciliary

Conjunctival congestion can be
- Generalized (all over the conjunctiva)
- Localized

Causes of Generalized Redness of the Conjunctiva

1. Acute conjunctivitis
2. Chronic conjunctivitis

Causes of Localized Redness of the Conjunctiva (see Fig 8.1)

1. Injury
2. Phlycten
3. Episcleritis
4. Scleritis
5. Pterygium
6. Allergic conjunctivitis

Causes of Bright Red Color of the Conjunctiva

Commonest cause is subconjunctival hemorrhage (see Figs 8.3, 8.4 and 8.6 to 8.8).

It can be
- Generalized
- Localized
- Scattered

Characteristics of Conjunctival Congestion (see Fig. 8.2)

1. It starts away from the cornea.
2. It is bright red in color.
3. The blood vessels are irregular.
4. There is no pain on pressing the globe.
5. It is generally associated with discharge.

Commonest cause is conjunctivitis (Fig. 1.60).

Circumciliary Congestion

Circumciliary congestion develops round the cornea hence, it is called **circumcorneal congestion** also. It starts from the limbus and spreads away. It does not reach periphery. The conjunctival congestion starts from the periphery and does not reach the limbus (see Fig. 8.2).

Circumciliary congestion generally associated with pain, and watering. The eyeball pains when pressed (this is called **ciliary tenderness**).

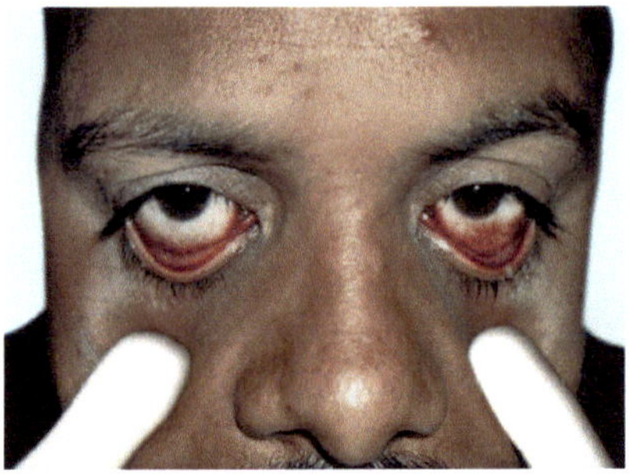

Fig. 4.60: Conjunctival congestion

The common causes of circum ciliarycongestion are—keratitis, acute and chronic iridocyclitis and acute congestive glaucoma, absolute glaucoma.

Itching in the Eyes

Itching in the eyes is a very common symptom in children.
The common causes are:

1. Spring catarrh
2. Allergic conjunctivitis
3. Seasonal allergic conjunctivitis

Cause of Dryness of the Conjunctiva

Normal conjunctiva is always wet due to a layer of tear on it.
The causes of dryness are:

1. Xerophthalmia—Vitamin A deficiency
2. Dry eye syndrome

In xerophthalmia, Bitot's spot may develop on the conjunctiva.

Bitot's Spot

Bitot's spot is a round or triangular spot situated on the temporal side of the conjunctiva between the limbus and the outer canthus. The base of the triangle is towards the cornea. It is foamy in nature and stains with Kajal. Commonest cause is vitamin A deficiency. It is generally associated with night blindness.

Dry Eye Syndrome

When the quantity of the tear is less than normal or it has changed quality, dry eye syndrome develops. Total tear present in the eye is measured by Schirmer's Test (Figs 4.61 and 4.62).

Normal reading is more than 30 mm, reading less than 15 is suggestive of dry eye syndrome.

Reading less than 10 mm is definitely dry eye.

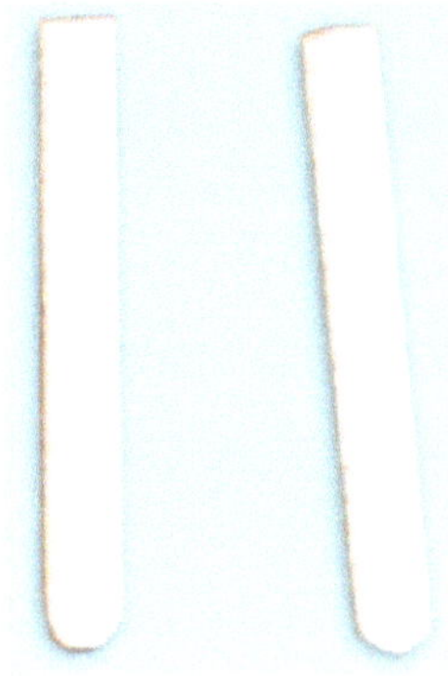

Fig. 4.61: Schirmer strips

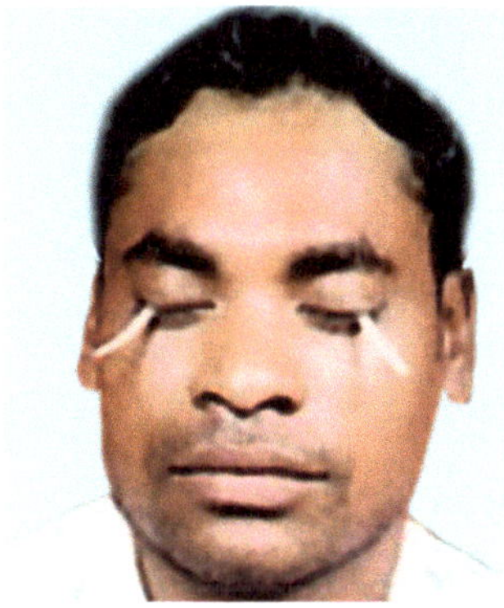

Fig. 4.62: Schirmer test

Examination of Globe

The globe (eyeball) consists of two structures:

1. The cornea
2. The sclera

The **cornea** is colorless and transparent. Its main function is optical (focussing) and second function is protective. The sclera is opaque. It is white in color. Its main function is protective. It does not have any optical property. It keeps the interior (inside) of the eye dark. The extraocular muscles are attached to the sclera. The nerves and arteries enter the eye through the sclera. The veins leave the eye through the sclera.

The junction of the cornea and sclera is called **limbus**. The cornea is more curved than the sclera. Hence, the junction of the two is not smooth. The cornea forms an angle with the sclera at limbus.

The sclera is covered by the conjunctiva anteriorly (in front). The posterior part is in contact with orbital fat.

The Tenon's capsule covers the sclera from the optic nerve to the limbus. The optic nerve leaves the globe through **posterior sclera foramen**.

The globe is examined for its size, color and surface irregularity.

Changes in Size and Shape of the Globe

The size of an adult globe is 24 mm. Absence of globe at birth is called **anophthalmos**. This is very rare condition. A small refracted globe is called **enophthalmos**. A small soft irregular globe is called **phthisis bulbae**.

A congenitally small globe is called **microphthalmos**. The cause is poor development of the eye.

A large eye is called **buphthalmos** (eye of an ox). The cause is **congenital glaucoma** present at birth.

Bulging of the globe is called **proptosis/exophthalmos**.

Proptosis is caused due to growth behind the globe while exophthalmos is due to disease of thyroid.

Signs of Microphthalms

- The eyes has very poor vision.
- There is pseudoptosis.
- The interpalpebral fissure is narrow.
- The globe is small but the curvature is maintained.
- The cornea is small.
- The anterior chamber is very shallow.
- The pupil is key hole shaped.

Signs of Phthisis

- Pseudoptosis
- Narrow interpalpebral fissure
- The eyeball is sunken
- The curvature of the cornea and sclera are lost.
- The anterior chamber depth is variable. It may be absent or even deep if the lens is absent.
- The intraocular tension is very low.
- The vision is very poor.

The common causes are:

1. Prolonged pan uveitis
2. Perforation of the globe

Signs of Buphthalmos

- There is pseudoproptosis due to increased length of the eye.
- The cornea is larger than 13 mm in diameter.
- The sclera is stretched
- The angle between the cornea and the sclera at the limbus is lost.
- The cornea may show deep opacities.
- The anterior chamber is deep.
- The vision is poor.
- Intraocular tension is very high.
- The child has photophobia
- The commonest cause is congenital glaucoma.

Signs of Proptosis

- Any growth behind the globe pushes the eyeball forward.
- The interpalpebral fissure is wide.
- The eye bulges beyond the orbital margin
- The amount of bulge is measured by an instrument called **exophthalmometer**.
- The movements of the eyeball may be normal or absent depending on position of the growth.

The term **exophthalmos** is used only in case of bulging of the eye due to disease of the thyroid gland.

Changes in Color of the Sclera

The normal sclera is white. There may be small, scattered black spots on the surface. They are due to deposit of **melanin** on the sclera. These spots are harmless (Fig. 4.63)

The sclera becomes yellow in **jaundice**. **Subconjunctival hemorrhage** gives red color to the sclera.

White raised area over the sclera, under the conjunctiva is due to **depot steroid injected** under the conjunctiva. Black irregular bulging in the sclera is caused due to **scleral staphyloma**.

Staphylomas

The staphylomas are abnormal bulging in the outer coat (sclera and cornea) of the eyes. The bulge is lined by uvea inside. The staphyloma can be **scleral** or **corneal**. The corneal staphylomas are also known as **anterior staphyloma**. In total corneal staphyloma whole of the cornea is replaced by scar tissue which is lined by iris. The color of the staphyloma is white. The areas where the iris is attached look black. The surface is irregular, have raised intraocular tension. Generally these eyes have no vision. If total corneal staphyloma develop in childhood, it starts squinting, may have nystagmus. Scleral staphylomas can be congenital (present at birth) or acquired:

	Name of staphyloma	Location of staphyloma
1.	Intercalary	Limbus
2.	Ciliary staphyloma	Away from limbus but in front of the equator
3.	Equatorial	At the equator of the globe
4.	Posterior	Posterior pole of the globe

Only intercalary and ciliary staphyloma are visible on external examination. The equatorial and posterior staphylomas are visible only on indirect ophthalmoscopy or exposing the globe after the conjunctiva has been cut during squint or detachment surgery.

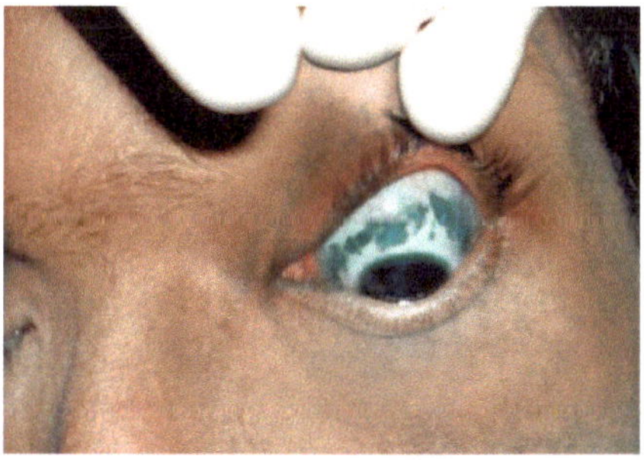

Fig. 4.63: Black discoloration of sclera

Examination of Cornea

Cornea is examined under following heads:

1. Shape
2. Size
3. Curvature
4. Surface
   a. Irregular
   b. Ectasia
   c. Staphyloma
5. Transparency
6. Sensation
7. Staining
8. Thickness
9. Vascularization
10. Deposits

Shape of the Cornea

The cornea looks circular but in fact it is horizontally oval. Its horizontal diameter is 11 mm and vertical diameter is 10.5 mm but this is not appreciated clinically unless measured by a corneal calliper. Gross changes in cornea are seen in microcornea, soft eye and phthisis.

Size of Cornea

A cornea with diameter more than 13 mm is called megalocornea and a cornea with diameter less than 9 mm is called microcornea.

Causes of Megalocornea

1. Buphthalmos—Primary and secondary
2. Congenital megalocornea

Primary buphthalmos and congenital megalocornea are present at birth. The former has raised intraocular tension (glaucoma) and may cause blindness. The second has normal tension and does not cause blindness.

Examining the Corneal Curvature

The average curvature of the cornea is 8 mm. The vertical curvature is slightly more than horizontal curvature.

Excess of increase in corneal curvature as in **keratoconus** or excessive flattening of corneal curvature as in **phthisis** and **microcornea** can be detected by oblique illumination but minimal changes which are vital for contact lens fitting, IOL power calculation and radial keratotomy require special instrument called **keratometer**.

The front surface of the cornea acts as a convex mirror that forms an erect, small, virtual image of an object in front of it, the image moves with the movement of the object. If the following are known, i.e. distance of the object from the convex mirror, the size of the object and the size of image formed is known, the curvature of the convex mirror can be calculated. More is the curvature, smaller is the image. Farther is the object, smaller is the image.

The phenomenon of image formation by convex mirror is utilized in keratometry.

A keratometer is a calibrated instrument that measures the corneal curvature at two meridians at right angles. The keratometer not only measure the corneal curvature but also denote its corresponding readings in dioptre. The keratometer measures only central 3 mm of the cornea. Different readings between the two meridians beyond normal physical limits denote astigmatism. The keratometric reading in each meridian is uniform but differ in two meridians. The condition is called regular astigmatism. If the keratometric values differ in the same meridian, the condition is called irregular astigmatism.

Causes of irregular astigmatism are—Pterygium, keratoconus, corneal opacities, limbal dermoid, iris prolapse.

The keratometers are used for contact lens fitting and IOL power calculation.

Examination of Corneal Surface

The cornea acts as a convex mirror. It forms a virtual, erect, small image of the object from sharp image. The surface of the cornea should be smooth, regular in curvature and wet. Loss of any of these distorts the image formed.

The examination of the corneal surface is called **keratoscopy** that can be done by various types of keratoscopes which may be self, illuminated or have to be illuminated by external source of light. They may have attached arrangement for photography. The cameras may be simple photographic cameras or digital cameras.

The commonly used keratoscopes are:

1. Placido disc
2. Ophthalmoscope mounted keratoscope
3. Photokeratoscope
4. Computerized corneal topography

Placido disc is a circular disc of ten inches diameter. It has a handle at one end. There is a hole in the center of the disc, through which the examiner looks at the cornea.

A plus two lens incorporated in the hole relaxes the accommodation of the examiner. Round the hole are concentric rings of increasing diameter. They are black and white in color. They are of equal width and alternate with each other. The disc has to be illuminated from outside.

To use the placido disc, the patients sits with his back towards a source of light. The light falls on the surface of the disc which is held by the examiner.

One eye is examined at a time. The examiner looks at the cornea through the peep hole and moves towards the cornea till the rings are seen on the cornea.

In a normal cornea the rings are circular. The distance between the adjoining rings are same. Any distortion of the rings mean uneven surface of the cornea.

The causes of distortion of the rings are:
1. Corneal opacities
2. Corneal ulcer
3. Pterygium
4. Irregular astigmatism
5. Keratoplasty
6. Soft eye
7. Keratoconus
8. Growths at the limbus
9. Keratectasia
10. Staphyloma

Ophthalmoscope mounted keratoscopes are self-illuminated discs similar to placido disc that works on the same principle as that of placido disc. The keratoscope is used after removing the head of the ophthalmoscope. The instrument is used like any direct ophthalmoscope. The cornea is seen through the hole in the center of the keratoscope. Some of the ophthalmoscopes have in built rings that can be projected on the corneal surface and examined by adding plus lenses.

Photokeratoscopes are specialized keratoscopes mounted on a table. They can detect small irregularities on the corneal periphery. They are used to examine the cornea for refractive keratotomies, before and after surgery. The photokeratoscopes can photograph the corneal changes. The method of photography is called **keratography**.The photokeratoscopes may have digital video, attachment with different color code. They are mostly used for lasik surgery.

Corneal Transparency

For sharp focus, the cornea has to be transparent. Any loss of transparency causes blurred vision. The loss of transparency of cornea are called **corneal opacity**. The opacity may develop at any level of cornea from epithelium to endothelium. More than one layer may be involved at the same time. According to level of involvement, corneal opacities can be—**Nebula**, **macula**, **leukoma** and **leukoma** adherent (see Figs 9.2 to 9.5).

Nebula is faintest opacity not visible in diffuse illumination. It is best seen on slit lamp.

The macula is denser than nebula and visible on focal illumination without magnification.

Leukoma is visible on diffuse illumination. Leukoma adherent is any corneal opacity in which iris is incarcerated (trapped) or was incarcerated.

It is possible to have more than one grade of opacity in the same cornea. The opacities do not stain with fluorescein. The sensation on the opacity is generally dull. They do not increase in density except in corneal dystrophy.

Causes of Corneal Opacity

1. Congenital (present at birth)
2. Injury
3. Infection—Corneal ulcer
4. Interstitial keratitis
5. Vitamin A deficiency
6. Vascularization
7. Dystrophy
8. Encroachment

All the above causes can cause either unilateral corneal opacity or bilateral corneal opacity.

Causes of Bilateral Corneal Opacity

1. Congenital (rare)
2. Injury
   - Cracker injury
   - Blast injury
   - Chemical injury
3. Keratomalacia
4. Ophthalmia neonatorum
5. Trachoma
6. Leprosy
7. Smallpox (not seen now a days)
8. Pterygium
9. Phlycten
10. Spring catarrh
11. Arcus senilis
12. Arcus juvenilis
13. Corneal dystrophy
14. Band keratopathy
15. Deposits on cornea

Examination of Level of Lesion in the Cornea

The cornea is **five-layered** structure. They are **epithelium**, **Bowman's membrane**, **stroma**, **Descemet's membrane** and **endothelium**. A disease may involve single-layer or it may involve more than one-layer. Each has separate slit lamp appearance. For this reason, it is essential to locate the level of the disease. This is done on slit lamp.

The commonly used methods are:
1. Examination with wide beam and low magnification.
2. Direct illumination—This is done by using a narrow beam, moderate magnification, the source of light is angled.
3. Retroillumination—Here the light beam is focused on the iris and the cornea is examined by the light reflected from the iris.

Examination of Corneal Sensation

Examination of corneal sensation is very simple, yet it is not done as frequently as it should be done.

To examine the corneal sensation, it must be assured that no anesthetic agent has been used during past 48 hours and the patient has not used contact lens for twenty-four hours because both of the above diminish corneal sensation.

To test corneal sensation—The patient sits comfortably and fixes a distant object, keeping both eyes open. One eye is tested at a time. A wisp of cotton is brought from the temporal side to touch the cornea. If corneal sensation is normal, the patient reflexly close both the eyes. When one eye has poor sensation, the other eye acts as control.

Causes of Diminished Corneal Sensation

1. Use of anesthetic agent (xylocaine 4%)
2. Prolonged used of contact lens
3. Herpes simplex keratitis
4. Herpes zoster keratitis
5. Absolute glaucoma
6. Corneal scar

There is no condition where corneal sensation is more than normal.

Corneal Stain

Intact corneal epithelium does not stain with any stain. Only the tear film in front of the epithelium is stained. Cornea is stained when the corneal epithelium is broken (breached) as following surgery, corneal ulcer and superficial keratitis.

There are **three stains** by which the cornea is stained. They are (Fig. 4.64):
1. Fluorescein
2. Rose bengal
3. Lissamine green

To stain with **fluorescein**, one drop of one percent fluorescein is put in the conjunctival sac and the patient is asked to keep the eye closed for a minute. After that excess of fluorescein is washed with normal saline and the eye is examined first under white light and then under a cobalt blue filter. Under white light, the stained area looks bright green and under cobalt blue the stained area looks yellow.

It is better to use single use sterilized **fluorescein strip** than drops. The drops are contaminated when kept in bottle for more than few days.

Besides staining, the fluorescein drops are used in:

1. Applanation tonometry
2. Contact lens fitting
3. Tear break up time
4. Locate leaking wound
5. Patency of nasolacrimal duct
6. Treat pediculosis

Intravenous fluorescein is used for **fluorescein angiography**.

Rose bengal is another stain used to stain cornea as well as conjunctiva. It is also available either as one percent drop or in single use sterilized strip. Rose bengal when instilled in conjunctiva causes intense burning, hence the conjunctiva is anesthetized prior to instillation of rose bengal. It stains damaged corneal and conjunctival epithelium. The stain is seen under white light.

When both the fluorescein and rose bengal are used together, the procedure is called **differential staining**.

Examination of Thickness of Cornea

The curvature of cornea is not equal on both the surfaces. The front (anterior) surface is less curved than the back (posterior) surface. This makes the center of the cornea thinner in the center and thicker on the

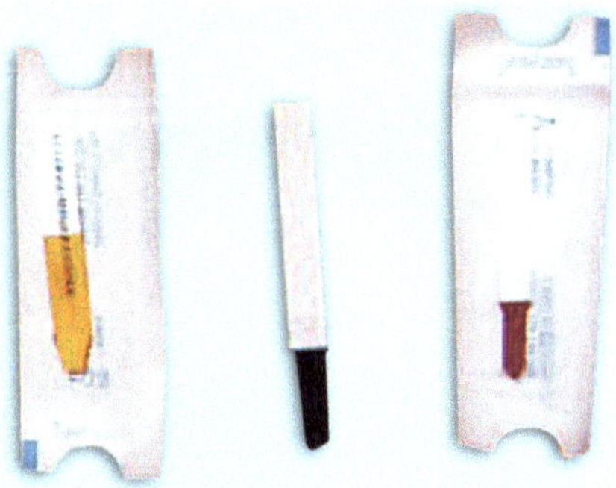

A B C

1. Fluorescein strip
2. Rose bengal
3. Lissamine green

Fig. 4.64: Strips used to stain cornea

periphery. The cornea at limbus is 1 mm thick while in front of the pupil, it is only 0.6 mm. Hence, perforation of central cornea is more common in the center than periphery (near the limbus). The corneal thickness is reduced in **keratoconus**, **keratectasia** and **buphthalmos**.

Causes of Thickened Cornea

- Corneal scar
- Disciform keratitis
- Swelling of the epithelium

Corneal thickness is required to be measure in cases where radial keratotomy and lamellar corneal grafts are planned and diagnosis of narrow angle glaucoma. The method is called **pachometery** and the attachment required is called **pachometer**. There are two types of pachometers, i.e. optical and ultrasonic. The first is used with slit lamp while the second is used along with biometer which is used to calculate IOL power.

Recording of Corneal Opacities

It is better to draw a diagram of the corneal lesions and following points are noted –

1. Number of opacities
2. Position (see Fig. 9.12)
3. Size of opacities
4. Grades of opacity (see Fig. 9.6)
   - Nebula
   - Macula
   - Leukoma
5. Staining – Positive/Negative
6. Vascularization (see Fig. 9.10 and 9.11)
7. Pigment in opacity—Adherent leukoma

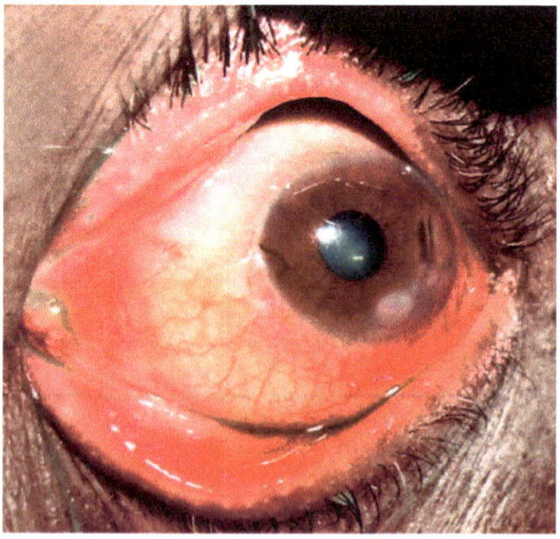

Fig. 4.65: Positive stain of corneal ulcer (*courtesy:* Dr Santosh patel)

Position of opacities is noted in relation to limbus, pupil, or clock number. For example, the opacity is 1 mm x 1 mm, 2 mm away from the limbus between 10 O'clock and 2 O'clock. Simple Leukoma neither stains nor is vascularized. There is no iris pigment in the opacity. The sensation over the opacity is less.

Corneal Vascularization

Normal cornea does not have vessels in it except peripheral 1 mm. Presence of vessels in the cornea means disease of cornea.

Vessels may be:

1. Superficial (in the epithelium)
2. Deep
   i. Interstitial (in the stroma)
   ii. Retro corneal (on the endothelium)

Causes of Superficial Vascularization of Cornea

1. Trachoma
2. Leprosy
3. Fascicular ulcer
4. Chronic corneal ulcer
5. Vascularization of leukoma
6. Pterygium
7. Chemical burn

The superficial corneal vessels are conjunctival in nature. They are large, irregular and join each other. They are visible over the limbus. Their presence is called **pannus**.

Causes of Deep (Interstitial) Vascularization

1. Interstitial keratitis
2. Disciform keratitis
3. Alkali burn
4. Vessel growing under lamellar keratoplasty

The deep vessels are ciliary vessels. They are not visible at limbus. They are straight, parallel to each other. They do not join each other. They are generally seen in sectors.

Retro Corneal Vascularization (on the Back of Cornea)

They are of two types:

1. Corneal
2. Retinal
   a. Conjunctival vessels grow behind the cornea only when the conjunctiva with its blood supply enter the anterior chamber following penetrating injury and the condition is called **epithelial down growth**.

b. Retinal—These vessels grow on the ciliary body → back surface of iris → pupil → front surface of iris → angle of iris → back of cornea (endothelium)

The Causes are

i. Advanced diabetic retinopathy
ii. Central retinal vein thrombosis
iii. Intraocular tumors

Corneal Deposits

Corneal deposits can be:

1. Superficial
2. Deep
3. On the back of the cornea

The superficial deposits are:

1. Foreign bodies—Single, multiple, one eye or both eyes
2. Band keratopathy
3. Mucus plaque
4. Tattoo

Causes of Opacities Between Bowmen's Membrane and Descemet's Membrane

1. Foreign bodies
2. Krukenberg spindle
3. Hudson stahli line
4. Fleischer ring (keratoconus)
5. Kayser, Fleischer ring (copper—brass)
6. Siderosis (Metallic iron ferrous salt)

Examination of Anterior Chamber

Anterior chamber is a space between the back surface of the cornea and front surface of iris and lens (Fig. 4.66).

It is examined for its depth and contents.

The depth of the anterior chamber is maximum in front of the pupil, i.e. 3 mm. It gradually decreases on the periphery and become absent where the cornea meets the iris. The junction of the cornea and iris is called angle of the anterior chamber.

The depth of the anterior chamber is increased in:

- Keratoconus—Conical cornea
- Aphakia—Lens is absent
- Buphthalmos—Congenital glaucoma

The depth is decreased in:

- Microphthalmos
- Narrow angle glaucoma
- Swollen lens

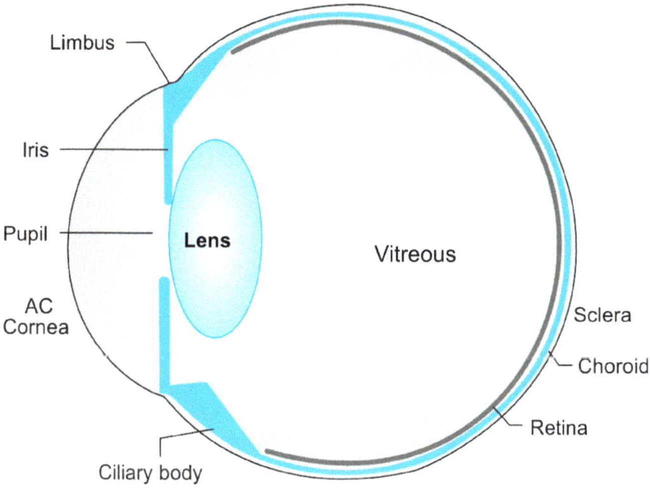

Fig. 4.66: Diagram showing normal depth of AC

The depth of anterior chamber is irregular in:
- Iris prolapse
- Adherent leukoma
- Iris bombe
- Tumors of the iris

The **angle of anterior chamber** is measured by an instrument called **gonioscope**.

The angle can be normal, wide or narrow. Narrow angle causes acute primary glaucoma. Wide angle is associated with chronic simple glaucoma.

Contents of Anterior Chamber

The normal contents of the anterior chamber is **aqueous**, which is a clear field.

The abnormal contents are:
1. Hypopyon—Pus in anterior chamber
2. Hyphema—Blood in anterior chamber
3. Lens in anterior chamber
   i. Whole of lens
   ii. Nucleus of lens
   iii. Cortical material of lens
4. Anterior chamber intraocular lens
5. Tumors of iris and ciliary body
6. Parasites in anterior chamber

Pseudohypopyon—White material other than pus in AC is called pseudo hypopyon. Causes of pseudohypopyon are **corticalmatter, opaque nucleus, malignant cells**.

Examination of Uvea

Uvea is the middle coat of the eyeball. It comprises of **iris**, **ciliary body** and **choroid**. Out of the three only iris is visible with torch. The rest are examined by special instrument like direct and indirect ophthalmoscope. The examination of iris consists of examination of iris proper and the pupil.

The iris is examined for:
1. Color
2. Its surface
3. Coloboma
4. Nodules
5. Examination of pupil

The color of the iris ranges from brown to black. It is light colored in albinism. There may be white patches of atrophy on the iris surface. They are generally due to trauma caused by instruments during lens extraction or due to some type of inflammation of iris like herpes zoster.

The surface of the normal iris is rough. Surface looses its roughness when the iris is swollen as in acute iritis or acute glaucoma.

Coloboma

The term coloboma means absence of iris. It can be **congenital** or **acquired**. The acquired colobomas can be peripheral or broad based. If the papillary margin is cut, it is called sphincterotomy. Peripheral iridectomies can be single or two. They are generally seen at the upper part. They may be triangular.

Broad based iridectomy removes the iris from the root of the iris up to papillary margin. It is wider at the root of the iris.

The nodules can be:
1. Inflammatory
   - Tuberculosis
   - Leprosy
   - Syphilis
2. Foreign body
3. New growths

Examination of the Pupillary Margin

Examination of iris is not complete without examining the pupil.
Pupil is examined for:
- Its position, size, shape, color and reaction.
- Normal pupil is central, circular and reacts to light.
- The position of the pupil may shift in chronic iridocyclitis, prolapse of iris and adherent leukoma.

- Normal pupil is about 2.5 mm in diameter.
- It becomes small in iritis and iridocyclitis.
- It becomes large following instillation of mydriatic and cycloplegic.
- The normal pupil is circular, when its shape is distorted, it is called irregular pupil.
- The commonest cause of irregular pupil is formation of posterior synechia.

Posterior Synechia

Normal iris moves smoothly over the normal lens as the pupil constricts and dilates. In **iridocyclitis**, the iris gets attached to the anterior lens capsule and the area that is attached to the lens does not move, this forms a notch at the papillary margin. The adhesion between the iris and the lens is called **posterior synechiae**.

The number of synechiae vary from single to many. Sometimes the whole of the iris is attached to the lens capsule all-round. This is called **ring synechia**.

The synechiae may be very small and break with mydriatic in acute iridocyclitis or may be broad and strong not breaking with mydriatic. When mydriatic is put in an eye with posterior synechiae, the pupil dilates in between the synechiae, giving a flower petal appearance to the pupil. This is called **festooned pupil**. After few instillation of mydriatic the pupil dilates fully, leaving patches of iris on the anterior lens capsule.

The ring synechiae do not dilate with mydriatic. It separates the anterior chamber from the posterior chamber, hence is called **seclusio pupillae**. The aqueous is prevented from entering the AC. This pushes the iris forward and a condition called **iris bombe** develops. In iris bombe, the iris is attached to the lens capsule at papillary margin and firmly fixed at the angle so the central part bulges forwards. The anterior chamber becomes irregular. It is shallowest in between the papillary margin and root of the iris. The peripheral part of the iris touches the cornea at the angle, thus preventing aqueous drainage and causing rise of tension.

Adhesion of iris to the posterior surface of the cornea is called **anterior synechia**.

Causes of anterior synechia are—Chronic iridocyclitis, chronic glaucoma and adherent leukoma.

Examination of Pupil

Pupil is a circular hole in the iris, in front of the lens. Its functions are to control the light entering the eye and allow flow of aqueous from posterior chamber to the anterior chamber. When the light is bright, it constricts as in day light. When the light is dull, it dilated as at night.

The pupil is examined for:
1. Its position—Central or not central
2. Shape of pupil—Circular or irregular
3. Size of the pupil
4. Color of the pupil
5. Reaction of the pupil

Causes of irregular pupil are
1. Congenital
   i. Persistent papillary membrane (see Fig. 12.7)
   ii. Coloboma of iris (see Fig. 12.4)
2. Iritis
3. Iris prolapse (see Fig 12.12f and 12.7g)
4. Adherent leukoma
5. Iridodialysis
6. Broad-based iridectomy
7. Sphincterotomy

   Size of pupil—Normal pupil is 2 to 2.5 mm in size.

   A small pupil is called miotic pupil. A dilated pupil is called mydriatics pupil.

Causes of small pupil are
1. Bright light
2. Iritis
3. Drugs that make the pupil small and called miotics. They can be local, i.e. pilocarpine or may be taken orally, i.e. opium.
4. Trauma

Causes of large pupil are –
1. Dull light
2. Glaucoma
3. Optic atrophy
4. Drugs: Drugs that dilate the pupil are called mydriatics. They can be local like atropine, hom atropine, tropicamide, cyclopentolate, adrenaline, phenylephrine.

   There are some oral medicines that also dilates the pupil.
5. Trauma
6. Blind eye

Color of Pupil

The normal color of the pupil with transparent lens is **black**. In case of albinism, it is **pink**. (see Fig. 12.8).

In case of cataract, it is **white** (Fig. 4.67).

In case of aphakia when the lens has been removed, it is **jet black**.

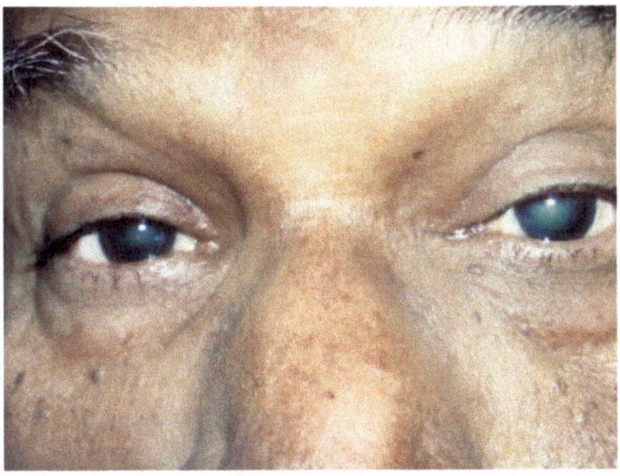

Fig. 4.67: Immature cataract

It is also white in case of **retinoblastoma**, a cancer of retina which is seen in children. Such a white color of the pupil is called **white reflex** in papillary area.

Reaction of Pupil

Normal pupil becomes small as soon as light falls on the pupil. Light may fall in one pupil but both the pupil constrict at the same time and equally. Constriction of pupil when light is thrown on the same pupil is called **direct pupillary reaction**. Constriction of the other pupil when light is thrown on the opposite pupil is called **indirection reaction**. In normal persons both direct and indirect papillary reaction should be present and equal.

Other causes of constriction of pupil are:

a. When a person sees small objects at 30 cm, this is called **accommodation**.
b. When a patient turns both eyes at an objects kept at 30 cm, this is called **convergence**.The pupil constricts both m accommodation and convergence.

The pupil should constrict to almost 1 mm size in presence of bright light and remain small so long the light falls on the pupil. As soon as the light is removed, the pupil dilates to reach its normal size. This is called **brisk pupillary reaction**. This is normal. If the pupil constricts slowly, does not constrict fully or dilate in presence of light, it is called sluggish pupil. This is abnormal.

The causes of sluggish pupil are:

- Dull light thrown on the pupil
- Recent use of mydriatic
- Ingestion of drugs that dilate the pupil
- Optic atrophy
- Advanced glaucoma

Examination of Lens

Lens is situated behind the iris in the pupillary area in front of the vitreous. It is suspended by zonules which attaché the lens to the ciliary body.

The normal lens is transparent.

Its front surface acts as a convex mirror and forms a small virtual image that moves with the movement of the object.

The back surface acts as a concave mirror and forms a real inverted image that moves against the movement of the objects.

These images are called **Purkinje image**. In case of complete cataract (when the lens becomes white), the small image is not formed. Both the images are lost when the lens is absent but are present when an IOL is put in place of cataract. When the light is thrown obliquely at an angle, the iris casts a shadow on the front surface of the lens, this is called **iris shadow**. This is present and well, visible in immature cataract (when whole of the lens is not white) but is not seen in case of mature cataract (when whole of the lens is white). The iris shadow is also absent when the lens is removed fully.

Any opacity in the lens is called **cataract**. It is white in color. If it extends from front surface to the back surface, it is called **mature cataract**. When only some fibres are white, it is called **immature cataract**.

Immature cataract can be:

1. Cortical—When the opacity is on the periphery.
2. Nuclear—When the opacity is in the center of the lens.
3. Posterior polar when a small opacity is present at the central part of the back of the lens.
4. It is possible to have both cortical as well as nuclear cataract in the same eye.

The opacities look white when seen by a torch but look black when seen on retinoscope.

Immature cataract must be differentiated from other causes of gradual diminished distant vision, i.e.

- Error of refraction
- Chronic simple glaucoma
- Retinopathies
- Maculopathies

Subluxated and Dislocated Lens

Normal lens is suspended from the ciliary body by the suspensory ligaments (zonule) behind the iris and in front of the vitreous.

If only some fibers of the zonules are broken, the lens shifts away from the break of the zonule, i.e. if the upper zonules are broken, the lens will shift down and if the lower zonules are broken, the lens will shift upwards (Fig. 4.68).

Table 4.3: Comparison between age related immature cataract and chronic simple glaucoma

	Immature cataract	Chronic simple glaucoma
Age	Generally past fifty years	Generally past fifty years
Laterality	Bilateral	Bilateral
Vision	Diminished	Diminished
Cornea	Bright	Bright
AC	Normal	Normal
Pupillary reaction	Brisk	Sluggish
Pupil	Central circular, normal in size	Central circular, large
Lens	Opaque	May be opaque
Fundus	Normal when visible	Glaucomatous change
Tension	Normal	Raised
Diurnal variation	Negative	Positive
Water drinking test	Negative	Positive
Difference in tension between the two eyes	Not more than 5 mm	More than 7 mm
Field changes	No change	Typical change

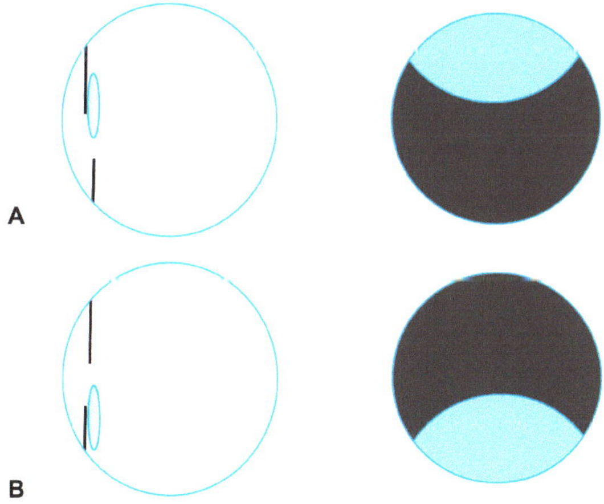

Figs 4.68A and B: Subluxation of lens; A. Subluxation upwords, partial, absence of lens from the pupillary area, lower part of the pupil is aphakic; B. Subluxation dowan words, upper part of the pupil aphakis

Table 4.4: Comparison between immature cataract and mature cataract

	Immature cataract	Mature cataract
Vision	6/60 to CF and good projection	H.M. to PL and good projection
Color of pupil	Grey	Pearly white
Iris shadow	Present	Absent
Retinoscope	Pink glow from side of the opacity	No glow

When only few zonules are broken, the condition is called **subluxation** of lens. The lens remain between the iris and the vitreous.

The pupil is divided into two parts:

1. Phakic where the lens is present
2. Aphakic where the lens the absent. The shift of the lens may be gross enough to be seen by torch without dilatation or small enough to be seen with fully dilated pupil.

The causes of subluxation can be **congenital** or **acquired**. **The acquired causes of subluxation** are blunt trauma, chronic iridocyclitis, buphthalmos.

Features of Subluxation of Lens

1. Vision—Generally low but if the subluxation is not visible with normal pupil, then the vision may be normal.
2. Anterior chamber – The anterior chamber is deep over the aphakic part and shallow over the lens.
3. Iris is tremulous over the aphakic part.
4. The aphakic part of the pupil is jet black. The phakic part shows lens. It looks white if the lens is cataractous.
5. On retinoscopy, the aphakic part is highly hypermetropic, the phakic part is either emmetropic or myopic.

Dislocation of the Lens

When all the fibers of the zonule are broken, the lens dislocates and is not visible in the papillary area. The lens can dislocate in the **vitreous** or in the **anterior chamber** or may be **thrown out of the globe**. A dislocated lens may be transparent or cataractous (Fig. 4.69).

The commonest cause of dislocation of lens is blunt injury to the eye. Sometimes a subluxated lens of long standing may also dislocate.

Signs of dislocation of the lens

1. In case of dislocation in the anterior chamber, the lens is visible in the anterior chamber.
2. The anterior chamber is deep in all cases of dislocation.

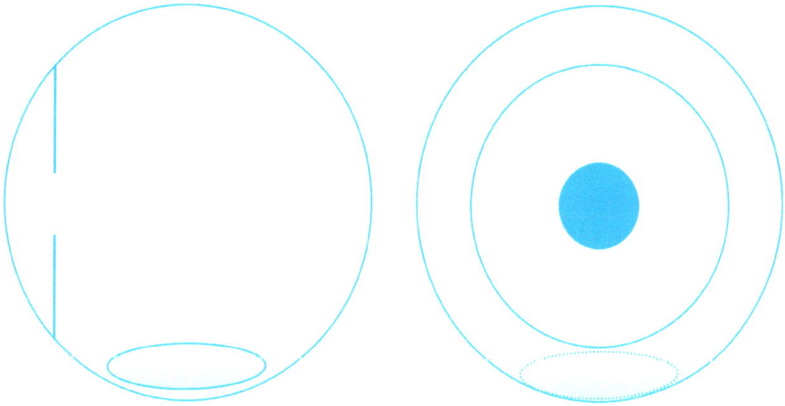

Fig. 4.69: Dislocation of the lens

3. Iris is tremulous.
4. Pupil is jet black.
5. The refraction is highly hypermetropic.
6. The vision is reduced to counting fingers.

Aphakic

Total or partial absence of lens from the papillary area is called aphakia. Commonest cause of aphakia is surgical removal of the lens. When the lens is removed completely inside the capsule, it is called **intracapsular cataract extraction** (ICCE). If the capsule is left and only the nucleus and cortex are removed, the condition is called **extracapsular cataract extraction** (ECCA). When an artificial lens (IOL) is put inside the eye after removing the lens, the condition is called **pseudophakia**. The IOL can be put in the anterior chamber, in the pupil or in the posterior chamber.

Symptoms of Aphakia

1. There is history of surgery or trauma.
2. Distant vision is reduced to CF2′.
3. The near vision is almost absent.
4. In case of surgery the mark of surgery is always present.
5. The anterior chamber is deep.
6. The iris is tremulous.
7. In case of surgery, generally an iridectomy or two are visible.
8. The pupil is jet black in case of intracapsular cataract extraction. It has a faint grey color in case of ECCE. This is called **after cataract**.
9. The error of refraction is high in hypermetropia with astigmatism.
10. There is total absence of accommodation.

Pseudophakia

The term pseudophakia means that the lens has been removed and an artificial lens (IOL) has been put in its place.

Features of IOL

1. There is history of surgery.
2. The scar of surgery is very small.
3. Anterior chamber is deeper than normal but not as deep as aphakia.
4. The iris is not tremulous.
5. Generally there is no iridectomy.
6. The lens can be either in front of the iris or behind the iris.
7. The pupil is central circular.
8. The papillary area has a glassy look.
9. The Purkinje images are brighter than normal transparent lens.
10. The distant vision may be normal or less than normal that requires glasses.
11. The accommodation is absent and requires correction.

Examination of Squint

Squint is a condition when one eye always deviates from point of fixation. There are two types of squints (Flow chart 4.2):

1. Latent—These are called **heterophorias**.
2. Manifest—These are called heterotropias.
   Manifest squint is again divided into two types:
   - **Concomitant** (Figs 4.70 and 4.71)
   - Paralytic (Fig. 4.72).

Symptoms of Squint

Symptoms differ in latent and manifest squint.

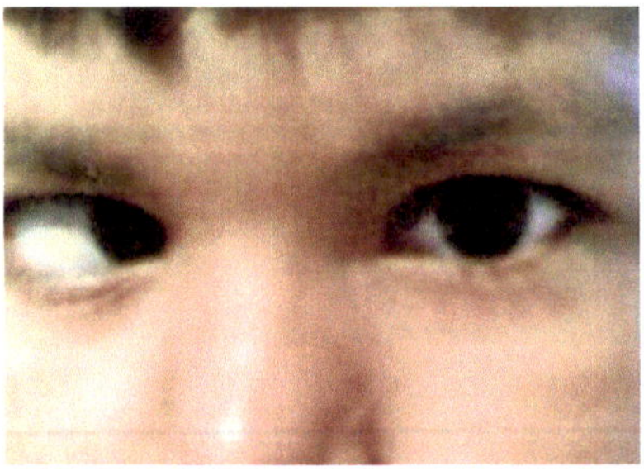

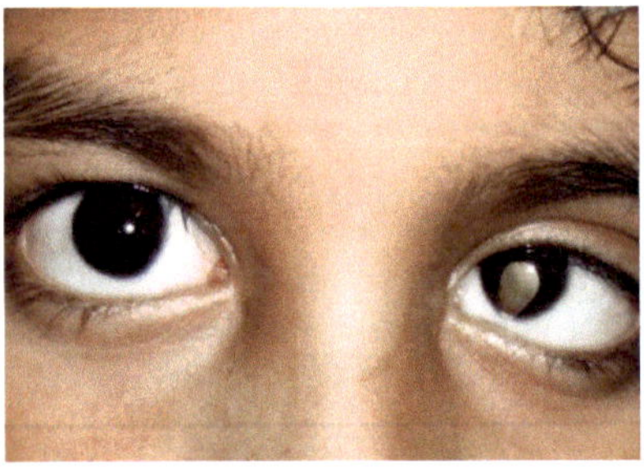

Fig. 4.70: Concomitant convergent squint

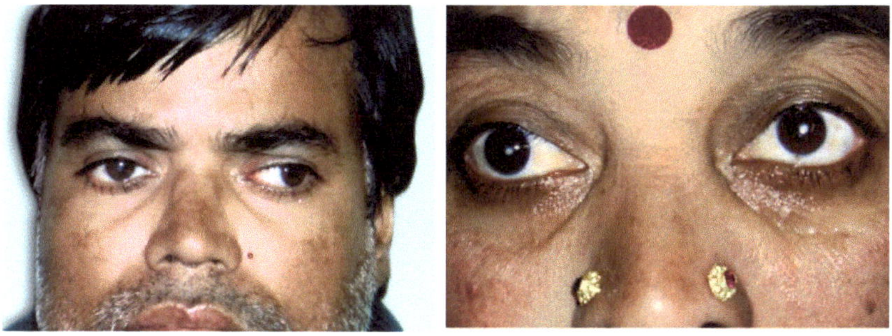

Fig. 4.71: Concomitant divergent squint

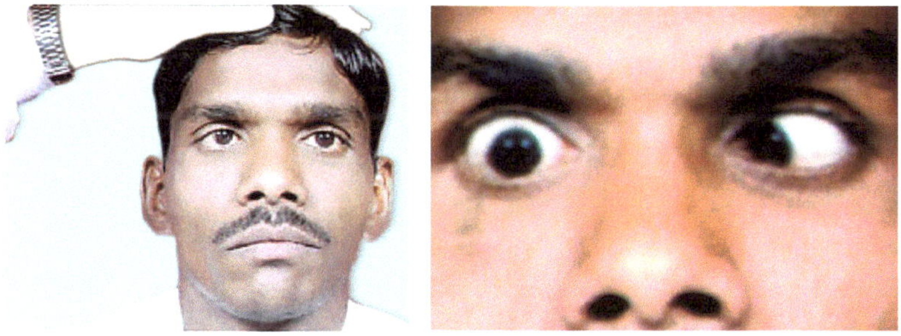

Fig. 4.72: Paralytic squint right lateral rectus palsy

Symptoms of Latent Squint

1. Patient as well as onlooker can not see any squint.
2. No symptom
3. Asthenopia (tiredness of eyes)
4. May have diminished vision

Symptoms of Manifest Squint

1. Manifest squint is an **obvious squint**. The onlooker can see the squint. Most of the time the patient is also aware of the squint.
2. In some cases only one eye squints always, this is called squinting eye and the other eye fixes and is always straight. This is called fixing eye. This condition is called **constant uniocular squint**, right or left.
3. In some cases the squint changes sides. The patient may have right eye squint for sometimes and the left eye is straight and fixes. After sometime the left eye squints and the right eye fixes. This is called **alternate squint.** The deviation in two eyes is equal.
4. The squint may be present at some hours of the day and straight at other hours. This is called **intermittent squint**.

Flow chart 4.2: Classification of squint

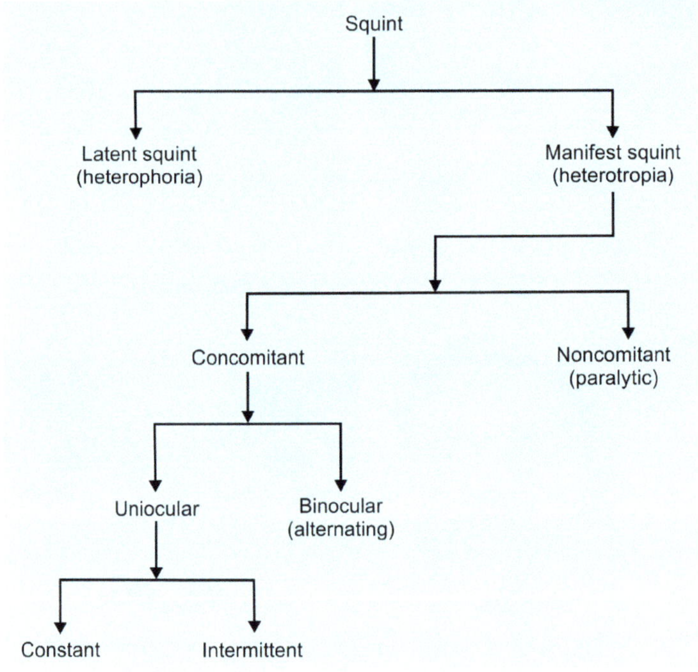

5. Diminished vision:
   a. Generally the squinting eye in uniocular concomitant squint has diminished vision.
   b. In alternate squint, either there is no visual loss in any eye or the visual loss is small and equal in both eyes.
6. Diplopia—Diplopia is a prominent symptom in paralytic squint.

Detection of Latent Squint

1. The patient does not show any deviation when both eyes are open and fixing.
2. When one eye is covered, and kept covered for few seconds, the following changes are seen:
   a. None of the eyes move when the cover is removed—This shows there is no latent squint and the condition is called **orthophoria**.
   b. When the eye under cover moves, it has latent squint and the condition is called **heterophoria**.
3. According to movement of eye under cover, it can be:
   a. **Exophoria** if the eye under cover has moved out.
   b. **Esophoria** if the eye cover under has moved in.

Examination of Manifest Squint

Manifest squint can be **concomitant** (nonparalytic) or **paralytic**. Both have distinct characteristics, which must be differentiated because treatment of the two conditions are different.

To Examine Manifest Squint

1. Ask the patient to keep both eyes open and look straight.
2. Observe which eye is squinting.
3. Note direction of deviation—Esotropia, exotropia, hypertrophia.
4. Roughly measure the angle of deviation by corneal reflex. If the corneal reflex is in the center of the pupil, there is no deviation. If it is at the papillary margin, it is 20°. If it is on the limbus, it is 45° and beyond limbus, it is more than 45° (Fig. 4.73).
5. Cover the straight eye.
6. The squinting eye will take up fixation and will become straight.
7. At the same time the eye under cover will deviate in the same direction by the same angle.
8. Remove the cover, the deviating eye under cover will go back to the straight position.
9. The originally squinting eye will start squinting again.

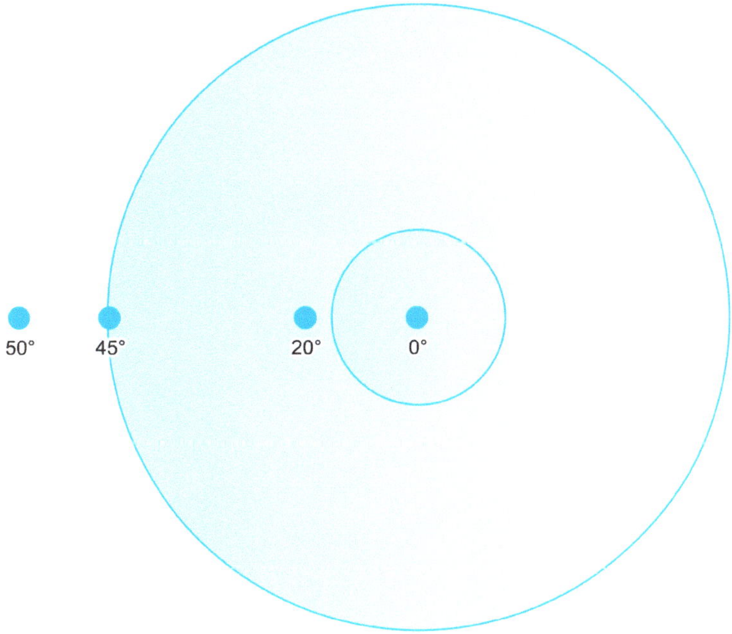

Fig. 4.73: Angle of deviation as measured by corneal reflexes

Characteristics of Paralytic Squint

1. Sudden onset.
2. Diplopia.
3. Obvious deviation of the effected eye.
4. Inability to move the eye equally in all direction.
5. Turning and tilting of the head.
6. Elevation and depression of the chin.
7. Headache, vomiting, giddiness.
8. May be associated with paralysis of hand or legs.

Charting of Diplopia

To chart diplopia, the patient wears a pair of red green diplopia glasses. Red in front of the right eye and green in front of the left eye (Fig. 4.74).

A patient is asked to keep his head straight.

A lighted candle is held at 1 meters distance in front of the patient.

The light looks red through the red glass, i.e. right eye and green through the green glass, i.e. left eye.

The candle is moved in the nine quadrants of gaze.

The patient moves the eyes to follow the candle.

No diplopia happens in nonparalytic squint.

Diplopia occurs in paralytic squint.

The two images, i.e. red and green may be separated only horizontally (paralysis of horizontal muscles).

The two images may be separated vertically and tilted (paralysis of cyclo vertical squint).

Various types of diplopia is shown in Fig. 3.1.

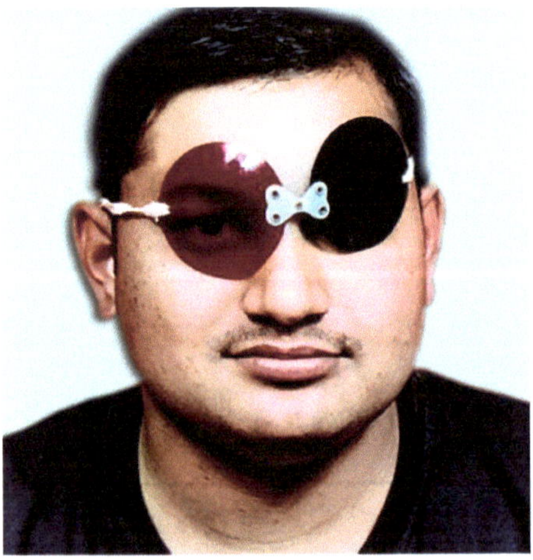

Fig. 4.74: Use of diplopia glass

Examination of Eye with Raised Intraocular Tension

Raised intraocular tension causes glaucoma which can be painful (narrow angle) or painless (wide angle).

Person with painful glaucoma has pain, redness of the eye and greatly reduced vision. These three symptoms make a person with painful glaucoma to seek medical help which gives him prompt relief.

A person with painless glaucoma (chronic simple glaucoma) rarely seeks medical treatment because there are no alarming symptoms. The loss of vision is so gradual that the patient may not be aware unless it is reduced very much.

Difficulty with painless glaucoma is that vision once lost is lost forever. Hence, persons with painless glaucoma should be detected early.

Signs of Painless Glaucoma (Chronic Simple Glaucoma)

1. Diminished, uncorrectable distant vision
2. Bright cornea
3. Normal anterior chamber
4. Wide angle of anterior chamber (seen by gonioscope)
5. Large sluggish pupil
6. Raised intraocular tension (recorded by tonometer) (Fig. 4.75).
7. Positive diurnal variation
8. No rise of tension by mydriatic
9. Glaucomatous field changes
10. Glaucomatous change in optic nerve

Symptoms of Painful Glaucoma (Narrow Angle Glaucoma)

1. Colored halos
2. Pain in the eye
3. Redness of the eye
4. Fast fall of vision

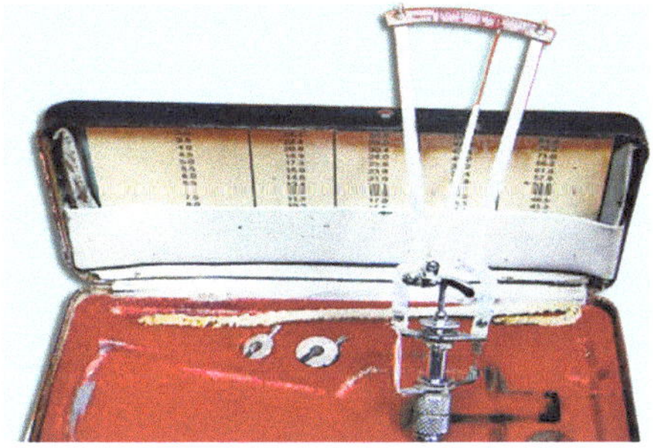

Fig. 4.75: Tonometer

Signs of Painful Glaucoma

1. Swelling of the lids
2. Circumciliary congestion
3. Hazy cornea
4. Shallow anterior chamber
5. Semidilated sluggish pupil
6. Raised intraocular tension more than 50 mm
7. Greatly reduced vision

Internal Examination of the Eye

There are various instruments that are used to examine the different internal areas of the eye, which are not visible ordinarily by oblique illumination and even by slit lamp. The slit lamp has to be modified to see the internal areas.

Internal part of the eye examined	Instrument
Depth of AC	Pachometer, ultrasound, biometer
Angle of anterior chamber	Gonioscopes
Periphery of the fundus	Indirect ophthalmoscopes, three mirror gonioscope
Fundus	Ophthalmoscope—Direct/indirect Slit lamp – 55 Hruby lens +60 to 90 D Operating microscope
Length of the eyeball	Biometer
Calculation of IOL power	Biometer

Special Examination

Instrument	Part examined
x-ray	Orbit, para nasal sinuses, skull, intra-ocular calcification
Ultrasound	Depth of AC, thickness of lens, position of lens, vitreous, retina, intraocular growth, orbital tumors
Fluorescein angiography	Retinal, choroidal, vascular disorder
OCT	Diseases of the macula and optic nerve

Synoptophore—Evaluation of squint

CHAPTER

5

Disorders of the Lids

The disorders of the lids can be present at birth (congenital) or develop after birth (acquired). They may involve one side (unilateral) or involve both sides (bilateral). When bilateral they are not always equal on both sides.
The causes of disorders of the lids are:
1. Congenital
2. Acquired—The acquired causes are:
   - Trauma
   - Infection
   - Allergy
   - Neoplasm (Tumor)

The common congenital conditions in order of frequency are:
1. Ptosis
2. Epicanthus
3. Blepharophimosis
4. Ankyloblepharon
5. Coloboma
6. Distichiasis

PTOSIS

Ptosis is the commonest congenital disorder (birth defect) of the upper lid. It is the drooping of the upper lid. Normally the upper lid covers the upper two millimeter of the cornea and drops down when the eye looks down.

If the upper lid covers more than two mm of the upper cornea, it is called **ptosis**. According to the level of upper lid in relation to the upper cornea the ptosis can be **mild**, **moderate** or **severe** (Fig. 5.1).

It is more commonly unilateral, when bilateral the drooping is not always equal in both eyes. A lid is said to be ptotic if the action of the levator is less than normal. The causes of subnormal action can either be in the muscle itself or in the nerve supply to the levator (Figs 5.2A and B).

Drooping of upper lid with normal function of the levator is called **pseudoptosis** (false ptosis).

Thus a drooped upper lid can either have **true ptosis** or **false ptosis**.

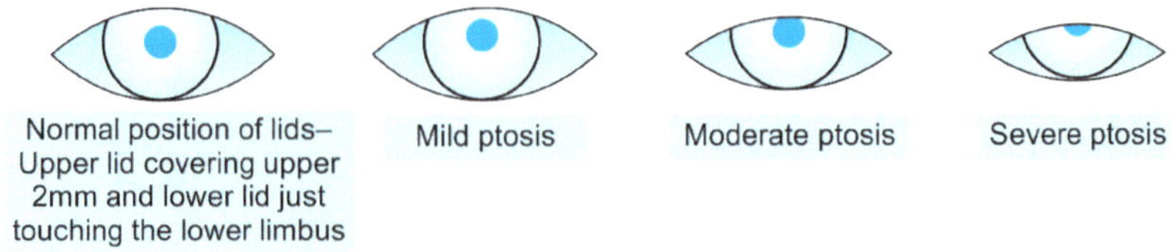

Fig. 5.1: Various grades of ptosis

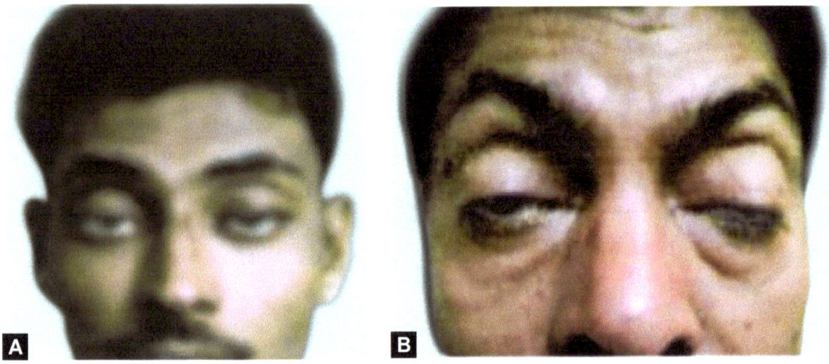

Figs 5.2A and B: Bilateral ptosis

Pseudoptosis

Pseudoptosis is due to increased volume of the upper lid. The action of the levator is normal (Fig. 5.3).

The common causes are

- Edema of the lid
- Inflammatory
- Allergic
- Infiltration by tumor

CONGENITAL PTOSIS

Simple Congenital Ptosis

This is generally present at birth but the parents become aware of it only when the child is few months old. It is generally unilateral. The child does not complain of any visual loss. It may be very mild or moderate. The child keeps the head tilted back. The eyebrow on the affected side is raised and the furrows of the forehead well-marked. The lid crease is absent. The vision is good, if the lid does not cover the pupil. Association of astigmatism is common. The levator function is fairly good (Fig. 5.4).

There is no medical treatment. Errors of refraction when present should be corrected by glasses. Only treatment is surgical correction of ptosis.

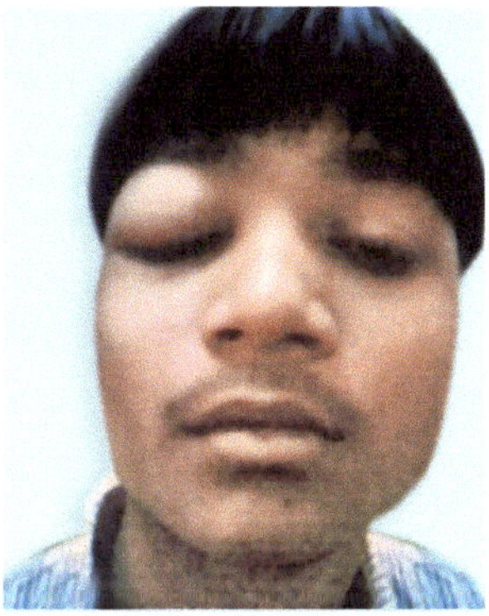

Fig. 5.3: Pseudoptosis cellulitis lid

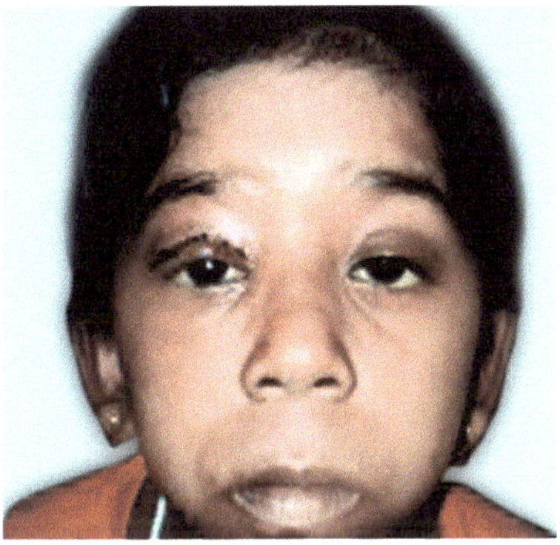

Fig. 5.4 Bilateral congenital ptosis (*Courtesy*: Dr Santosh patel)

Complicated Ptosis

1. Association of **poor action of superior rectus** is very common because both the superior rectus and levator develop from same mesodermal mass and both have common nerve supply, i.e. upper division of third nerve.
2. Ptosis with **blepharophimosis syndrome**: This is less common than above condition. It is bilateral. It consists of **epicanthus**, **bleparophimosis** and telecanthus (distance between the two eyes is more than normal. This gives an impression of divergent squint).
   The treatment consists of surgical correction of ptosis, epicanthus and blepharophimosis by multiple operation.
3. Ptosis with **jaw winking** (Marcus Gunn ptosis): This is an unilateral congenital ptosis of moderate degree where the ptosis disappears when either the mouth is opened or moved to the other side. In some cases the condition disappears as the child grows.

ACQUIRED PTOSIS

This can develop any time after birth. The causes can be:

1. Trauma to the levator or third nerve
2. Neurogenic:
   i. Third nerve palsy
   ii. Horner's syndrome
3. Myogenic:
   i. Myasthenia gravis
   ii. Ocular myopathy
4. Mechanical: This is pseudoptosis due to increased weight of the lid caused by edema (swelling) of the lid, growth of the lid.

Ptosis in third nerve palsy is generally unilateral (on one side). It can be complete, i.e. no action of levator is left or is poor. It is generally associated with paralysis of other extraocular muscles and paralysis of pupil except in diabetes where the pupil is normal.

The common causes of ptosis due to third nerve palsy are:

- Trauma (Injury)
- Diabetes
- Intracranial (inside the brain) aneurysm
- Infection

Horner's syndrome is unilateral. It consists of:

- Mild ptosis
- Miosis (small pupil)
- Enophthalmos (eye retracted back)
- Absence of sweating on the side of ptosis

The condition is caused due to defect in sympathetic chain in the neck.

MYOGENIC PTOSIS

Commonest myogenic ptosis is due to **myasthenia gravis**. This is a bilateral disease. The commonest symptom is **diplopia** in the evening and drooping of the upper lid. The ptosis is mild. Multiple extraocular muscles are also involved. The pupil is normal. The treatment is medical.

Epicanthus is a congenital fold of skin over the medial canthus. The fold covers a part of sclera on the nasal side more than normal. This gives an appearance of false squint (**pseudoesotropia**). It is a bilateral condition. It may be the only congenital anomaly or may be associated with **ptosis** or **blepharophimosis**. Isolated epicanthus without ptosis is fairly common which disappears without any treatment as the child grows. Epicanthus with ptosis does not improve without surgery when present with ptosis. The epicanthus should be corrected before ptosis (Fig. 5.5).

Ptosis with Blepharophimosis

This is a **severe** form of **bilateral ptosis** with **epicanthus** and **telecanthus**. In blepharophimosis both horizontal and vertical dimension of the inter-palpebral fissure is reduced. It is corrected by surgery. The epicanthus and blepharophimosis should be corrected before the ptosis is corrected.

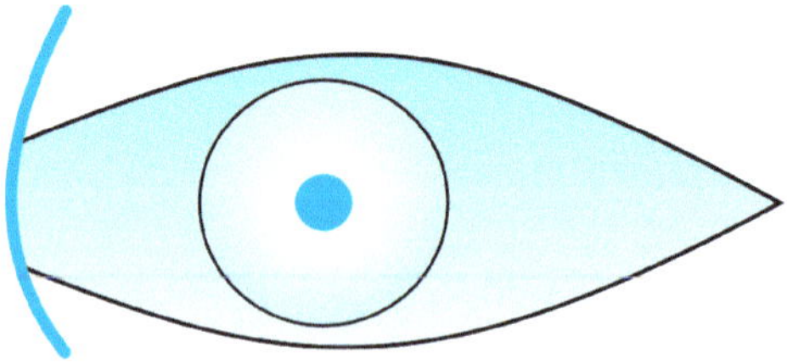

Fig. 5.5: Epicanthus

Ankyloblepharon

This is a minor congenital anomaly of the lids in which there are small strands of skin that join the two lids preventing the lids to open. There is no ptosis. The treatment is simple cutting of strands (Fig. 5.6).

Coloboma of the Lid

These are congenital notches in the lid margin. The notch may extend few milimeters into the substance of the lid. Coloboma of upper lid is more common than lower lid. The coloboma of upper lid is present at the junction of medial (towards the nose) one third with lateral two-third (towards ear) of the lid. The coloboma of the lower lid is situated on the lateral side and is broader and shallower. The coloboma is corrected surgically (Figs 5.7 and 5.8).

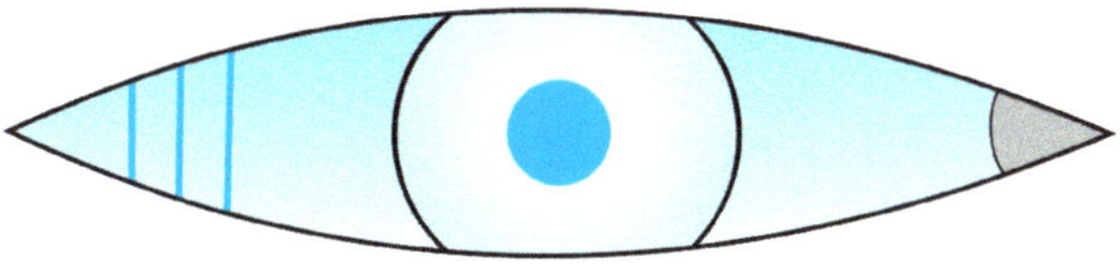

Fig. 5.6: Congenital ankyloblepharon

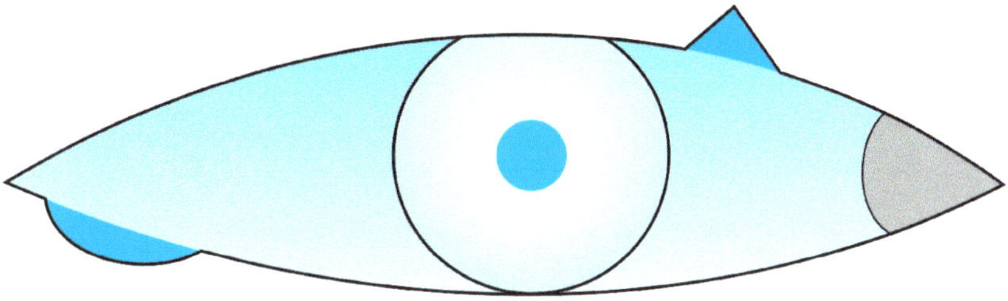

Fig. 5.7: Congenital coloboma—Upper and lower lid

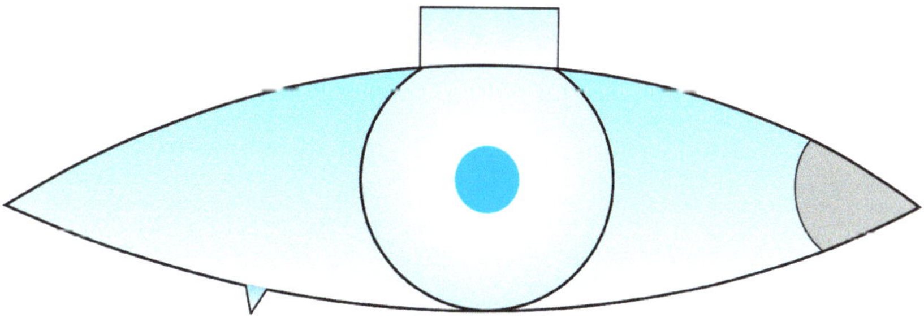

Fig. 5.8: Acquired total coloboma of the upper lid at the center and a notch coloboma of the lower lid

DISTICHIASIS

This is a **rare** congenital anomaly of lid margin. Normal lid has two to three rows of lashes arising in front of the opening of the tarsal gland (Fig. 5.12). In distichiasis an additional row of lashes develop in place of tarsal opening. They rub against the cornea and conjunctiva. They should be differentiated from more common condition of trichiasis (Fig. 5.9).

Trauma (Injury) to the Lids

The lid can be involved either mechanically or chemically.
The mechanical injuries are:

- Abrasion
- Lacerated
- Punctured

Abrasions are caused due to rubbing of the superficial layers of the skin against hard object. They are mild in nature, cause roughening of the skin with small areas of bleeding. They cause burring of the lid and mild pain. They are treated by cleaning the area and dusting the rough surface with antibiotic powder. They heal in four to five days.

Laceration (Tearing) of Lid (Fig.5.10)

Laceration is produced by blunt object. It is of two types:

1. Involving the lid margin
2. Without involving the lid margin

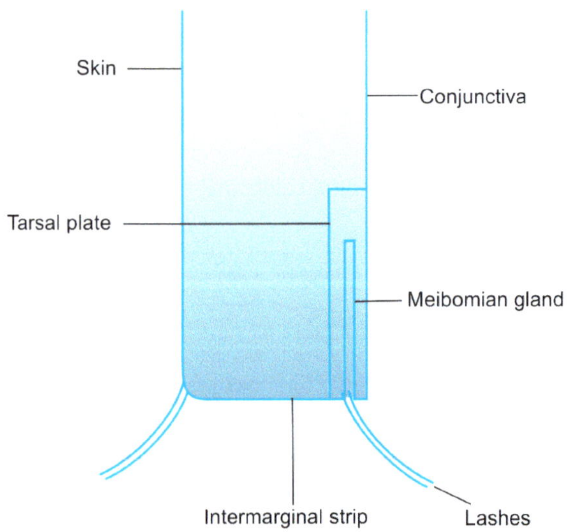

Fig. 5.9: Distichiasis

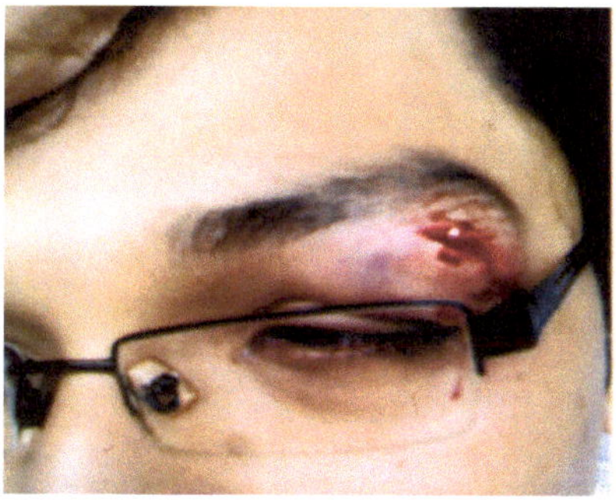

Fig. 5.10: Lacerated wound

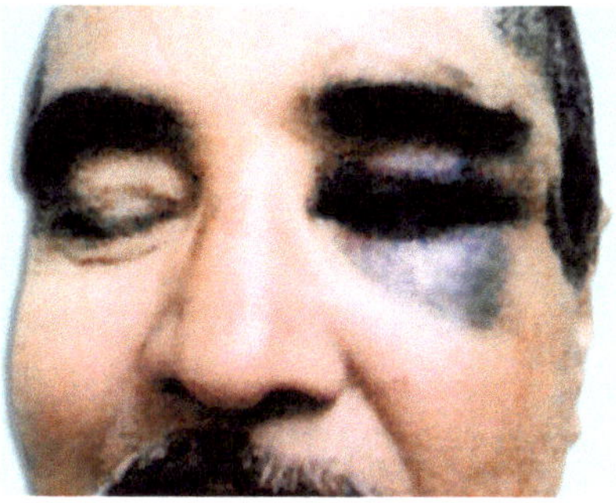

Fig. 5.11: Black eye

Those involving the lid margin tear all the structures from the skin to the conjunctiva. They are generally triangular in shape with broad base at the lid margin and narrow apex away from the lid margin. The wounds that do not involve the lid margin may involve only the skin or may involve all the structure. Both types of injuries may be associated with various degrees of injury to the globe. The treatment is surgical repair. Those involving the lid margin require more skill to repair.

Punctured wounds are caused by shart-hard pointed objects like thorn, needle, knife, arrow, etc. They are small in length but are more likely to penetrate the globe.

Blunt injury of the lid is caused by hard objects larger than the diameter of the orbit like fist, cricket ball, etc. It may abrade the lid. More common is **ecchymosis** (black eye) of the lid (Fig. 5.11). The black color is due to change in the color of blood under the skin. The color changes from pink to black over next few days. The ecchymosis may develop within few hours to few days after the injury. The lid is swollen and there is **pseudoptosis**. It is commonly associated with **subconjunctival hemorrhage**. The globe should always be examined for associated injury.

Treatment of simple ecchymosis is cold compress immediately following injury. The patient should be told that it takes seven to eight days for the ecchymosis to disappear.

ABNORMALITIES OF LID MARGIN

The abnormalities of the lid margins are (Fig. 5.12)

1. Distichiasis
2. Trichiasis
3. Entropion
4. Ectropion
5. Madarosis
6. Tylosis
7. Coloboma
8. Ankyloblepharon

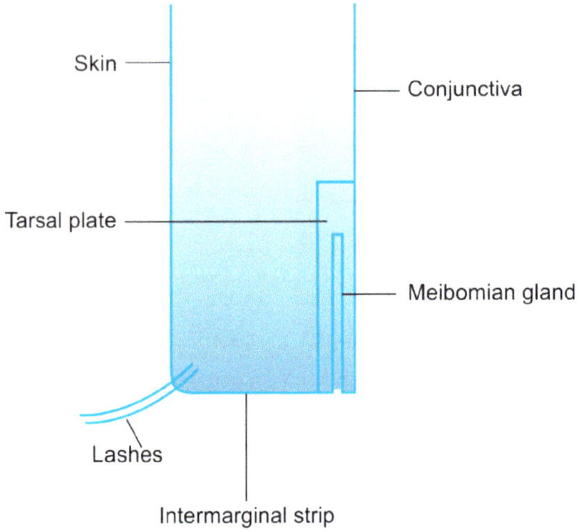

Fig. 5.12: Diagram showing normal lid margin

Distichiasis

Please see above.

Trichiasis

In turning of a few or all lashes is called trichiasis. It may be in one lid only, may involve more than one lid. The lashes rub against the conjunctiva and cornea causing constant watering and redness. There may be ulcers on the cornea. New vessel formation on the cornea is very common. It may be associated with entropion. It is a common cause of corneal opacity (Fig. 5.13)
The common causes of trichiasis are:
1. Trachoma
2. Leprosy
3. Chronic blepharitis
4. Scar on the lid margin

Treatment

If only few lashes are turned in, they are **plucked (epilated)** regularly but if many lashes are turned in they are best corrected by surgery. They may also be destroyed by laser or cryo.

Entropion

This is in-turning of the lid margin. It may be mild, moderate or severe. It may involve one eye or both eyes. It may be present only in one lid or both the lids.

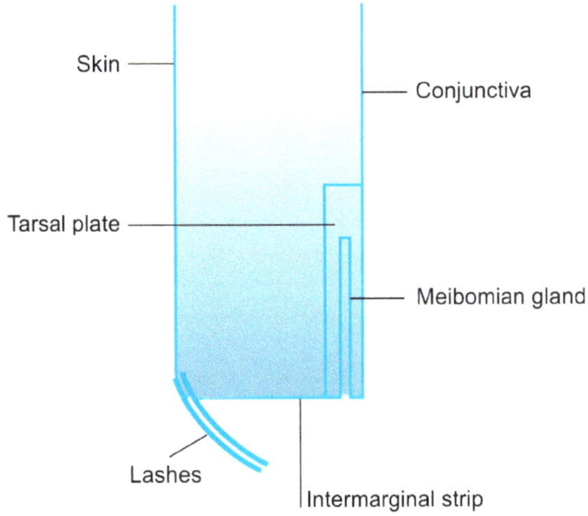

Fig. 5.13: Trichiasis

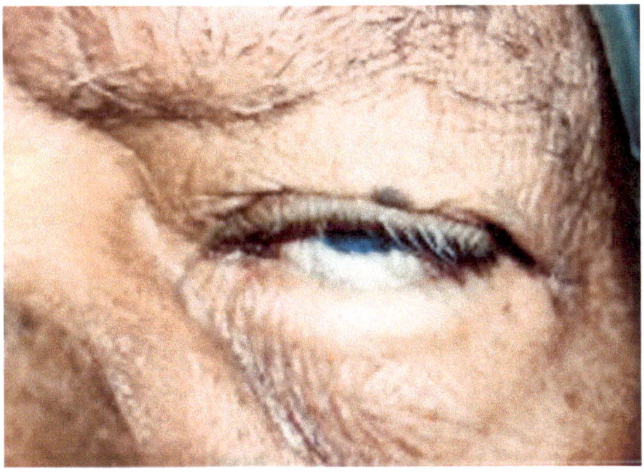

Fig. 5.14: Senile entropion (*Courtesy:* Professor Sanjay Shrivastava)

There are two types of entropion:

1. Senile (old age)—This is also called spastic entropion.
2. Cicatricial

Senile entropion is seen in lower lid only. Initially it develops in one eye, the other eye is also involved soon. This is seen generally in aged, thin, malnourished patient. The cause of entropion lies in the laxity of the skin and orbicularis. Loss of orbital fat plays an important role. The symptoms are watering from the eye, recurrent redness in the eye (Fig. 5.14).

The treatment is surgical shortening of the orbicularis.

Cicatricial entropion is seen in both lids but is more marked in the upper lid due to scarring of the tarsal conjunctiva and tarsal plate. The commonest cause is **stage four trachoma**. The other causes are leprosy and alkali burn (Fig. 5.15).

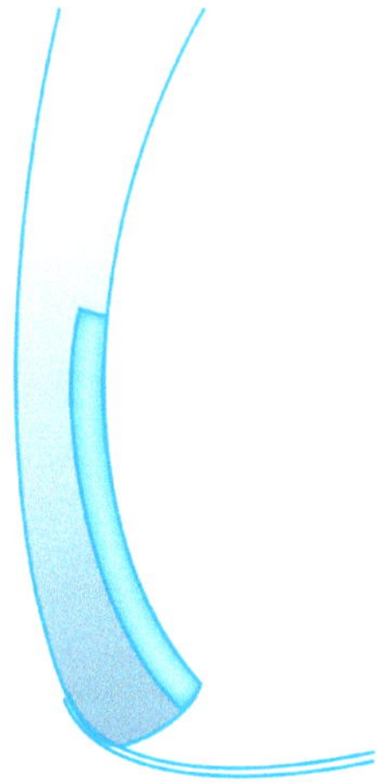

Fig. 5.15: Cicatricial entropion

The symptoms are similar to spastic entropion but more serious in nature, i.e. watering, redness, photophobia. cicatricial entropion is responsible for superficial vascularization of cornea and severe corneal opacity, which is main cause of blindness in trachoma where all the four lids may be involved. Treatment consists of:

1. Management of trachoma in initial (beginning) stage by chemotherapy (medicine).
2. Surgical repair of entropion in late stages.

Once entropion has developed:

1. Medicine will not correct entropion.
2. Medicine (antibiotic) is given to control secondary infection.
3. In early stages repeated epilation may be helpful.
4. Surgical correction from conjunctival surface is the only treatment.

Ectropion (Fig. 5.16)

This is outward turning of the lid margin.
There are three types:

1. Senile
2. Paralytic
3. Cicatricial

Senile ectropion is generally bilateral and mild, causing troublesome epiphora (Fig. 5.17).

Paralytic ectropion is caused due to paralysis of orbicularis (involvement of seventh nerve):
The common causes are:

- Leprosy (Both sides and chronic)
- Bells palsy (One side only and acute)
- Injury to the facial nerve
- It is confined to lower lid only.

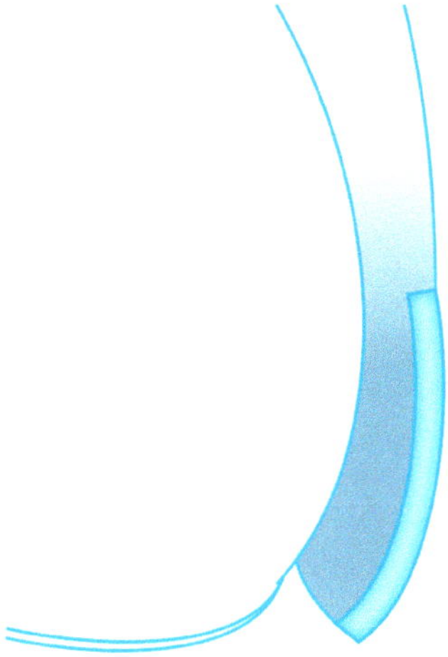

Fig. 5.16: Ectropion

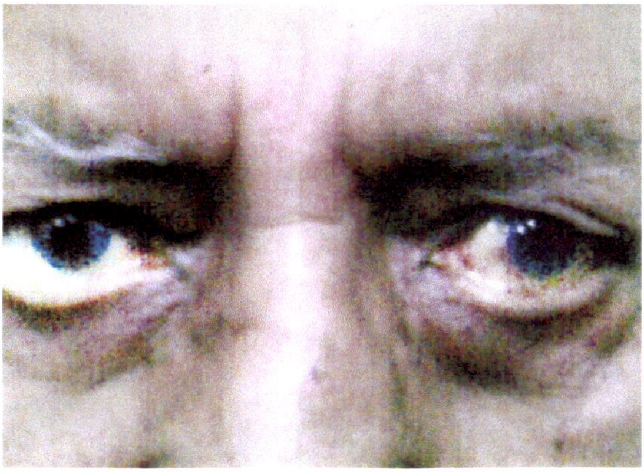

Fig. 5.17: Senile ectropion (*Courtesy:* Professor AK Chandrakar)

The lid margin is everted. The margin of the lid becomes visible without applying pressure. In severe cases the lower tarsal conjunctiva is exposed and thickened. The symptoms are watering from the eye, discharge, corneal ulcer.

Treatment—Acute cases do not require any treatment except local antibiotic.

In chronic cases the treatment is tarsorrhaphy (stitching of the lid margin).

Cicatricial Ectropion

This is due to scar formation over the skin of the lid. The causes are acid and alkali burn, thermal (heat) burn. Both the lids may be involved. In severe cases the conjunctiva is everted, thickened and red. The patient may not be able to close the lid properly. The symptoms are watering, pain, redness. Treatment consists of removal of the scar, followed by skin graft.

Madarosis

This is loss of eye lashes. It may involve only a patch of eye lashes or there may be loss of lashes all along the lid margin. It may be localized to one lid or may involve multiple lids. **The common causes of madarosis are**— Ulcerative blepharitis, trachoma, leprosy, thermal burn, chemical burn. It is generally associated with tylosis.

There are hardly any symptoms.

The treatment is treatment of the cause.

Tylosis

The term denoted thickening of the lid margin. The lid margin is rounded and looses contact with the globe. This is generally associated with madarosis. The cause of tylosis is same as that of madarosis. The treatment is directed towards the cause (Fig. 5.18).

Coloboma

The term coloboma of the lid means loss of the lid margin. It can either be **congenital** or **acquired**. The common acquired causes are trauma that may be accidental or surgical. The accidental colobomas may be very small or may involve the whole of the lid. Loss of large part of upper lid is an emergency that require early reconstruction of lid, otherwise the exposed cornea will develop ulcer and the eye will be lost. All colobomas must be repaired in layers and should be made to prevent knotching of the lid margin (Figs 5.7 and 5.8).

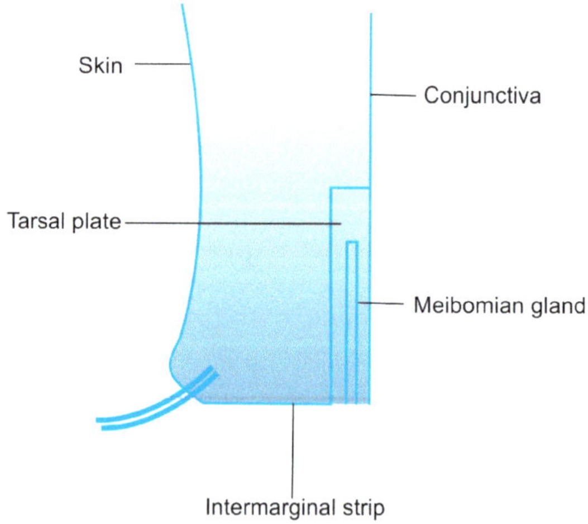

Fig. 5.18: Tylosis

Ankyloblepharon

This is a congenital condition. This should not be confused with surgical tarsorrhaphy (stitching of lid margin) (Fig. 5.6).

Motility (Movement) Disorders of the Lid

They are **ptosis, lagophthalmos, lid retraction** and **blepharospasm.** Lagophthalmos (Fig. 5.19) is not a disorder of lid margin. This is paralysis of orbicularis. The result of paralysis of orbicularis are:
1. The patient can not close the lids completely.
2. In an attempt to close the eye, the eyeball role up (Bell's phenomenon)
3. The interpalpebral fissure is wider than normal.
4. The lines on forehead are abolished.
5. The nasolabial fold is abolished.
6. The lower lid is everted.
7. The lower part of the bulbar conjunctiva and the cornea are exposed.
8. There is excessive watering from the eye.

The lagophthalmos is unilateral more often. **The commonest cause of bilateral lagophthalmos is leprosy.**

The common causes of unilateral lagophthalmos are: Bell's palsy, leprosy, trauma to facial nerve outside the skull, extensive cicatricial ectropion, proptosis.

Symptoms

Symptoms of lagophthalmos depend on severity and duration of lagophthalmos. In mild cases of recent (few days) origin only symptom is inability to close the eye and watering. In severe cases besides above there is deviation of the angle of mouth.

Treatment

Initial treatment consists of instillation of antibiotic drops during day and ointment at bed time.

If the lagophthalmos does not improve in a month, a **tarsorrhaphy** is required. In mild cases only lateral tarsorrhaphy is enough. In severe cases median tarsorrhaphy is required. In case of proptosis, total tarsorrhaphy is

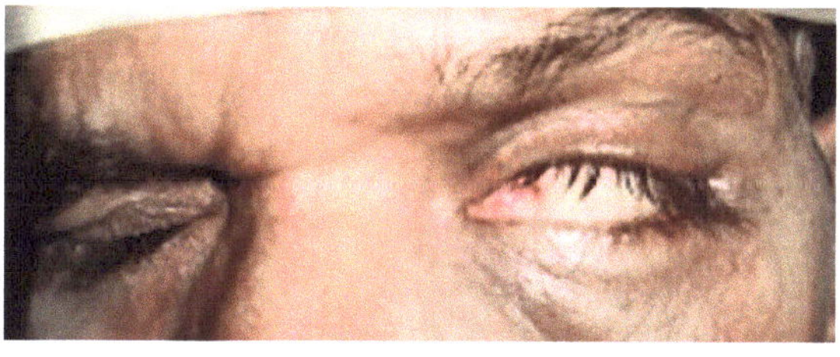

Fig. 5.19: Lagophthalmos left eye (*Courtesy:* Professor Sanjay Shrivastava)

needed. In cases of leprosy transplantation of temporalis or palmaris longus is helpful.

Bell's palsy is acute (sudden) paralysis of seventh (facial) nerve. The exact cause is not known, most probably this is due to swelling of the facial nerve in the stylomastoid canal. It is unilateral, seen in all ages. The patient suddenly realizes that he can not close the lid on affected side. There is watering from the eye and in few hours, he develops foreign body sensation. On examination, it is found that the orbicularis is not contracting well, i.e. partially paralyzed. There is lagophthalmos.

The management is same as any case of lagophthalmos. Oral administration of steroid under supervision of ophthalmologist helps to recover in few days. If no improvement is noticed in few days, a tarsorrhaphy may be required.

Lid Retraction

Normal lid covers two millimeters of the upper lid and touches the lower border of the cornea. No part of sclera is visible above or below the cornea. When the person looks down the normal lid follows the globe and keeps the cornea covered. In case of lid retraction a part of the sclera is visible above the cornea when the patient is looking at a distant object. Sometimes the lower sclera is also visible. The condition may be unilateral (one sided) or bilateral. The eyes have a staring look. The causes of lid retraction are stimulation of the Muller's muscle, thyroid diseases instillation of phenylephrine in the conjunctiva. The patient may not be aware of the condition unless pointed out or there may be lacrimation, and redness of the eye. Treatment is treatment of the cause (Fig. 5.20).

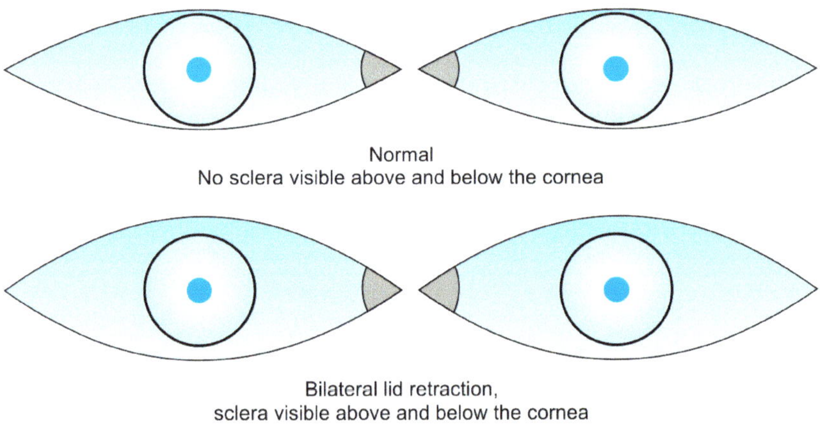

Fig. 5.20: Lid retraction

Blepharospasm

This is involuntary closure of the lids. It generally involves both the eyes. It has two forms:

1. Reflex (secondary) blepharospasm
2. Essential blepharospasm

Reflex blepharospasm is very common in children. Any cause that irritate the fifth nerve in the globe (mostly cornea) cause blepharospasm.

Common Causes of Blepharospasm

- Phlyctenular keratoconjunctivitis (commonest)
- Corneal abrasion
- Corneal foreign body
- Tarsal foreign body
- Corneal ulcer
- Interstitial keratitis
- Severe anterior uveitis

Blepharospasm is associated with photophobia that is intolerance to light.

Reflex blepharospasm is abolished by instillation of local four percent xylocaine in the eyes.

The management is management of the cause.

Essential blepharospasm is a chronic bilateral condition seen in elderly persons, more common in females. It is due to neurological cause. The eyes are normal. It starts as frequent blinking and gradually reaches a stage when the time between two blinks is so long that the eyes close for sometime. This makes momentary loss of vision. The patient finds it difficult to cross the road, board a train or bus. There is no specific treatment. Injection of botox (botulinum) toxin in the orbicularis gives relief that may last for few months.

Infections of the Lid

Infections of the lid can be divided into two parts:

1. Infection of the skin and subcutaneous tissues of the ...
2. Infection of the lid margin:
   i. Skin of the lid margin
   ii. Glands of the lid margin
      a. Gland of Zeis and Moll
      b. Meibomian (tarsal) glands

The infection of the lid may be acute (sudden) or chronic (many days old). They may be recurrent developing one after another. They may be unilateral or bilateral. They may involve only one lid or may involve many lids. Acute infection of the lid is associated with various degrees of edema (swelling) of the lid.

Causes of Lid Edema are

1. Infection of the skin on the lid—Boils, cellulitis, abscess.
2. Infection of the lid margin, stye and infected chalazion.
3. Eruptions on the lids, chickenpox, herpes zoster.
4. Allergic dermatitis.
5. Inflammation of conjunctiva—Ophthalmia neonatorum, acute purulent conjunctivitis, membranous conjunctivitis.
6. Inflammation of lacrimal sac, acute dacryocystitis, lacrimal abscess.
7. Inflammation of orbit—Orbital cellulitis, acute dacryoadenitis (inflammation of lacrimal gland)
8. Inflammation of eyeball—Acute iridocyclitis, endophthalmitis, panophthalmitis.
9. Other causes—Cavernous sinus thrombosis, acute paraorbital sinusitis, angio neurotic edema (severe acute allergic edema).
10. Injury—Craniofacial injury (injury to the skull and face).
    Infection of the skin and subcutaneous tissue may cause vescicle, boils, cellulitis and abscess.

They are caused by many organisms. Main among them are—Bacteria (staphylococci) and viruses—Herpes zoster, chickenpox, herpes simplex and molluscum.

Boils: Boils are infection of hair follicle. They are acute in onset, caused by many pus forming organism but most commonly by staphylococci. It may be a single boil or there may be many of them (Fig. 5.21).

They are more common in summers and in children but can develop at any age. In adults with recurrent boils the first investigation is to exclude diabetes. They may involve single or more than one lids, may be associated with boils on forehead and face. They are painful, tender, red, raised areas with white center. The surrounding skin may be swollen. They may subside without any treatment or may pass into cellulitis lid and abscess of the lid or may evacuate without leaving any scar.

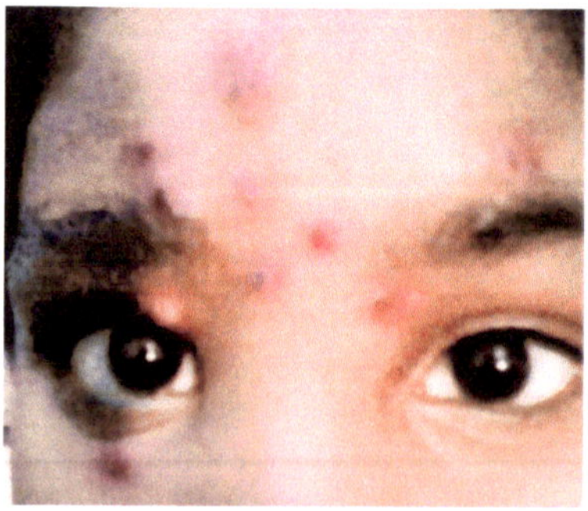

Fig. 5.21: Boils of face and lid (*Courtesy:* Professor ML Garg)

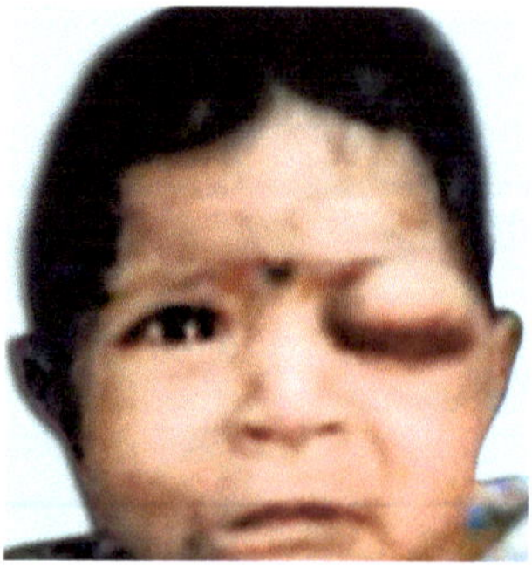

Fig. 5.22: Cellulitis lid (*Courtesy:* Dr Nidhi Pandey)

Cellulitis lid: This is infection of subcutaneous tissues. The lid is swollen but does not fluctuate. It causes **pseudoptosis**. Once it starts fluctuating the condition is called **lid abscess**. There develops a weak spot, from where the pus may drain out if not surgically drained. The treatment consists of draining of the pus by a stab incision at the softest part of the swelling and expressing the pus out (Fig. 5.22).

Treatment of cellulitis consists of warm dry fomentation, systemic antibiotic and analgesic. Local antibiotic drops and ointments are not effective.

Herpes Zoster Ophthalmicus

Herpes zoster is caused by a virus called **vericella zoster virus**. This virus causes chickenpox in children and herpes zoster ophthalmicus in adults. It does not mean that children do not develop herpes zoster ophthalmicus. Percentage of children developing herpes zoster is far less than in adults. Similarly adults developing chickenpox is rare.

Herpes zoster ophthalmicus is an acute disease. It is unilateral. The lesions do not cross the midline of face.

It starts suddenly with feeling of unwellness (malaise), fever and severe pain on one side of the head and face. The pain is felt mostly on the distribution of fifth cranial nerve. The disease most commonly involves the first division of the fifth cranial nerve. The second division is less commonly involved. The third division is least effected (Fig. 5.23).

The pain is followed by redness of the skin, swelling of the lids and development of vesicles (clear fluid filled blister). The fluid gradually becomes turbid (white) which after few days burst and start healing by crust formation which leave punched out scars. Even when all the lesions have healed the pain persists and may last for months to years. This is called **postherpetic neuralgia**. Chances of involvement of cornea and iris are more when the vescicles develop at the tip of the nose.

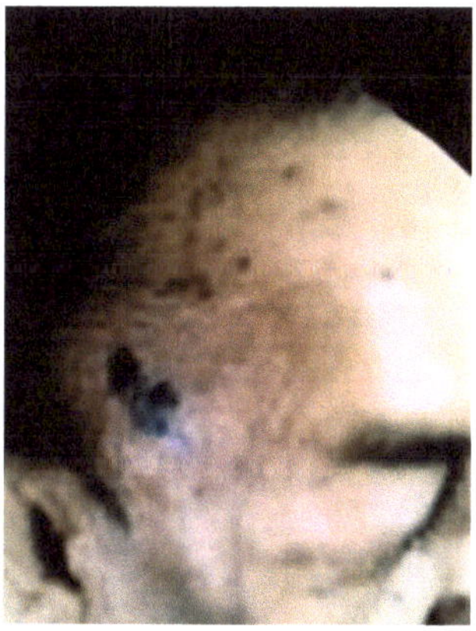

Fig. 5.23: Herpes zoster ophthalmicus (*Courtesy:* Dr Nidhi Pandey)

The other parts of the eye that are involved in Herpes zoster besides lids are:

1. Conjunctiva—Acute conjunctivitis and vescicles.
2. Cornea—Superficial and deep keratitis
   —Loss of corneal sensation. This may last forever.
3. Iris—Iritis, atrophy of iris
4. Sclera—Scleritis
5. Intra ocular tension is low in the beginning but may rise to cause glaucoma.
6. Neurological
   a. Cranial nerve
      i. Optic nerve—Optic neuritis
      ii. Third, fourth and sixth nerve paralysis
      iii. Fifth nerve—Loss of sensation
      Postherpetic neuralgia
      iv. Seventh nerve—Facial palsy, pain in ear.
   b. Spinal cord—Paralysis of the opposite limb—Herpes zoster opthalmicus in patient with AIDS is a serious problem, it not only leads to blindness but may cause death of patient.

Management is divided into two parts:

1. Ocular (for eyes)
2. Systemic—For skin and nervous system

Treatment of Ocular Involvement

- Acyclovir ointment three times a day.
- Broad spectrum antibiotic drops three times a day.
- Acyclovir skin ointment to be applied over the vesicles three times a day.
- Atropine eye ointment once a day
- Analgesic tablets for pain.

  Systemic treatment is best left to physician.

Vericella (Chickenpox)

Vericella is caused by the same virus that causes herpes zoster (varicella zoster) but differs from its clinical presentation. The lesions of chickenpox are vesicles all over the body on both the sides of midline. It generally develops in children. Most of the time it is self-limiting and subsides without treatment but sometimes it may be serious enough to cause infection of the lungs (pneumonia) or brain (meningitis and encephalitis). It is preventable by vaccine given after age of one year.

The ocular involvements consist of vesicles similar to those seen in herpes zoster that heal by scab formation but do not leave scar. It does not cause postherpetic like neuralgia. The corneal sensation is normal. The cornea is rarely involved. The conjunctiva may develop vesicles that look like phlycten.

Herpes Simplex

Herpes simplex type one virus causes multiple vesicles on the lid. It may be present in neonates as well. Lid infection does not require any specific treatment but the patient may develop corneal and uveal lesions months or years later. No specific treatment is required for lid lesion.

Molluscum Contagiosum

This is a chronic disease of the skin anywhere in the body. It is caused by a **poxvirus**. It spreads by close body contact. In the lid it starts as a painless translucent nodule. The number of nodules vary from one to many. The nodules are raised, dome shaped with a central depression. A thick milky material comes out when the nodule is ruptured. The milky material is infectious and contains the virus. A nodule near the lid margin causes **toxic conjunctivitis** and **keratitis**. The disease is **self-limiting** and does not require active treatment unless it is causing conjunctivitis or keratitis. The infection is severe and seen all over the body in AIDS. The specific treatment is removal of the nodule or destruction by cryo.

Warts (Verruca)

Warts are common. They are seen in adults. They become more common as age increases, are caused by **papovavirus**. They are raised, rough, dry, painless growths seen both on the skin of the lids or at the lid margin. There number varies between one to many. Growth on the lid margin cause **toxic conjunctivitis**. They do not respond to antiviral drugs. They are best destroyed by **cryo, laser or bipolar diathermy**. They may surgically removed as well.

Infections of the Lid Margin

Infection of the lid margin may involve the skin of the lid margin or the glands of the lid margin.

Blepharitis

Infection of the skin of the lid margin is called blepharitis. The lid margin is partly covered by skin and partly conjunctiva. The lid glands open in the lid margin so the lid margin is infected from all the three sources. Blepharitis are never acute. They are generally bilateral and involve all the four lids. They are more common in children and young adults. Blepharitis has a long course and is difficult to treat.

Blepharitis is divided into two main types:

1. Squamous (Nonulcerative)
2. Ulcerative (Table 5.1)

Table 5.1: Difference between squamous and ulcerative blepharitis

	Squamous blepharitis	Ulcerative blepharitis
Age	Children and young adult	Children and young adults
Side	Both	Both
Lids	All	All
Complaints	Powder like, dry white scales in the lashes	Matted lashes, yellow coarse wet flakes
	Can be removed with ease	Difficult to remove
	No ulceration on removal of scales	Small ulcers on removal of scales
	Mild	Progressive
	Loss of lashes less frequent	Loss of lashes more frequent
	Lashes grow back after loss	Lashes may not grow after loss
Complication	None	Tylosis, madarosis, trichiasis
	Dandruff of scalp	Chronic conjunctivitis, staphylococcal infection

Parasitic Infestation of Lid Margin

This disorder is caused by a common parasite the lice. There are two types of lice. The head lice and body lice. It is the second type that infests the eye lashes. The scientific name of lice that involves the lashes is **phthiriasis palpe brum** or **crab lice**. It can occur at any age. The children get it from infected parents and attendants. The adults get it as sexually transmitted disease. The organism clings at the base of the lash and cause irritation, redness and itching. They involve all the lashes. The parasites are visible in naked eye.

Inflammation of Glands of the Lid Margin

There are two types of glands at the lid margin. They are:

1. Sebaceous or sweat glands: They are situated at the base of the lashes. They are called glands of Zeis and Moll.
2. Meibomian glands or tarsal glands: They are present in the tarsal plate and open on the lid margin behind the lashes.

Acute infections of the glands of Zeis and Moll are called **stye** or **hordeolum externum**. The chronic infection of meibomian glands is called **chalazion**. (Fig. 5.24).

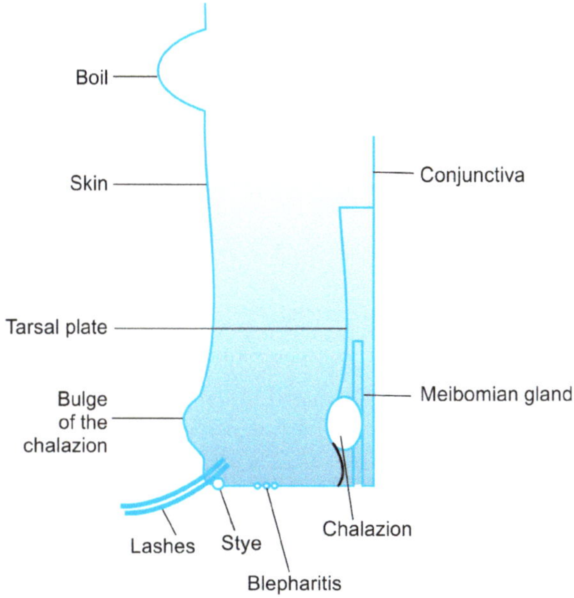

Fig. 5.24: Inflammation of the lid margin

Stye

Stye is an acute suppurative (pus forming) inflammation of glands of Zeis and Moll. Styes are very common in children. They may involve any of the lids. They have a short course and may resolve without treatment. Recurrences are common. A stye starts as a painful tender spot on the lid margin where a small red painful nodule develops with in a day or two. The surrounding area may be swollen. The interpalpebral fissure is narrowed in case of stye of the upper lid. The **preauricular lymph glands** are enlarged. The pain and swelling subsides with in a few days when pus drains out. There may be more than one stye in one lid or they may develop in crops. The styes stop developing after few episodes of recurrence. They are best treated by hot fomentation, analgesics and local antibiotics. The adults with stye should be investigated for diabetes. Stye may cause cellulitis lid. They never develop malignancy (Fig. 5.25).

Chalazion (Meibomian Cyst, Tarsal Cyst)

Chalazion is as common as stye, seen in all ages, in both sexes, all over the world. It may be present only in one lid or more than one lid, may be involved either as multiple nodules or single nodule. Chalazion is a **chronic granuloma** of tarsal gland. It is painless and slow growing. It develops as a small pinhead nodule which is better felt by finger than seen. It gradually enlarges may become as big as 1 cm across. It develops away from the lid margin. The skin can be moved over the nodule but the nodule can not be

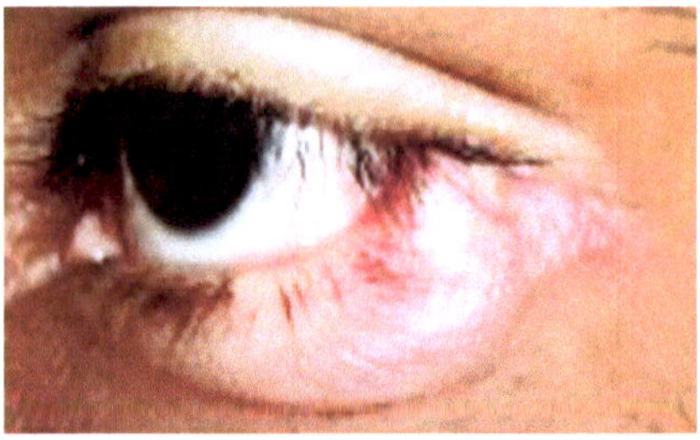

Fig. 5.25: Stye
(*Courtesy:* Professor Sanjay Shrivastava)

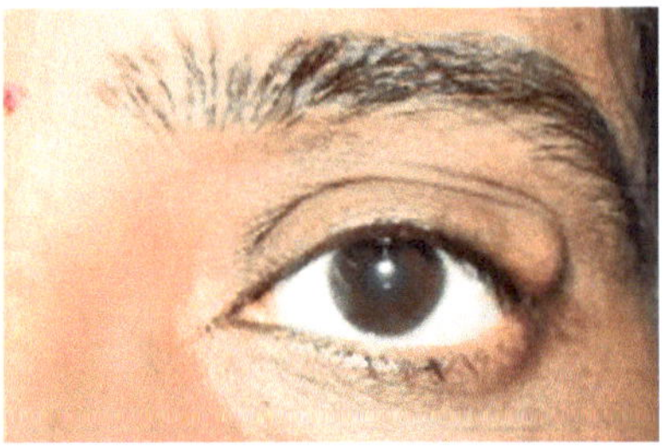

Fig. 5.26: Chalazion uper lid
(*Courtesy:* Dr Santosh Patel)

moved over the tarsal plate. On everting the lid, the conjunctiva over the nodule has a bluish pink color. The preauricular glands are not involved (Fig. 5.26).

The exact cause of chalazion is not known. Most probable explanation is that there is low grade infection in the duct of the tarsal gland that blocks the duct. This leads to accumulation of meibomian secretion giving rise to a nodular swelling.

There are some predisposing factors. They are –

- Errors of refraction, chronic blepharitis, family history of chalazia, diabetes (in adults). Some of the chalazia resolve without treatment. The chalazia that do not resolve have following course.
- They may get infected and result in **hordeolum interna**.
- Burst on the conjuctival surface
- Converted in tarsal cyst

There is no medical treatment for chalazia. Repeated hot fomentation is supposed to help in resolution. The specific treatment is surgical drainage of the granuloma and scrapping of the lesion.

Recurrences are common even after surgery. However after four to five recurrence the chalazia stop developing.

If an adult develops a granuloma at the same side following surgery. The excised disease should be examined to exclude malignancy (cancer). Malignant changes are not seen under thirty years of age.

Hordeolum internum is acute infection developing on a chalazion. Its features are similar to stye but more painful. The lid can not be everted due to severe pain. It requires strong painkiller, and broad spectrum antibiotic. Occasionally after few days the pus drains automatically with great relief. All adult patients with hordeolum internum should be investigated for diabetes.

New Growths of the Lid

The new growths of the lid are slowly progressive, painless, swelling that may arise from:

1. Skin: Warts, molluscum xanthelasma, basal cell carcinoma, squamous (Fig. 5.28), cell carcinoma, malignant melanoma
2. The meibomian glans—Tarsal cyst, adenocarcinoma (Fig. 5.27)
3. Blood vessels—Hemangioma
4. Nerves—Neurofibroma

The growth can be

1. Benign (noncancer)
2. Malignant (cancer)

The benign growths are:

1. Xanthelasma
2. Hemangioma
3. Neurofibroma
4. Nevus

The malignant growths are:

1. Basal cell carcinoma
2. Squamous cell carcinoma
3. Adeno carcinoma
4. Xeroderma pigmentosa
5. Malignant melanoma
6. Kaposi sarcoma

Xanthelasma (Xanthoma)

They are very common lesions developing slowly in the skin of the upper lid on medial side. They are yellowish in color. The surfaces are wrinkled, they move with the skin, they are not painful. They are seen mostly in obese (fat) women over forty years. Generally there is a positive family history. These women have raised lipid (fat) in their blood. They are often diabetic

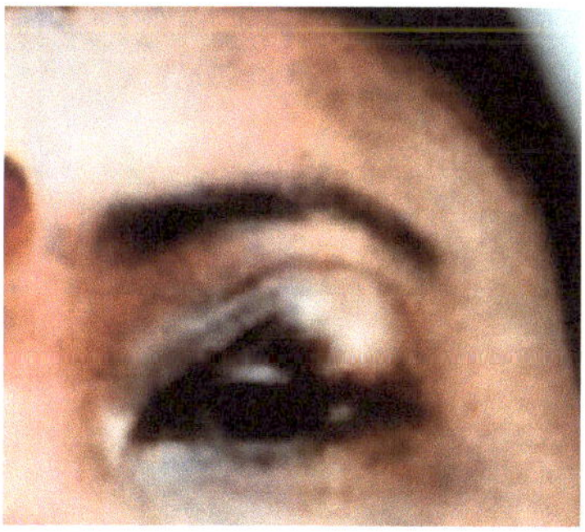

Fig. 5.27: Adenocarcinoma tarsal gland *(Courtesy:* Professor AK Chandrakar)

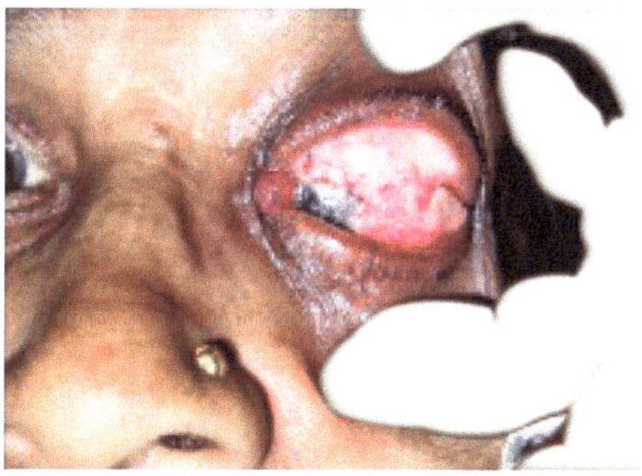

Fig. 5.28: Squamous cell carcinoma upper lid *(Courtesy:* Dr Santosh Patel)

also. The condition does not require any treatment unless the patient wants to get them removed. In such cases they are removed surgically or by laser. Recurrences are common (Fig. 5.29).

Hemangioma

These are congenital (present at birth), seen in **children**. They are **unilateral**, may be present at birth either as frank growth called **strawberry nevus** (capillary hemangioma) or as birth mark called **port-wine stain**. They become prominent when the child cries. Third variety is **cavernous** hemangioma. Most of the capillary hemangiomas are either stationary and disappear after six to seven years or they grow slowly during first four or five years and regress over next three-four years except cavernous hemangioma.

If the hemangioma is large, it cause pseudo ptosis, anisometropia, astigmatism and amblyopia.

There is another type of hemangioma that involves half of the upper part of face and hemangioma of uvea associated with secondary glaucoma and convulsion (fits). The condition is called **Sturge-Weber syndrome**.

Most of the capillary hemangiomas do not require any treatment. If they are causing amblyopia they should be treated by injecting corticosteroid in the growth.

Neurofibromatosis

This is a congenital (present at birth). They develop in the **peripheral nerves**. They may be localized in the lid and orbit or may be seen in brain and spine also. They may be present all over the body as small round nodules.

In the lid, it causes diffuse swelling of the lid with a S shaped curve. Whole of the lid the thickened. It causes **pseudoptosis**. The skin of the lid may have **coffee colored** stain. Sometimes it is associated with **glaucoma**. There may be small **nodules on the iris**. Treatment is plastic reconstruction of the lid.

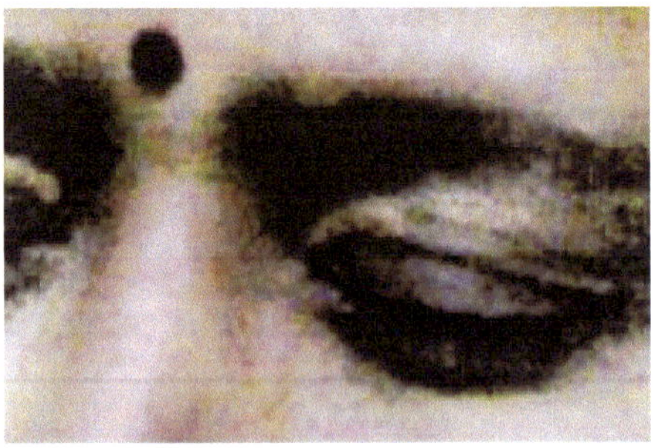

Fig. 5.29: Xanthelasma (*Courtesy:* Dr Santosh Patel)

Nevi

Nevi are common skin lesions of the lid. They may develop anywhere in any lid. A nevus may be single or there may be more than one nevi. They generally develop in young adults and frequency of incidence increase as age advances. They may be flush with the skin with less pigment or may be raised over the surface. Sometimes there may be two nevi one in each eye on the same side. Nevi do not cause any ocular problem and do not require any treatment unless the patient wants to get them removed by surgery.

Malignant Growth of the Lids

Basal Cell Carcinoma

This is the **commonest malignant tumor** of the lids. About 50% of all malignant tumors of the lids are basal cell carcinoma. It is seen after fifty years of age. Commonest site for development of the tumor is lower lid. Upper lid is less frequently involved. It is **slow progressive** tumor that does not metastasie (spread to distant parts). There are two forms—the first is **nodular** that starts as a nodule on the skin with fine blood vessels on the surface. There is generally a small depression at the center of the growth. The growth ultimately breaks down as ulcer but does not invade surrounding tissues. The second is **flat ulcerative form** that has everted borders which are pigmented (black in color) and the ulcer invades the deeper as well as surrounding tissue.

The treatment consists of confirmation of diagnosis by biopsy. Once diagnosis has been confirmed the specific treatment is surgical excision of the growth and plastic repair of the gap. The second line of treatment is radiation but this is less effective than surgery. There are no drugs that are effective against basal cell carcinoma.

Squamous Cell (Epidermoid) Carcinoma

This is **less common** than basal cell carcinoma but **more malignant**. It may develop in any lid. It also develops after 50 years of age. The tumor starts as a nodule which soon enlarge in size, may or may not ulcerate. **Metastasis is more common**. Treatment consists of local excision with plastic reconstruction (Fig. 5.28).

Adenocarcinoma of the Lid

This is rarer than squamous cell carcinoma. It most commonly develops in the tarsal glands, hence this is also referred to as **meibomian gland carcinoma**. It may develop from glands of zeis, sebaceous glands in caruncle or sebaceous glands in the eyebrow (Fig. 5.27).

The meibomian gland carcinoma is the commonest type of **adenocarcinoma** of the lids. It may develop from any lids. Involvement of upper lid more common than lower lid. It develops more frequently in

females past fifty years of age. The commonest mode of presentation is a chalazion like growth in any of the lids. It not only looks like a chalazion but also behaves like a chalazion. The only difference is that a chalazion once removed surgically does not recur at the same place but a meibomian gland carcinoma always recurs at the same site. Moreover lymph nodes are not involved in chalazion but they are commonly involved in meibomian gland carcinoma. Hence, it is essential that material removed from any chalazion like growth in adults should always be sent for histopathological examination to rule out possibility of meibomian gland carcinoma.

The treatment is excision of growth with plastic reconstruction.

Xeroderma Pigmentosa

This is a rare condition of **generalized malignant pigmented growths** all over the body. It has very high percentage of death. The condition is seen in children who die before they reach twenty five years of age. The condition is genetic. There may be more than one in the family who may suffer from this disease. The growths start as little brown spots (freckles) over the parts of the body that are exposed to direct sun rays. The lids are effected in early stages. The freckles develop fine blood vessels on the surface, nodules soon become malignant. The malignancies can be any of the following, i.e. basal cell carcinoma, epidermoid carcinoma or malignant melanoma.

There is no treatment for the condition. Life can be prolonged by keeping the child away from the sun.

Malignant Melanoma

This is a rare tumor, seen in elders. They are **highly malignant** hence fatal (cause death). They may develop anywhere on the skin. They are generally black. In the beginning they look like moles (nevi) but grow faster. Any pigmented growth that increases fast in size should be considered to be malignant and biopsy should be taken to exclude the malignancy. All malignant melanomas are not pigmented. There is no known treatment for malignant melanoma.

Kaposi Sarcoma

This malignant tumor was previously thought to be rare but with spread of HIV infection it has become more frequent. It is also a fatal condition. It is a vascular tumor that may start either in the skin of the lid or conjunctiva. There is no specific treatment. Main attention is directed to treat AIDS. The conjunctival lesions are treated by excision. Small skin nodules are treated by cryotherapy and large areas are treated by external beam radiation.

CHAPTER

6

Disorders of the Lacrimal System

The lacrimal system is divided into **two parts**—(Fig. 6.1). The first is called **secretory system** that consists of lacrimal gland and accessory lacrimal glands. Its main function is to produce tear. The second is called **drainage system** and it consists of lid, puncta, canaliculi, lacrimal sac and naso lacrimal duct. The function of these parts is to drain the tear. The tear is an important fluid that forms a thin layer over the conjunctiva and cornea. It has three layers: (Fig. 6.2).

1. The lipid (fat) layer, the aqueous layer and mucus layer. These layers are produced by different parts of the eye and have different functions.
   i. **The lipid layer** is produced by the meibomian glands in the lids. It is very thin, prevents evaporation of the aqueous layers which is the thickest layer. It is the most superficial layer of the tear film.
   ii. **The aqueous layer**—This forms 90% of the tear film. It is produced by lacrimal and accessory lacrimal glands. Besides aqueous (water) it contains sodium chloride, glucose, proteins and urea. One of the important components of the aqueous part of the tear is lysozyme that has antimicrobial properties which prevents microbial infection to some extent. This is the middle layer of the tear film (Fig. 6.3).

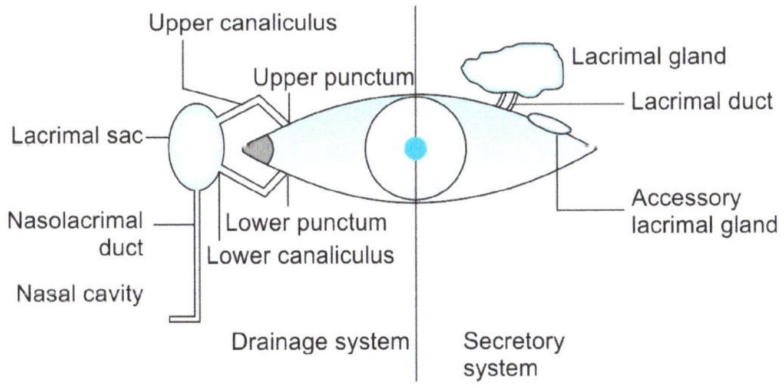

Fig. 6.1: Diagram showing lacrimal system

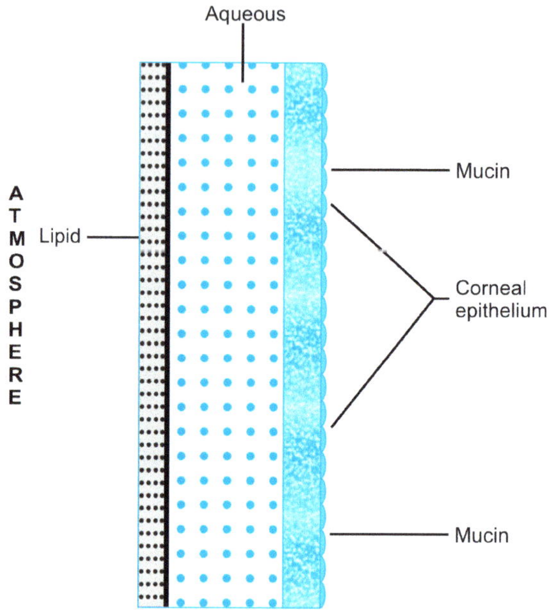

Fig. 6.2: Diagram showing various layers of tear film

iii. **The mucus layer** is produced by goblet cells of conjunctiva. It anchors the aqueous layer to the ocular surface. This is the inner most layer of the tear film.

The tear is produced at a constant rate and drained at an equally constant rate. This prevents overflow of tear in normal condition and hardly any tear is seen in the eyes. This requires a tear of optimum quality, quantity and a good drainage.

DRAINAGE OF TEAR

The main bulk of tear is produced in the lacrimal gland in superotemporal part of the orbit. To this is added lipids from meibomian gland and mucous from goblet cells in the conjunctiva. The tear spreads all over the globe by capillary action, gravity and squeezing action of orbicularis. This drives the tear towards the inferonasal part of the conjunctiva. From there it passes into the puncta. **75% of the tear is drained by lower puncta**. From the puncta the tear passes into the two canaliculi to the lacrimal sac, and nasolacrimal duct that open inside the nose. Failure of any part of this passage will cause obstruction of tear flow and tear will spill (overflow) over the lower lid margin even in presence of normal tear production. This overflow of normal amount of tear is called **epiphora**.

Excess production of tear is called **lacrimation,** where there is an overflow of tear in presence of normal outflow. Epiphora is worsened if lacrimation is added to defective drainage.

Decreased production of tear or abnormal composition of tears is called **ocular surface disorder** or **dry eye syndrome**.

The functions of the tear are:
1. It keeps the ocular surface moist (wet).
2. It flushes out any external particle.
3. It forms an optical layer over the cornea.
4. It prevents microbial infection.

The disease of lacrimal system can be any of the following –
1. Abnormal tear
   a. Watering
   b. Dry eye
2. Disease of drainage system
3. Diseases of lacrimal gland

WATERING OF THE EYES

Watering of the eyes is a very common symptom (complaints) of eye diseases, either external or internal **diseases**. It can be acute (sudden) or chronic (of many days). It can happen in one eye or both eyes. It may be associated with redness, discharge from the eyes, itching, pain and diminished vision in various combinations.

There are two types of watering of the eyes:
1. Lacrimation
2. Epiphora

Lacrimation

Lacrimation is over production of aqueous part of the tear due to irritation of the fifth nerve or psychogenic cause. The irritation can be in the ocular structures like conjunctiva, cornea or anterior uvea and extraocular muscles. The nonocular structure can be paranasal sinuses and nasal mucosa. It can be unilateral or bilateral. Lacrimation is mostly acute in onset but may last for sometime unless the cause has been removed.
The common causes of lacrimation are:

Table 6.1: Shows various cause of lacrimation and their location in various structures

Structures involved	Causes
1. Lid	Trichiasis, entropion, ectropion, lagophthalmos, foreign body in the tarsal conjunctiva
2. Conjunctiva	Acute conjunctivitis, allergic conjunctivitis, phlycten
3. Cornea	Corneal foreign body, corneal abrasion, phlyctenular kerato-conjunctivitis, corneal ulcer, keratitis, buphthalmos, acute keratoconus
4. Uvea	Acute iridocyclitis, endophthalmitis

Epiphora

This is overflow of normal tear due to malfunction of tear flow anywhere between lid to nasolacrimal duct. It can be unilateral or bilateral. Generally epiphora is chronic. The causes of epiphora are:

Table 6.2: Shows causes of epiphora and their location in various structures

Structures involved	Causes
1. Lid	Ectropion of lower lid, lagophthalmos, coloboma of lower lid
2. Puncta	Absence of puncta, pin-point puncta, obstruction of puncta by foreign body, eversion of puncta
3. Canaliculus	Absence of canaliculus, obstruction of canaliculus due to infection, laceration of canaliculus
4. Lacrimal sac	Chronic dacryocystitis, absence of sac (surgical removal of sac), granuloma of sac
5. Nasolacrimal duct	Congenital obstruction, acquired obstruction due to fracture of nasal bone

Dryness of the Eyes

A normal eye should have a wet conjunctiva and cornea. Any condition that reduces this wetness of ocular surface is designated as dry eye syndrome or ocular surface defect. This is brought about in two ways:

1. Deficiency of any of the components of tear, i.e. aqueous lipid or mucous
2. Defect in ocular surface, i.e. in the lid conjunctiva or cornea

Deficiency of Components of Tear

Commonest type is due to hyposecretion (less production) of tear in the lacrimal gland. This is brought about by age, menopause, thyroid disease, Sjögren's syndrome, many drugs taken orally or instilled locally.

The lipid deficiency is produced due to chronic blepharitis and meibomiantis. The mucous defect is brought by reduced goblet cells in the conjunctiva.

Defect in Ocular Surface

This is produced due to—coloboma of lid, ectropion of lid, lagophthalmos, pterygium, growth of conjunctiva, vitamin A deficiency, trachoma and many types of keratoconjunctivitis, chemical burns.

Symptoms

Symptoms of dry eye are many: Most of the persons do not complain of diminished tearing unless this is pointed to them.

More common features are: Recurrent redness of both the eyes, foreign body sensation, mucus secretion, fluctuating vision, intolerance to light. On examination the eyes look normal unless examined carefully.

1. The height of tear between the lower lid and the lower end of cornea (tear meniscus) is reduced. This is seen on slit lamp after staining the tear with fluorescein dye under cobalt blue filter.
2. The Schirmer test is less than 20 mm.
3. Tear break-up time is less than 15 seconds.
4. Fluorescein staining of corneal defect but not conjunctiva.
5. Rose Bengal staining—This stains both cornea and conjunctiva.
6. Lissamine green (stain cornea)

Treatment

Dry eye syndrome once developed stays for rest of the life. The treatment only reduces the symptoms. The treatment consists of prescribing tear substitutes (artificial tear) frequently.

Sjögren's Syndrome

This is a systemic condition seen mostly in women after menopause. Besides bilateral aqueous deficiency dry eye, they have dryness of mouth and pain in joints.

Diseases of Lacrimal Drainage System

The **main symptoms** of diseases of lacrimal drainage system is **epiphora**. The other symptoms are pain, tenderness, swelling over the sac, positive regurgitation and conjunctival congestion on the medial side.

Any part of the drainage system from puncta to nasolacrimal duct may be involved. They are diseases of:

1. Puncta—The puncta may be either absent or very small (pin-point) by birth or may be closed by foreign body. In both the condition the symptom is watering from the eye.
2. Canaliculi—Similarly the canaliculi may either be absent or very narrow by birth. More common is tearing on the lower canaliculus due to laceration. Less common is infection of canaliculi by fungus.
3. The lacrimal sac—The lacrimal sac is most commonly infected part of tear film draining system. It is involved in maximum number of disorders. They are:
   i. **Absence of the sac**, due to surgical removal. The process of removal is called **dacryocystectomy** or DCT in short.
   ii. **Infection:**
      a. Chronic dacryocystitis—This can be in newborn or adults.
      b. Acute dacryocystitis in any age.
      c. Granuloma of the sac—Rhinosporidiosis, tuberculosis, syphilis.
   iii. New growth—These are very rare.

4. Nasolacrimal duct:
   Obstruction
   - Present at birth
   - Acquired in adults
   - Following injury to face

Congenital Nasolacrimal Duct Obstruction

This is commonly known as **congenital dacryocystitis**. The nasolacrimal duct must be patent (open from one end to other) at birth. In 30% children it is not patent at birth and takes about a week to open. Out of these, about 10% children of the duct will not open even after few weeks. These are the children who suffer from congenital dacryocystitis.

In majority of the cases, it is found on one side only. Family history is positive in twenty percent cases.

As the nasolacrimal duct has an obstruction, the tear does not drain in the throat resulting in epiphora and distension of the sac and positive regurgitation from the sac.

The lacrimal glands do not start functioning before three weeks after birth, hence the watering starts only after three weeks. So any watering from the eye before two weeks after birth in not due to nasolacrimal duct obstruction. Other causes like **injury** during birth and **ophthalmia neonatorum** should be excluded.

Treatment of nasolacrimal duct obstruction in newborn is simple and successful provided done properly, otherwise it is a failure.

The treatment consists of pressing the sac, so the contents are forced down the nasolacrimal duct. This forces the obstruction to open. The correct method should be demonstrated to the mother. This is followed by instillation of antibiotic drop in the conjunctiva. The process must be repeated four to five times a day every day for about ten days. 90% of the children will be cured by this method. Children who do not respond will have to undergo **probing of nasolacrimal** duct under general anesthesia.

CHRONIC DACRYOCYSTITIS

There are two types of chronic dacryocystitis according to age of the patient. They are:

1. Chronic dacryocystitis in adults.
2. Chronic dacryocystitis in children.

Chronic Dacryocystitis in Adults

This is the commonest cause of epiphora in adults. It is mostly unilateral but can be bilateral. It is more common in **females** because they have narrower nasolacrimal duct which predisposes obstruction following spread of infection from the nose. Other causes are swollen inferior turbinate, deviated nasal septum and nasal polyp.

Infection from the nose cause swelling of the mucosa of nasolacrimal duct which blocks the flow of tear and conjunctival secretion which accumulates with in the sac causing it to distend. To this is added infection from the conjunctiva. The commonest cause of infection is **pneumococcus**.

The result is epiphora, redness of conjunctiva and visible swelling over the sac. If pressure is applied over the sac mucopurulent discharge regurgitates from the puncta. This is called **positive regurgitation test**. Chronic dacryocystitis is clinically divided into four stages. They are:

Stage I

- There is constant epiphora.
- There is mild conjunctivitis at the inner canthus.
- No or very little regurgitation on pressing the sac.
- There is no visible swelling.

Stage II

- Epiphora persists
- There is a visible diffuse swelling over the sac which is called **mucocele of the sac**.
- Pressure applied to the sac results in regurgitation of thick discharge.

Stage III

- The findings are same as in stage II but the swelling is larger and tense. The regurgitation is frank pus. This is called stage of **pyocele**.

Stage IV

Stage IV is the stage of complication. They are:

a. Both the canaliculi are blocked, so is the nasolacrimal duct. The sac shows a large tense swelling which does not reduce in size on pressure. There is no regurgitation. This is called **encysted mucocele** of the sac (Fig. 6.3).

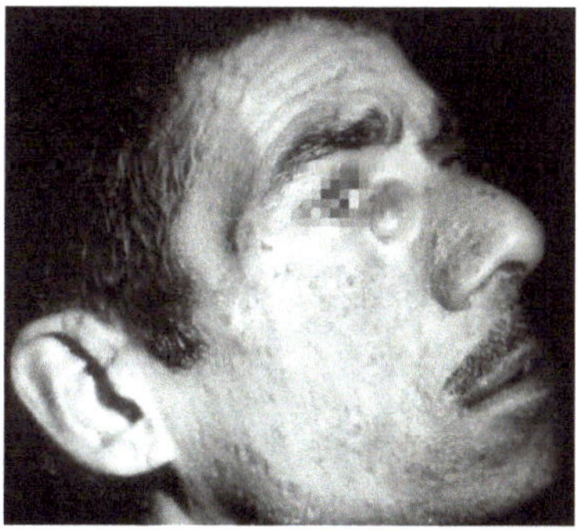

Fig. 6.3: Encysted mucocele of the sac

b. The infection passes through the sac wall and infects the tissue round the sac. This is called **acute dacryocystitis** or **pericystitis of the sac**. This is a painful condition. The skin over the sac is red and warm. The area is tender.
c. The stage of **lacrimal abscess**—An abscess develops over the sac.
d. The abscess burst, the pus is evacuated and a **fistula develops**. Fistula is a hollow tract that joins the inside of the sac to the skin surface. This results in sudden diminished pain and swelling. The epiphora disappears but tear drains from the sac through the track.
e. The sac is infected by pneumococci which is a dangerous organism. It can invade intact cornea and result severe **corneal ulcer with hypopyon** (pus in anterior chamber). This is a serious condition.
f. Acute dacryocystitis can cause:
   i. Preseptal orbital cellulitis
   ii. Cavernous sinus thrombosis—This is again a serious condition.

Management

Treatment depends on stage of dacryocystitis.
The stage I, II and III require surgery.

The definite surgery is **Dacryocystorhinostomy** (DCR) where sac wall is joined to nasal mucosa.

This can be done through:
i. The skin—The procedure is called **external DCR**.
ii. Through the nose by endoscope. This is called **endoscopic DCR**.
   The stage of complication require large doses of broad spectrum antibiotic orally or by injection till the acute stage has subsided which is followed by usual DCR.

Chronic Dacryocystitis in Children

Chronic dacryocystitis in children is **less common**. It is seen as often in boys as in girls. It is more **often bilateral**. The clinical features are similar to those seen in adults, the difference lies only in the causes. The causes are –
- Untreated or partially treated congenital dacryocystitis
- Following measles and chickenpox
- Facial injury
- Rhinosporidiosis

The management is same as in adults.

Diseases of Lacrimal Gland

Diseases of lacrimal gland are less common than diseases of lacrimal sac. The three common disorders of lacrimal glands are:
1. Hyposecretion (less production of tears)
2. Inflammation
3. Tumors

Inflammation of lacrimal gland (**dacryoadenitis**) can be:
- Acute
- Chronic

Acute Dacryoadenitis

Acute dacryoadenitis is more common than chronic dacryoadenitis. Common organisms causing them are:
i. Viruses—Mumps, measles, influenza
ii. Bacteria—Gonococcus, staphylococcus and streptococcus

Commonest cause of acute dacryoadenitis is mumps which is a systemic condition. It is seen in children and adolescents who have not been immunized against mumps. The condition starts with fever, rigor (shivering), pain all over the body.

The dacryoadenitis is generally unilateral. The gland is swollen, tender and painful. The upper lid is swollen. There is drooping of the lid. The lid has a S shaped curve. The conjunctiva is congested.

Acute dacryoadenitis in mumps is associated with painful swelling of parotid glands and submandibular gland.

The condition is self-limited but can cause serious complication.

Treatment

Mumps is a fully preventable disease by a vaccine given at nine months of age along with measles and rubella.

There is no specific treatment for acute dacryocystitis.

The pain is controlled by oral analgesic for three four days.

Dry hot fomentation two times a day for three four days.

Broad spectrum antibiotic drop in the conjunctiva.

Chronic Dacryoadenitis

Chronic dacryoadenitis is less common than acute dacryoadenitis. It is generally seen in adults, commonly bilateral and not painful. The condition is caused by tuberculosis, leprosy, syphilis. The glands are swollen. There is mild-ptosis. There may be slight proptosis.

The treatment is treatment of primary disease, i.e. tuberculosis, etc.

Tumors of the lacrimal system

There are no known tumors on lacrimal drainage system.

The tumors of the gland can be:
1. Benign (noncancer)
2. Malignant (cancer)

Out of the two, the benign tumors are more common than malignant tumors. The commonest benign tumor is called **mixed tumor** of the gland.

The clinical features are—It develops after 50 years of age, is unilateral and slow growing tumor.

The features are—Ptosis, S shaped curve of the lid margin, visible and palpable growth at the superior outer part of the orbit, the eyeball is pushed down and towards the nose. There may be slight proptosis and diplopia. Lymph glands are not enlarged. Treatment is surgical removal of the whole gland. **Malignant tumor** is **adenocystic carcinoma** which has the same features as of mixed tumor. The only difference is that it progresses fast and preauricular lymph nodes are enlarged. The treatment consists of removal of all the contents of the orbit including the eye.

CHAPTER

7

Disorders of the Orbits

Orbits are two spaces one on each side of the nose. The main contents of the orbit are- the eye ball, extraocular muscles, cranial nerves, blood vessels, and orbital fat. **There are no lymphatics in the orbit**. The blood vessels and the nerves communicate with the brain. Hence, it is very common for infection and inflammation to spread from the brain to the orbit and from orbit to the brain.

The commonest finding of orbital disorder is displacement of the globe forward. Backward displacement of the globe is less common. The forward displacement of the globe can either be—(1) **proptosis** or (2) **exophthalmos**. The backward displacement of the globe is called **enophthalmos**. The term **anophthalmos** is used to denote congenital absence (at birth) of the eyeball. This is very rare. More common is **microphthalmos** that means a small eye by birth. Surgical removal of the eye is called **empty socket** of the orbit.

PROPTOSIS

When an eyeball bulges outside the orbit due to a mass behind the eyeball or due to small orbit, the condition is called proptosis. Proptosis is not associated with systemic disease (thyroid).

Proptosis can be:

1. Congenital (present at birth) or
2. Acquired (develops after birth)

Second is more common than the first.

Congenital Proptosis

It is bilateral and almost always equal in both sides. It is due to faulty development of base of the skull that results in small orbit. The skull itself is also deformed (tower skull) (Crouzon syndrome, Aperts syndrome). Associated deformities of the face are also common.

The children with such proptosis have mental retardation. The eyes are too large for the orbit hence, they are pushed out of the orbit. The children have poor vision due to associated optic atrophy. Squints are common. Rarely there may be a congenital mass in the orbit to cause proptosis.

Acquired Proptosis

These are generally by unilateral. Rarely, they can be bilateral. The masses that cause acquired proptosis are **tumors, hematomas** (accumulated blood), **abscess** (accumulated pus), **pseudotumor** (inflammatory mass), **parasitic cysts, dermoids, mucoceles of paranasal sinuses, meningoencephalocele, meningocele**.

Common tumors causing proptosis in children are: (Figs 7.1A and B)
- Retinoblastoma
- Neuroblastoma
- Ewing's tumor
- Wilm's tumor
- Leukemia
- Rhabdomyosarcoma
- Optic nerve glioma
- Hemangioma

Common tumors that cause proptosis in adults are:
1. **Secondaries from**
   a. Bronchus
   b. Breast
   c. Prostate
   d. Kidney
   e. Lymphomas
2. **Primary tumors** (Fig. 7.2)
   a. Optic nerve meningioma
   b. Neurofibroma
   c. Orbital varices
   d. Dermoids
   e. Cavernous hemangioma

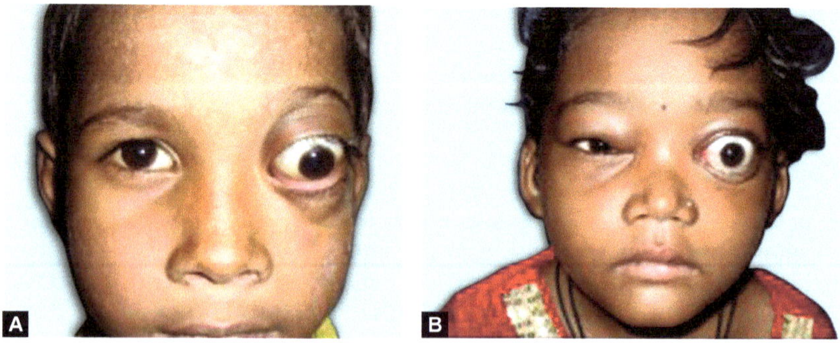

Figs 7.1A and B: Proptosis in children (*Courtesy:* Dr Santosh Patel)

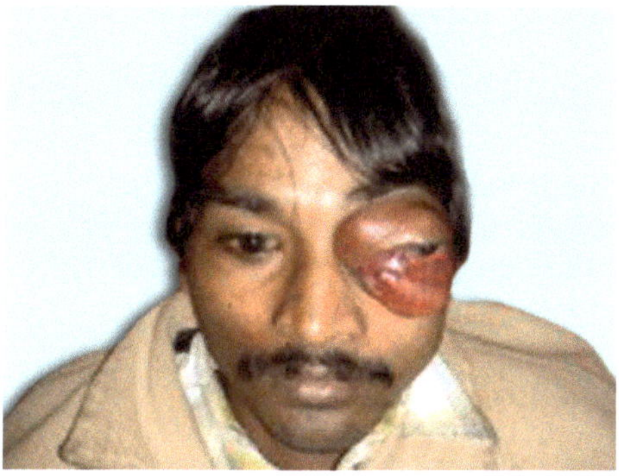

Fig. 7.2: Malignancy (cancer) of the orbit (*Courtesy:* Dr Santosh Patel)

3. Extension from surrounding structures
   a. Globe (eyeball)
      - Retinoblastoma
      - Malignant melanoma
   b. Lacrimal gland
      - Mixed lacrimal tumor
   c. Paranasal sinuses
      - Mucocele
   d. Brain
      - Meningocele—meningoencephalocele
4. Others
   a. Parasitic cyst
   b. Pseudotumor orbit
   c. Foreign body in orbit
   d. Hematoma

Causes of Unilateral Proptosis

1. Congenital—Meningocele, encephalocele, dermoid
2. Tumors
   i. Primary tumors: Retinoblastoma, neuroblastoma, rhabdomyosarcoma, hemangioma, glioma of optic nerve, meningioma of optic nerve, lacrimal gland tumors, leukemia, lymphomas.
   ii. Extension of tumors from surrounding structures
   iii. Secondaries from distant organs
3. Infective condition
   Orbital cellulitis, cavernous sinus thrombosis
4. Inflammatory—Pseudotumors of orbit.
5. Others—Parasitic cyst, foreign body, orbital varix.

Note: Some of these may become bilateral.

Pseudoproptosis

This is a condition where the eyes seem to be bulging out of the orbit without being so.

The conditions that produce pseudoproptosis are:

1. Unilateral (one sided) high myopia
2. Unilateral buphthalmos (glaucoma in children)
3. Unilateral large ciliary staphyloma
4. Retraction of the upper lid
5. Unilateral lagophthalmos
6. Contralateral microphthalmos and phthisis
7. Contralateral mild ptosis

Direction of Proptosis

1. Axial—Straight forward due to any growth inside the muscle cone. Common causes are **glioma of optic nerve**, **meningioma of optic nerve** sheath.
2. Downwards due to growth from roof of the orbit.
3. Upwards due to growth from floor of the orbit.
4. Down towards the nose—Lacrimal gland tumors
5. Down towards the ear—Growth from frontal sinus

Measurement of Proptosis

Proptosis can be measured either clinically or by various instruments called **proptometer** or **exophthalmometers**.

EXOPHTHALMOS

The term exophthalmos is used to denote bulging of the eye due to thyroids malfunction. This can happen even with normal thyroid function. It is more common in women. It is rare under ten years of age. It may start in one eye and the second eye develops exophthalmos afterwards. Bilateral exophthalmos is not always equal in two sides. Exact cause of exophthalmos is not known. Most probably this is due to chronic inflammation of extraocular muscle that enlarges the extraocular muscles pushing the eyeball out. In the beginning the patient may not be aware of exophthalmos, may just have redness of the eye, irritation in the eye and puffiness of the lids and diplopia (seeing two) later. There is lid retraction and lid lag. This is followed by exophthalmos that may be **mild**, **moderate** or **severe**. Severe exophthalmos is always associated with complication. The first complication is corneal exposure that may lead to keratitis and corneal ulcer. Second complication is pressure over the optic nerve leading to optic atrophy. Both may cause diminished vision and blindness.

Differentiation Between Exophthalmos and Proptosis

1. Clinical features: Exophthalmos has signs and symptoms of thyroid malfunction confirmed by T_3T_4 and Tsh.
2. X-ray does not show any change in orbit in exophthalmos but proptosis may be associated with:
   a. Enlargement of orbit, orbital fissure, optic foramen
   b. May show foreign body or intraorbital calcification.
3. Ultrasonography (USG) has limited value in both proptosis and exophthalmos. They are only good for lesions in the anterior (front) part of the orbit. It shows enlarged extraocular muscles in exophthalmos.
4. Computed tomography (CT) is one of the most useful diagnostic tools in diseases of the orbit both for proptosis and exophthalmos.
5. Magnetic resonance imaging (MRI)—This method outlines fine (subtle) changes that are not visible on CT but has a limited use in boney changes.

Infectious Diseases of the Orbit

The infectious diseases of the orbit may be present:
1. In the contents of the orbit—**orbital cellulitis**
2. In the walls and its covering of the orbit.

Common source of infection of orbit are:
1. From paranasal sinuses
2. From distant organs via blood
3. Penetrating injury

ORBITAL CELLULITIS

It can be acute orbital cellulitis or chronic orbital cellulitis.

Acute Orbital Cellulitis

This is an emergency requires urgent treatment by broad spectrum antibiotic given intravenous or intramuscular. It is more common in children. It is commonest cause of acute (fast growing) proptosis. It is unilateral (one side) in most of the cases. It is associated with fever, vomiting, headache and pain in and around the eye.

Types of Acute Orbital Cellulitis

1. Retroseptal (behind the orbital septum)
2. Preseptal (in front of the orbital septum)

Retroseptal acute orbital cellulitis is true orbital cellulitis. Preseptal cellulitis is a disease of lid. The commonest source of infection is acute or chronic untreated sinusitis.

The signs of acute orbital cellulitis consist of:
Edema of lids, pseudoptosis, chemosis of conjunctiva, mild to moderate proptosis, restricted movements of the globe, diminished vision, sluggish pupillary reaction suggests optic nerve involvement.

The orbital cellulitis should be differentiated from preseptal cellulitis, cavernous sinus thrombosis and retained foreign body by X-ray. This shows presence of sinusitis and intraorbital foreign body.

Ultrasonography shows involvement of muscles, presence of foreign body or pus.

CT gives better results than X-ray or ultrasonography.

Orbital abscess is accumulation of pus behind the orbital septum. This is generally due to unresolved orbital cellulitis. The commonest presentation is proptosis of moderate degree. The direction of proptosis depends upon position of abscess. If it is inside the muscle cone the proptosis is axial (straight forward), otherwise proptosis is eccentric (shifted to one side). Other features are—restricted movements, diminished vision. The diagnosis is confirmed by ultrasonography and CT.

Treatment is broad spectrum systemic antibiotic (antibiotic by mouth or injection). No attempt should be made to drain the abscess without proper localization and done by person trained in surgery of orbit.

ORBITAL PERIOSTITIS

Orbital periostitis is infection of either bones of the orbit or covering of the bones (periosteum). It produces diplopia, diminished vision, eccentric proptosis, tenderness (pain on pressure).

Diagnosis is confirmed by CT.

Treatment is systemic broad spectrum antibiotics.

Cavernous Sinus Thrombosis

It is an ophthalmic emergency. It should be managed in consultation with neurophysician. It is an acute infection (sudden) of **cavernous sinus,** which is situated behind the orbit on either side of the midline. Cranial nerves third, fourth, fifth and sixth pass through it, so inflammation of cavernous sinus involves these nerves.

The infection reaches the cavernous sinus via blood from many sources viz. face, lips, nose, lids, sinuses mastoid.

The disease starts on one side, the other side gets involved few days later. The patient has fever, headache, vomiting. The effected side has edema (swelling) of lids, conjunctiva is chemosed (swollen), hyperemic (red). The eyeball is proptosed. The movements of the eyeball are restricted. The vision may be diminished. There is tenderness over the mastoid (a bone of the skull behind the lower part of the ear). The other eye may develop paralysis of lateral rectus only or all the signs of the already effected eye may develop in this eye also.

The common conditions that have similar presentation are—Orbital cellulitis and panophthalmitis. Panophthalmitis is always associated with loss of vision.

The diagnosis is confirmed by CT of the orbit and cavernous sinus.

The best way to deal with the condition is administration of broad spectrum antibiotic by injection in hospitals where the patient gets specialized treatment. In all patients with diabetes should be excluded.

Chronic Inflammation of Orbit

A group of slowly developing diseases that produce proptosis and mistaken as malignant (cancer) are in fact chronic inflammatory masses. They are collectively called **pseudotumors** of the orbit. The disease may involve any of the soft tissues or all tissues of the orbit, i.e. blood vessels, extra-ocular muscles, lacrimal gland or nerves. The exact cause of the disease is not known. Most probably it is an **autoimmune disease**. Other causes are tuberculosis, syphilis, ruptured dermoid, ruptured parasitic cyst.

The disease is generally unilateral (one sided), seen equally in men and women after forty years of age. The disease is slow growing, causes mild to moderate proptosis, swelling of lids, puffiness of conjunctiva, redness of conjunctiva, restricted movements of the globe, diplopia and diminished vision.

The diagnosis is made by excluding other causes of unilateral proptosis. X-ray has little role in diagnosis. Better results are found by ultra-sonography, CT and MRI.

If the disease involves superior orbital fissure through which pass third, fourth, part of fifth and sixth nerve, the condition is called **superior orbital fissure syndrome** or **Tolosa Hunt syndrome**. It is associated with diplopia. If the disease involves the apex of the orbit, it is known as **orbital apex syndrome** that is associated with loss of vision and afferent pupil.

Tumors of the Orbit

The orbits contain tissues of various origin and is surrounded by many structures hence many tumors from surrounding structures can invade orbit.

The orbits have rich blood supply hence tumor cells from distant organs may get deposited in the orbits.

Classification of Tumors of Orbit Flow chart 7.1

The tumors of the orbit can be congenital (present as birth defect) or may be acquired (develop after birth).

The common congenital tumors of orbits are:

1. Dermoids
2. Encephalocele

Flow chart 7.1 The flow chart shows classification of orbital tumors

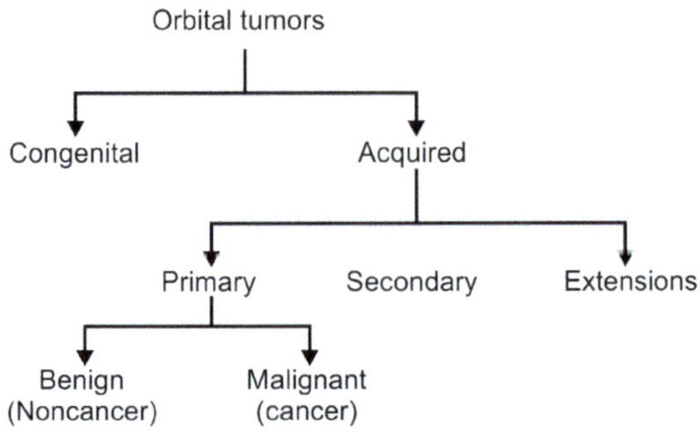

3. Meningocele
4. Meningoencephalocele
5. Hemangioma

The congenital tumors are benign (noncancerous). They are present from birth, become visible after few months to years.

Dermoids are slow growing cystic circular growth. They contain skin, hair, fatty tissue. They are commonly present at superotemporal aspect of the orbital rim, less commonly on the superomedial. Still less in the back of the orbit causing slow growing proptosis. The growth in front of the septum orbitale are visible and do not cause any symptom. They do not cause proptosis. Investigation required for dermoids are X-ray orbit, CT and USG. Treatment is surgical removal without breaking the cyst (Fig. 7.3).

Meningocele

The orbits do not contain meninges (covering of brain). In case of meningocele some part of the meninges get into the orbit and are converted as circular cystic swelling. They may be present in front or behind the

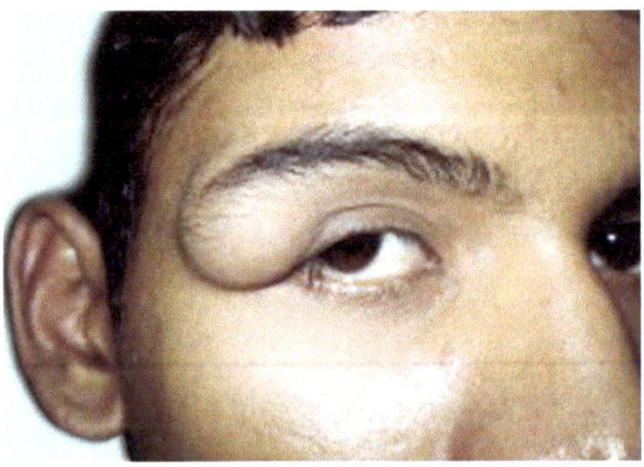

Fig. 7.3: Dermoid of superotemporal rim of orbit (*Courtesy*: Dr Santosh Patel)

septum orbitale. Those present in the orbit cause proptosis. They are best visible on CT and USG. Treatment is removal by surgery.

Encephalocele

When brain tissue gets into orbit, it is called encephalocele. If it is associated with meningocele it is called meningoencephalocele. The presentation is similar to meningocele.

Acquired Orbital Tumors

Acquired tumors of orbit can be:

Primary
- Secondary
- Extension from surrounding structure

Primary Orbital Tumors

1. Benign (noncancerous)
2. Malignant (cancer)

The common acquired orbital benign tumors are:

1. Hemangioma
2. Neurofibroma
3. Glioma of optic nerve
4. Meningioma of optic nerve
5. Mixed tumor of lacrimal gland

The benign tumors grow slowly, are generally seen on one side, do not spread outside the orbit.

The common primary malignant tumors of the orbit are:

- Rhabdomyosarcoma
- Orbital lymphoma
- Carcinoma of lacrimal gland

Common malignant tumors that extend from other structures:

1. Eyeball
   - Retinoblastoma
   - Malignant melanoma
2. From the neighboring structures
   - Paranasal sinus
   - Nasopharynx
   - Brain

Metastatic Tumors of Orbit

In children

1. Neuroblastoma
2. Nephroblastoma

3. Ewing's sarcoma
4. Leukemia (cancer of blood)

In adults
1. Breast
2. Lung
3. Prostrate
4. Stomach

Symptoms of Orbital Tumor

Symptoms depend upon:
1. Nature of tumor: Malignant/nonmalignant
2. Location of tumor
3. Size

The common symptoms of orbital tumors are:
1. Proptosis
2. Diminished movement
3. Diplopia
4. Diminished vision
5. Pain in and around the orbit
6. Symptoms of primary tumors

Signs of Orbital Tumor

1. **Proptosis:** Tumors inside the muscle cone produce axial proptosis (straight). Tumors outside muscle cone produce eccentric proptosis (the eyeball is shifted away from the growth)
2. Lagophthalmos (inability to close the eyes)
3. Diminished movements
4. Exposure of cornea
5. Diminished vision
   The proptosis can not be reduced by pressure.

Diagnosis of orbital tumors is confirmed by following investigation:
1. X-ray
2. USG
3. CT
4. MRI
5. Fine needle biopsy.
   A fine needle is inserted in the mass and tumor cells are aspirated (sucked out). The material is stained by special stains and examined under microscope.
6. Exisional biopsy—A small piece from the mass is removed and examined by specialist called histopathologist.

Treatment

1. Benign tumors are treated by surgical removal.
2. Primary malignant tumors are treated by
   i. Surgical removal
   ii. Chemotherapy
   iii. Radiation
   iv. Combination of above
3. Tumors extending from neighboring structures and metastatic tumors require treatment of primary tumor alongwith local treatment by oncologists (a person specializing in treatment of cancer).

Enophthalmos

In enophthalmos the eyeball is placed backward in the orbit in relation to normal position of the eye.

The causes of enophthalmos are:

1. The eyeball is small—Microphtlamos
2. The eyeball is soft—**Phthisis bulbi**
3. The eyeball is retracted back
   a. Fibrosis of the muscle
   b. Fracture floor of orbit
   c. Squint surgery
4. Neurological—Horner's syndrome

Signs of Enophthalmos

The intrapalpebral aperture is narrow. There is pseudoptosis. The curvature of cornea is less. Generally vision is poor that can not be corrected. Artificial eyes improve the appearance in enophthalmos.

CHAPTER

8

Disorders of Conjunctiva

Conjunctiva extends from the intermarginal strip of the lid to the cornea. It covers the tarsal plate and the visible part of the **sclera** (the white of the eye). The part that covers the lid over the tarsal plate is called **tarsal conjunctivitis** or **palpebral conjunctivitis**. The part that covers the sclera is called **bulbar conjunctiva**. The tarsal conjunctivitis is firmly attached to the tarsal plate and can not be separated from it. In normal conjunctiva the **tarsal glands** are visible as blue parallel lines. The bulbar conjunctiva is loose, it can be separated from the sclera. The conjunctiva at the junction of the tarsal and bulbar conjunctiva is very loose. It is called the **fornix**. The conjunctiva is well supplied by blood vessels. It has rich lymphatics.

The diseases of the conjunctiva are:

1. Congenital – Rare
2. Acquired – Infection
   – Allergy
   – Nutritional
   – Degenerative
   – Neoplastic (New growths)

The common features of conjunctival diseases are:

1. Hyperemia (redness)
2. Subconjunctival hemorrhage (blood under conjunctiva)
3. Chemosis (puffiness)
4. Discharge
5. Exudates
6. Itching
7. Xerosis
8. Pinguecula
9. Pterygium
10. Growth

HYPEREMIA

Normal conjunctiva is transparent. Few blood vessels are visible. In hyperaemia, the number of blood vessels increase, giving red color to the conjunctiva. This is known as conjunctival congestion. Conjunctival congestion starts at the fornix and spread towards the cornea.

The causes of conjunctival Congestion are (Fig. 8.1):

1. Trauma (injury)
2. Infection
3. Allergy
4. Pterygium
5. Growth

Conjunctival congestion can be unilateral (in one eye only) or bilateral (in both eyes). Congestion is generally associated with watering or watering with discharge.

The congestion can be generalized, i.e. a large part of the conjunctiva is congested.

The causes of generalized conjunctival congestion are:

1. Acute conjunctivitis
2. Chronic conjunctivitis
3. Allergic conjunctivitis
4. Chemical injury to the conjunctiva

Causes of local conjunctival congestion are:

1. Trauma (injury)
2. Pterygium
3. Phlycten
4. Episcleritis
5. Circumciliary congestion
6. Angular conjunctivitis
7. Growth of the conjunctiva

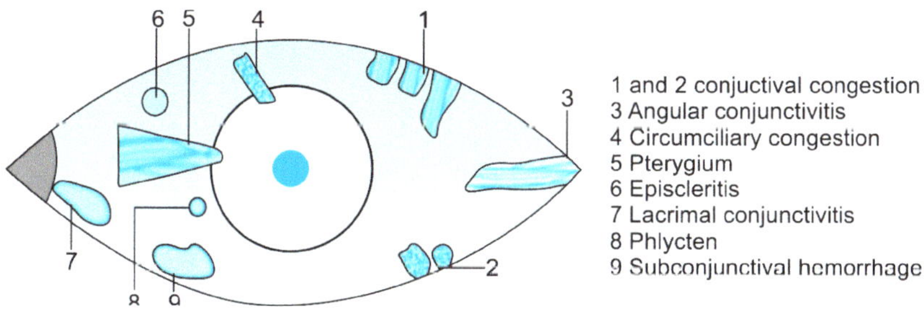

Fig. 8.1: Diagram showing localized conjunctival congestion

There are three types of conjunctival congestion (Fig. 8.2):

1. Conjunctival congestion
2. Circumciliary (corneal) congestion
3. Episcleral congestion

Conjunctival Congestion

Starts in the fornix and fade towards the cornea, may reach up to the cornea. They are bright red in color. The blood vessels move with the conjunctiva and disappear by putting a drop of weak solution of adrenaline. There is no pain on pressing the eyeball. It is generally associated with **conjunctival discharge**, are generally bilateral. The common causes are **infective conjunctivitis** and **allergic conjunctivitis**. The congestion disappears with treatment of conjunctivitis.

Circumciliary Congestion

The circumciliary congestion starts from the limbus and fades towards fornix. It does not extend more than two to three millimeters from the limbus. The color is pink. There is **ciliary tenderness** (pain on pressing the eyeball). The common causes are keratitis, iridocyclitis and acute glaucoma. They disappear with treatment of the cause.

Episcleral Congestion

It is less common than the above two. This is seen in **absolute glaucoma**. It is due to dilatation of episcleral vessels that start from the periphery, proceed towards the limbus, before reaching limbus they bifurcate and join the adjoining (nearby) vessels on each side and change the direction.

Subconjunctival Hemorrhage (Blood Under the Conjunctiva)

The subconjunctival hemorrhage are accumulation of blood under the conjunctiva. The color is bright red in the beginning and gradually becomes dark. A subconjunctival hemorrhage may develop anywhere in

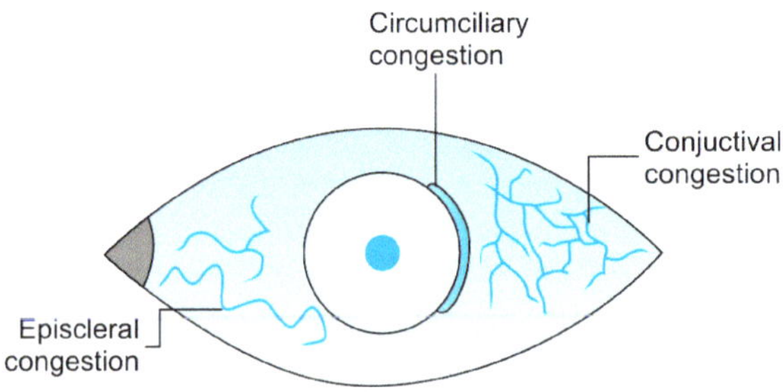

Fig. 8.2: Diagram showing three types of conjunctival congestion

the conjunctiva. The commonest place being in the bulbar conjunctiva. It may be (i) Localized, (ii) Generalized and (iii) In small spots (petechial hemorrhage) (Figs 8.3 to 8.8).

The causes of localized sub conjunctival hemorrhages are:
- Trauma
- Whooping cough (commonest cause in children)
- Idiopathic (when no cause can be found)
- Blood dyscrasia (abnormal blood)

Causes of generalized subconjunctival hemorrhages are:
- Head injury
- Orbital injury

The generalized subconjunctival hemorrhages develop few hours to two days after the injury start from the fornix, hence their outer edges are not visible.

Petechial hemorrhages are seen alongwith conjunctival congestion in pneumococcal conjunctivitis, acute viral **Hemorrhagic conjunctivitis and** in **epidemic keratoconjunctivitis**.

Subconjunctival hemorrhages do not require any treatment. They disappear in ten to fifteen days without any trace.

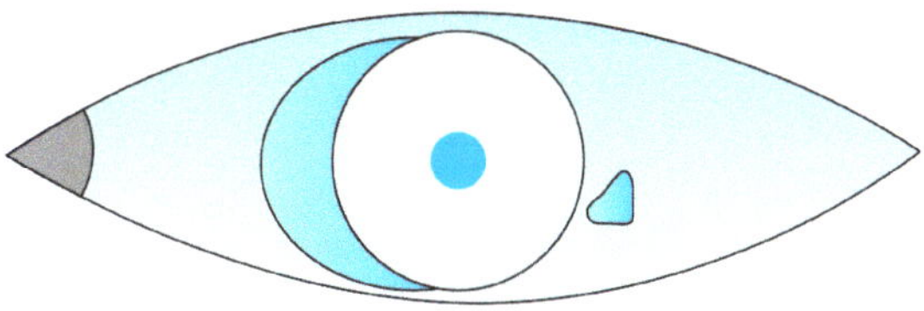

Fig. 8.3: Localized subconjunctival hemorrhage, periphery visible

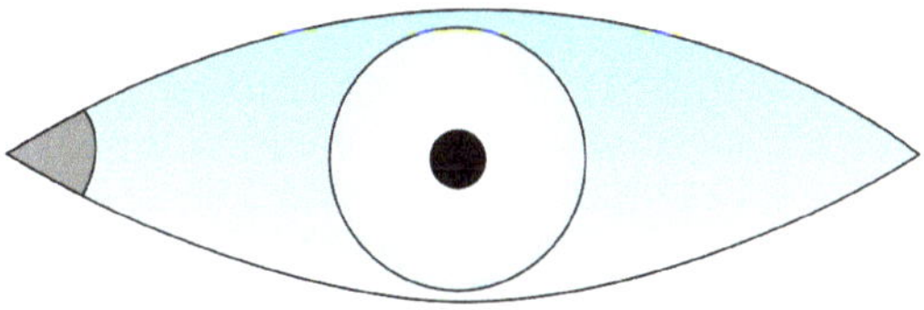

Fig. 8.4: Generalized subconjunctival hemorrhage, periphery not visible, may be due to head injury

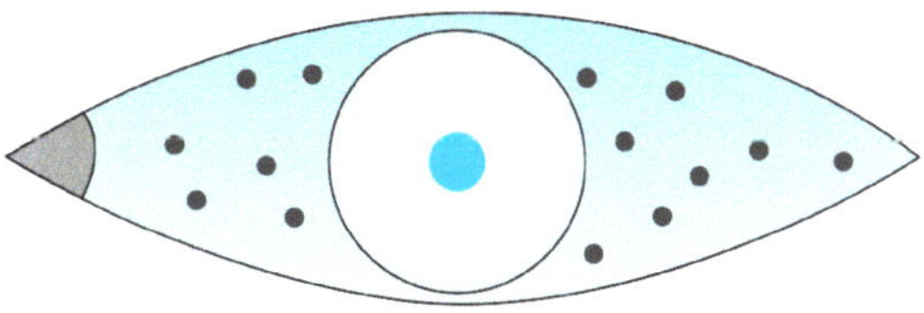

Fig. 8.5: Petichial hemorrhage

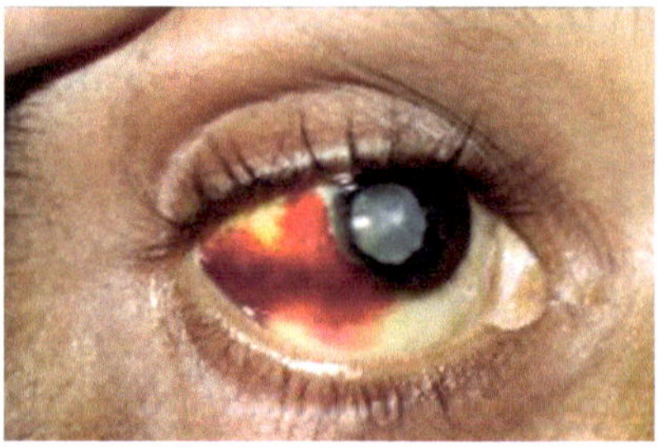

Fig. 8.6: Localized subconjuctival hemorrhage due to injury
(*Courtesy*: Dr Santosh patel)

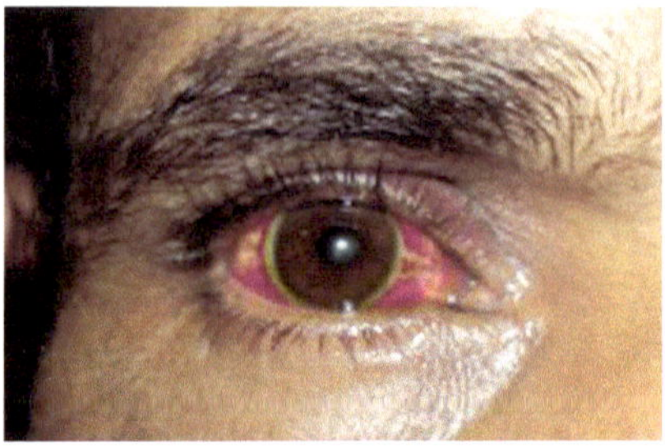

Fig. 8.7: Generalized subconjuctival hemorrhage in viral conjunctivitis
(*Courtesy*: Dr AK Chandrakar)

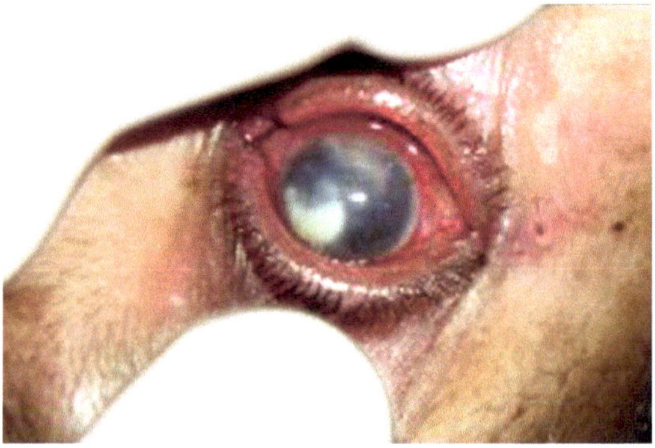

Fig.8.8: Generalized conjuctival congestion in corneal ulser (*Courtesy*: Dr Nidhi Pandey)

Lacrimation (Watering from the Eye)

Normal conjunctiva is moist (wet). There is sufficient tear to keep it moist. Excess of tear production is called lacrimation. Lacrimation should be differentiated from epiphora which is overflow of normal amount of tear.

The causes of lacrimation are:

1. Conjunctiva
   - Trauma (injury)
   - Viral conjunctivitis
   - Allergic conjunctivitis
2. Cornea
   - Injury
   - Foreign body
   - Keratitis
   - Buphthalmos

3. Uvea – Acute iritis
   – Acute iridocyclitis
   – Endophthalmitis
4. Reflex – Irritation of fifth nerve
5. Psychogenic
   Lacrimation starts in the effected eye. The other eye develops it reflexly. Lacrimation may be associated with conjunctival discharge and redness.

In all cases of lacrimation, following examination should be done:
1. Exclude epiphora
2. Examine the cornea for injury, keratitis and by fluorescein stain:
3. Examine tarsal plate for foreign body
4. Look for evidence of iritis

Conjunctival Chemosis

Conjunctival chemosis is accumulation of fluid under the conjunctiva. The conjunctiva is raised away from the sclera, disappears with pressure. The color of the conjunctiva is congested. It is not painful. The commonest cause is **acute allergic conjunctivitis**. It can be unilateral or bilateral. It disappears without treatment or with the treatment of allergy. The other causes are severe infection of conjunctiva like **gonococcal conjunctivitis** and **panophthalmitis**.

Xerosis of Conjunctivitis (Xero = Dry)

The normal conjunctiva is wet and glossy. When it looses its gloss (lustre) and becomes dry, it is called xerotic conjunctiva.

The commonest cause of xerosis of conjunctiva is vitamin A deficiency. **The xerosis in vitamin A deficiency** generally develops on the lateral side (towards the ear) of the conjunctiva as a localized lustre less dirty white area which is little raised. It is a bilateral condition and may be associated with **night blindness**. Xerosis due to vitamin A deficiency is seen in children. The xerosis may spread all over the conjunctiva and even involve the cornea. Such a condition is called **xerophthalmia**, which is a serious condition but fully preventable and treatable. The prevention is administration of 100,000 unit of oral vitamin A to every child every six months between six months to six years along with usual immunization under national plan for immunization.

The other causes of xerosis are:
- Defect in the lid (coloboma)
- Lagophthalmos
- Proptosis
- Trachoma
- Severe dry eye syndrome

Bitot's Spot

Bitot's spot is a triangular white spot on the bulbar conjunctiva on the lateral side away from the cornea. The base of the triangle towards the cornea. It is a bilateral condition, commonly seen in hypovitaminosis A but can be seen without it also. It does not disappear with administration of vitamin A and may last for many years.

Grades of Xerophthalmia

World Health Organization (WHO) has graded signs of xerophthalmia into two groups. They are: Primary and secondary.

The primary signs of xerophthalmia

X1A	Conjunctival xerosis
X1B	Bitot's spot with xerosis of conjunctiva
X2	Corneal xerosis
X3A	Corneal ulceration with corneal xerosis
X3B	Keratomalacia

The secondary signs of xerophthalmia

XN	Night blindness due to vitamin A deficiency
XF	Xerophthalmic fundus (rare)
XS	Corneal scar

Complication of Xerophthalmia

1. Night blindness. This is treatable by two intramuscular injection of 100,000 IU one on each day.
2. Corneal dryness
3. Non infective corneal ulcer
4. Perforation of corneal ulcer
5. Corneal opacity leading to blindness

Prevention of Xerophthalmia

1. Administration of vitamin A: All pregnant mothers should get 100,000 IU of vitamin A between six to nine months of pregnancy.
2. All children should be immunized as per national program.
3. All children should get 100,000 IU (55 mg retiny palmitate) orally every six months up to six years of age. Oral vitamin A syrup is available in all primary health centers and anganbadi free of cost.
4. All children suffering from measles should get 100,000 IU of injectable vitamin A.
5. Children suffering from chronic diarrhea should be treated by qualified persons.

Diet

1. All newborn should be fed the colostrum (the first thick yellow breast milk).
2. All children should be breast fed for first six months. Thereafter solid food should be added to the diet but breast feeding should continue till three years. If mothers milk is not sufficient, the child should drink cows or buffalos milk.

Conjunctival Exudation (Discharge)

In normal eyes there is no discharge from the conjunctiva. Presence of discharge always means disease of conjunctiva. The discharge varies from disease to disease and severity of the disease.

The conjunctival discharge contains tear, mucus, pus cells and organism.

The conjunctival discharge can be:

Type	Cause
Watery	Allergic conjunctivitis
Mucoid	Simple conjunctivitis
Mucopurulent	Severe bacterial conjunctivitis
Purulent (pus)	Gonococcal conjunctivitis

Itching

Normal eyes do not cause itching. Itching always means allergic conjunctivitis. Itching may be mild or severe.

The causes of itching of the eyes are:
1. Spring catarrh
2. Seasonal allergic conjunctivitis
3. Drugs and chemicals
4. Allergic dermatitis (itching of the skin)

Pinguecula

These are very common bilateral harmless nodule that develop on the conjunctiva on the medial side of the cornea little away from the limbus. They are two to three millimeters in size, circular in shape and pale white. They develop under the conjunctiva. There are no blood vessels on them. They are not painful or tender. They last for whole life, do not require any treatment. However pterygium may develop over them.

Pterygium

Pterygium is a very common disease of the conjunctiva that involves cornea also. It is a triangular, red, fleshy growth of the conjunctiva. It commonly develops after 30 years of age. It is more common in males than in females. It is common in persons who lead an outdoor life and exposed to dust and sun rays. It is bilateral condition. It develops on the nasal side more often, rarely it can be seen on temporal side. Pterygium on both sides of the cornea is very rare. The exact cause of the condition is nor known. In some cases it is familial, i.e. more than one person in the same generation or two-three generations may be seen. Role of pinguecula is development of pterygium has not been proved. Most probably causes are ultraviolet rays and fine dust.

The pterygium has an apex, a body and a base. The apex is on the cornea and the base is in the canthus. The body is a fleshy mass with prominent blood vessels. The body is fixed to the episclera, hence a probe can not be passed under it. It has three stages.

The stages of pterygium are:
1. Progressive
2. Stationary
3. Atrophic

Progressive

In the progressive stage, it grows fast over two to three years on the cornea. On the cornea it may stop growing before it reaches the pupil and converted into a stationary pterygium. Otherwise it grows to cover the pupil or may cross the pupil causing loss of vision. Pterygium never disappears without treatment. It atrophizes and is converted into a thin, pale triangular patch.

The commonest symptom of pterygium is cosmetic (look). The other symptom is diminished vision.

The cause of diminished vision in pterygium:
1. Obscuring (covering) the pupil
2. Irregular astigmatism

   The pterygium never develop malignancy (cancer). It frequently gets infected.

Treatment

1. There is no medical treatment.
2. The treatment is surgical removal with steps to prevent recurrence (growing again).
3. Small pterygium between the pupil and limbus does not require any treatment.
4. Pterygium if not operated well is bound to grow again. Recurrence is more severe than the original growth.

Episcleritis

Episcleritis is not a disease of conjunctiva. It is inflammatory condition of episclera (a tissue that fixes the conjunctiva to the sclera). It is a localized, raised and sometimes tender area generally in the interpalpebral aperture away from the limbus. It is generally confused either as pinguecula or phlycten.

Phlycten

Phlycten is a nodule of the conjunctiva due to endogenous allergy. It is seen in children. It may involve cornea.

Conjunctivitis

The term conjunctivitis denotes inflammation of conjunctiva. It can be infective caused by microbes and allergic.

Infective conjunctivitis are due to-
1. Bacteria
2. Virus
3. Chlamydia

Bacterial Conjunctivitis

They are very common, equally seen in men and women. They are more common in children. They begin in one eye and the other eye gets involved soon. The disease can be acute (sudden onset) or chronic (gradual onset and long duration).

The symptoms of acute bacterial conjunctivitis are redness in the eyes, watery or mucopurulent discharge, matting of lid margin at night, foreign body sensation. It is not painful. Vision is not diminished.

The sign of acute bacterial conjunctivitis are mild swelling of the lids, crusts on the lid margin, bright red color of conjunctiva, prominent blood vessels. The congestion is more in the fornixes. The discharge is watery or mucopurulent. Cornea is bright, AC and pupil are normal. Regurgitation test is negative.

The milder form is self limiting (it is cured even without treatment in few days), The moderate and severe form require treatment. Local antibiotic drops are sufficient. There is no need to give antibiotic by mouth or injection except in gonococcal and diphtheritic conjunctivitis.

Treatment

1. The lid margins are cleaned.
2. Remove the discharge.
3. There is no need to wash the conjunctiva.
4. Instil broad spectrum antibiotics at least every four hourly in both eyes, only one drop at a time. The ointment of same antibiotic is applied at night to prevent sticking of the lids together.

Commonly used antibiotics used in bacterial conjunctivitis are:

1.	Gentamycin	0.3% drop and ointment
2.	Chloramphenicol	0.4% to 1% as a drop and ointment
3.	Ciprofloxacin	0.3% drop and ointment
4.	Ofloxacilin	0.3% drops
5.	Tobramycin	0.3% drops

Special Types of Acute Bacterial Conjunctivitis

They are not only blinding (loss of vision) but can be life threatening (may kill).
They are:
- Pneumococcal conjunctivitis
- Gonococcal conjunctivitis
- Diphtheretic conjunctivitis
- Moraxella conjunctivitis (nonvision threatening and not life threatening)

Pneumococcal Conjunctivitis

This is acute bilateral mucopurulent conjunctivitis. The conjunctival congestion is associated with **petechial hemorrhage** (small hemorrhages). It can cause hypopyon (pus in anterior chamber). The main sources of the organism are throat, nose and lacrimal sac. The disease is easily treated by local instillation of antibiotic one drop each eye every hourly. Presence of pus in anterior chamber requires hospitalization and treatment under specialist.

Gonococcal Conjunctivitis

This is one of the most dangerous conjunctivitis that can cause not only blindness in both eyes but also death in new born. It is caused by organisms called gonococci. One of the dangerous feature of the organism is that it can pass through cornea even without injury. The disease is a sexually transmitted disease in adults. The new born gets the disease from the infected mother.

The conjunctivitis caused by the organism is acute and spreads fast. It is found in two forms:
1. In newborn
2. In adults

Gonococcal conjunctivitis in newborn is also known as ophthalmia neonatorum.

Ophthalmia Neonatorum

Ophthalmia neonatorum is an **acute** (fast developing,) **bilateral purulent** conjunctivitis. The conjunctival discharge is **pus**. The disease develops within first month of birth.

Gonococci are the commonest organism to cause ophthalmia neonatorum. Other organisms that can cause ophthalmia neonatorum are:

Bacteria	–	Pneumococci staphylococci
	–	Hemophilus
Virus	–	Herpes simplex
Chlamydia	–	Inclusion conjunctivitis
Chemical	–	Silver nitrate drops (Non-Infective)

Conjunctivitis neonatorum by gonococci is most dangerous. The rest of the organisms cause mild conjunctivitis which do not cause loss of vision or death.

Typical gonococcal conjunctivitis in new born develops within two to three days of birth. The child gets the infection from the mother who herself is infected. Both the lids are swollen, and have too much of pus like discharge. The conjunctiva is bright red. Cornea should be examined carefully from the first day because gonococci can penetrate intact cornea.

Management

Management of Ophthalmia Neonatorum

1. Prophylaxis (prevention)
   a. **Mother**: All mothers should be examined before delivery for any evidence of gonococcal infection in the birth passage and those found to suffer from gonococcal infection should be treated before the due date of delivery.
   b. **The newborn children**
      i. The eyes should be cleaned.
      ii. One drop of one percent freshly prepared silver nitrate drop once only in each eye or one percent **betadine eye** drop in each eye are instilled.
      iii. Any of the **broad spectrum antibiotic** eye drop—one drop in each eye may be an alternative.
2. Treatment of conjunctivitis
   i. Clean the lid margin
   ii. Remove the discharge
   iii. Instil one drop of any of the following in each eye –
   Gentamycin, ciprofloxacin, tobramycin
      One drop every five minutes for six times
      One drop every ten minutes for six times
      One drop every hour for first 24 hours
   This should control the infection, otherwise the child should get injectable antigonococcal antibiotic in consultation with pediatrician.
   iv. If the cornea is involved 1/2 percent atropine sulphate eye ointment is put in each eye, once only.

Complication of Ophthalmia Neonatorum

If not treated, the cornea develops a **central ulcer** that perforates leading to endophthalmitis or a **central perforation** that may heal, leaving an **anterior polar cataract**. This later leads to diminished vision and **nystagmus**.

Gonococcal Conjunctivitis in Adults

In adults, it is generally unilateral. The infection spreads from genitals to eye by contaminated fingers.

It takes less than two to three days for the infection to develop in the eyes. The lids are swollen, the conjunctiva is congested and chemosed. The discharge looks like pus. The cornea should be examined at the time of first examination for evidence of its involvement. The corneal involvement is in the form of corneal ulcer, iritis and hypopyon.

The infection may spread to the other eye by fingers.

Treatment

Local: 1. Atropine sulphate one percent drop once a day.
2. Antigonococcal antibiotic drop one hourly by day and two hourly by night.

Systemic: Injectable broad spectrum antigonococcal antibiotic in consultation with physician.

Diphtheretic Conjunctivitis

This is an acute, bilateral conjunctivitis that develops in children who have not been immunised (who have not received D.P.T. injection). It can cause blindness as well as death. It is caused by diphtheretic bacilli, which can pass through intact cornea.

The conjunctivitis is generally associated with diphtheria of throat.

The lids are swollen, the conjunctiva is congested. The tarsal conjunctiva develops a membrane (white cover) that may cover the whole of the tarsal conjunctiva in both lids or may be seen in patches. Sometimes the membrane may develop on the bulbar conjunctiva. It is difficult to remove the membrane. In an attempt to remove it, there is bleeding from the conjunctiva. The cornea may develop ulcer.

Besides diphtheria there are other organisms that also cause membrane formation. All cases of membrane on the conjunctiva should be considered due to diphtheria unless proved otherwise.

Management of Diphtheretic Conjunctivitis

Prophylaxis (prevention)—All children should get two doses of DPT as part of national immunization program. This saves the child from diphtheria of throat as well as eyes.

Treatment

Systemic: All cases of diphtheritic conjunctivitis should be treated by child specialist.

Local: Local treatment consists of instillation of one percent atropine sulphate once and frequent instillation of broad spectrum antibiotic one hourly.

No attempt should be made to remove the membrane.

Moraxella Conjunctivitis

Conjunctivitis is caused by organism Morax Axenfeld in persons with chronic disease and malnutrition. The conjunctivitis is chronic, bilateral, mild, seen in the outer angle of the conjunctiva. It causes **marginal keratitis** and **hypopyon**. The treatment consists of improvement of diet, personal cleanliness, administration of broad spectrum antibiotic drops three times a day and instillation of **zinc sulphate drop two** to three times a day. If hypopyon is present, **atropine sulphate one percent** as drop is instilled two times a day.

Viral Conjunctivitis

Viral conjunctivitis are very common. They may involve the eyes only or may be associated with similar infection of nose, throat and skin. Viral conjunctivitis may be mild and last for a few days and cured without treatment or may be severe but are not known to cause blindness unless the cornea is also involved.

The common types of viral conjunctivitis are –

- Pharyngo conjunctival fever
- Epidemic kerato conjunctivitis
- Acute hemorrhagic conjunctivitis
- Herpes simplex conjunctivitis
- Herpes zoster varicella conjunctivitis
- Conjunctivitis associated with measles

Pharyngo Conjunctival Fever

As the name suggest, it is associated with fever and pain in throat. It is generally seen in children and young adults, is bilateral, lasts for short period, self-limiting (does not require treatment). Antibiotics and anti-viral drugs have very little effect on conjunctivitis. Mild transient corneal involvement is seen in some cases.

Epidemic Keratoconjunctivitis

This is more severe than the above, involves **many members of the community**, seen in **children** and young adults, is **bilateral** with follicle formation. Sometimes there may be **pseudomembrane formation**. The eyes are bright red with watery discharge. Corneal involvement is common, generally develop after a week from the day of onset of conjunctivitis. The corneal involvement starts with diminished vision, watering and photophobia in the form of small multiple opacities scattered all over the cornea. They do not stain. They persist even after the conjunctivitis has subsided. The corneal involvement may last for weeks to months.

There is no known treatment. The antibiotics and antivirals have no role to play. Oral pain killers are given to reduce discomfort. Antibiotics ointment prevent secondary bacterial infection.

Acute Hemorrhagic Conjunctivitis

This also happens in epidemics almost every year. Both eyes are effected at the same time. The conjunctivitis is **severe**. **Subconjunctival hemorrhage** is the rule. It may be small and scattered or large and cover whole of the sclera. **Photophobia** and **foreign body sensation** are common. Corneal complications are rare. The subconjunctival hemorrhages may last for weeks after the conjunctivitis has subsided.

Herpes Simplex Conjunctivitis

This is seen in young adults and children. It can cause nongonococcal ophthalmic neonatorum. It is primary manifestation of herpes simplex. In young children, the disease is passed by healthy carriers (persons, who suffer from the disease but do not have symptoms). In newborn corneal involvement is rare. In young adults cornea may show microdendrite and require antiviral drops.

Herpes Zoster Varicella Conjunctivitis

This is seen in two forms:

1. Conjunctivitis in chickenpox
2. Conjunctivitis in herpes zoster ophthalmicus

First is bilateral acute mucopurulent conjunctivitis that develop in children with chickenpox. The conjunctiva is congested. There may be vesicle of chickenpox on the conjunctiva and lid margin. A vesicle near the limbus causes photophobia. The conjunctivitis subsides with chickenpox itself.

The second is seen in adults and unilateral, associated with eruption on the forehead and lids. It may involve cornea. Episcleritis is common.

Conjunctivitis in Measles

Conjunctivitis is very common in measles which is a disease of childhood. **Measles is fully preventable** disease. It presents as rashes all over the body including the lid. Small vesicle may develop on the conjunctiva and caruncle. **Koplik's spot** is a bright red spot with bluish white center. This spot is diagnostic of measles.

No treatment is required for conjunctivitis. However measles is associated with vitamin A deficiency. Hence, all children should get an extra dose of 100,000 IU of vitamin A.

Chlamydial Conjunctivitis

Chlamydia are a group of organisms that are larger than largest virus but smaller than smallest bacteria. There are many types of chlamydiae. Out of the chlamydia, trachomatous causes conjunctivitis.

Chlamydia involves the conjunctiva in three forms:

1. Trachoma
2. Inclusion conjunctivitis in adults
3. Ophthalmia neonatorum

Trachoma

Trachoma is one of the major preventable and treatable causes of blindness, so much so that WHO has included it among five important causes of blindness. It is a **chronic keratoconjunctivitis** that has an **acute onset** and a **chronic course**. It is seen in dry, hot climate in crowded locations with unhygienic surrounding. Many members of the community suffer from various stages of the disease at the same time.

The disease is caused by an organism **chlamydia trachomatis**. It has an acute onset, a long course and a longer duration of complication that may last for rest of the life and cause blindness unless treated. It starts in the conjunctiva and spread to cornea and tarsal plate.

The disease **starts in childhood**, the features of which are similar to bacterial conjunctivitis. It involves both the eyes. The attack may be cured without any complication. **Reinfection is common** which brings another subacute attack. This stage lasts for many months to years and involves the cornea first and the tarsal conjunctiva later. This is most infective stage. The symptoms of this stage are: Redness of the eyes, gritty sensation, watering, chemosis of the conjunctiva, follicles in the tarsal conjunctiva and discharge.

The cornea is involved few months after. The corneal changes are—**Superficial keratitis**, **superficial vascularization** called **pannus**, **follicles** at limbus which break to form small shallow pits that are called **Herbert's pits**. Herbert's pits are diagnostic of well established trachoma. It takes many years for the Herbert's pits to develop.

While these changes are progressing, changes develop in the tarsal conjunctiva in the formation of fibrosis. The fibrosis causes thickening of tarsal plate, development of star like scars under the conjunctiva, **trichiasis** and **entropion**. Trichiasis and entropion cause corneal vascularization, ulceration and opacity formation. This leads to diminished vision that may lead to blindness.

Due to different mode of presentation and prolonged course of the disease, it is not possible to cover them under one classification.

The currently used classification of trachoma is WHO classification of trachoma that is as follows:

- TF – Follicles in the upper tarsal conjunctiva
- TI – Papillary hypertrophy in upper tarsal conjunctiva
- TS – Trachomatous scarring
- TT – Trichiasis and entropion
- TCO – Corneal opacity

Trachoma is infectious in TF stage only, after which it becomes non-infectious (the disease does not spread from one person to other).

Trachoma spreads from one person to other by dirty infected fingers and flies. It is very common for trachomatous eyes to be infected by other bacteria which makes the eyes prone to develop corneal ulcer and deep opacities. This condition is called **blinding trachoma**.

Management of Trachoma

Treatment of trachoma is divided into:
1. Prophylaxis (prevention)
2. Management in acute stage
3. Management of blinding trachoma
4. Management of established trachoma
5. Management of complication

Prophylaxis

1. There is no vaccine that can prevent trachoma.
2. There is no chemoprophylaxis.
3. Prophylaxis is directed to persons at risks, i.e. those persons who do not suffer from trachoma but come in contact with persons suffering from infection (TF stage) of trachoma.

This comprises of two groups:
a. Those who suffer from the disease
b. Those who do not suffer

Those who are suffering from acute trachoma should get full antibiotic treatment. Those who are at risk should be given –

Antibiotic ointment 1% tetracycline, .5% erythromycin or 1% chloromycetin two times a day, five days a week for one month with gap of two months and the whole process is repeated till all the persons in the community have been fully treated.

The persons should be explained importance of personal cleanliness. Cleanliness of hands and face, the children are demonstrated simple method of washing the face.

The community should be explained dangers of open defecation and choked drains because they act as breeding ground of flies. The flies play an important role in spreading of trachoma.

Women and children should be asked not to share common boxes/pots of Kajal and Surma.

Management of Acute Stage

The acute stage is treated by administration of
1. 20–30 sulfacetamide three times a day.
2. Tetracycline 1%, erythromycin 0.5% or chloromycetin 1% ointment two times a day.
3. Broad spectrum antibiotic like .3% ciprofloxacin, .3% ofloxacin two times to prevent secondary infection.

Management of Blinding Trachoma Consists

1. Management of acute trachoma.
2. Intensive treatment of bacterial conjunctivitis with local broad spectrum antibiotic drops.
3. 1% atropine sulfate once a day if cornea is involved.

Management of Established Trachoma

This requires continuous treatment for at least three months.
It consists of:

   a. Capsule tetracycline 500 mg two times a day for three to four weeks. Children under ten years should not be given tetracycline.
   b. Tablet doxycycline 100 mg daily for 15 days.
   c. Tablet erythromycin 500 mg two times a day for 15 days.
   d. Azithromycin 1gm single dose.

2. Sulfacetamide drops 20% – 30% three times a day for 3 months.
3. Tetracycline ointment 1% or erythromycin ointment 0.5% two times a day.
4. Personal cleanliness.
5. Face wash

Treatment of Complication

It takes ten to fifteen years for complications to develop, so they are not seen under 20 years of age.

By the time complications develop, the person is no more infective.

The complications make the patient uncomfortable due to constant rubbing of the conjunctiva and cornea by lashes and lid margin. The eyes are red, have mucopurulent discharge, the vision is greatly reduced and there is constant watering. No medical treatment can undo the trichiasis or entropion. They require surgical correction for permanent cure. However, if there are only few lashes rubbing against the cornea, they can be **epilated** (pulled out).

The WHO model of treatment is called **SAFE** method where S stands for surgery, A for antibiotic, F for face wash and E for environment.

Adult Inclusion Conjunctivitis

This is an acute or subacute mucopurulent in young sexually active adults. It is most of the time bilateral but may start in one eye. It is always sexually transmitted disease. The infection is transferred to the eyes by hands. Corneal involvement is common. If untreated it passes into chronic conjunctivitis with superficial (on the surface) vessels on the cornea but never goes to stage of complication seen in trachoma.

Management

Local antibiotic drops four times a day. Oral antibiotics as in trachoma. If possible the sexual partner should also be treated.

Ophthalmia Neonatorum by Chlamydia (See Ophthalmia Neonatorum)

Allergic conjunctivitis

Allergy is the commonest cause of noninfective conjunctivitis. It is mostly seen in children and young adults.
Allergic conjunctivitis is of two types:

1. Exogenous (allergen reaches the eye from outside)
2. Endogenous (the allergen reaches the eye from the body itself) Flow chart 8.1

Acute Allergic Conjunctivitis

This is a bilateral conjunctivitis of sudden onset. The exact allergen may not be possible to pinpoint, which is always organic, may be microbial or of plant or animal origin. The patient suddenly develops excessive watering from both the eyes. The conjunctiva is greatly **chemosed**. The chemosed conjunctiva may protrude (come out of) through the lids. Running of nose is very common. The condition subsides without treatment within an hour or so. Instillation of weak steroid drops give prompt relief. Repeated attacks are common.

Chronic Allergic Conjunctivitis

Simple allergic conjunctivitis: This occurs many a times throughout the year in both the eyes. It is caused by recurrent entry of allergen which are commonly drugs or chemical, rarely organic allergens may also case the disease. The patient complains of constant but mild itching, constant redness, watering and discharge. It is treated by avoiding the allergen and instillation of mild steroid or drops containing antihistamine.

Flow chart 8.1: Exogenous allergic conjunctivitis can be acute or chronic

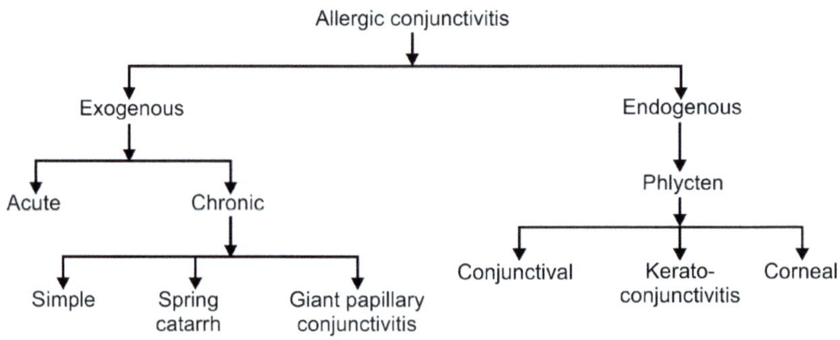

Spring Catarrh or Vernal Conjunctivitis

It is seen in **children** between five to ten years, more commonly in **boys** than girls. It is a **bilateral, recurrent**, chronic condition which develops at the onset of **summer** and passes off after the summer, only to appear next summer. However it may be seen to appear in different seasons as well. There **may be a family history**. The disease generally disappears after puberty. The exact cause is not known but external organic allergen like pollen are the commonest cause.

The main complaints are **intense itching, white thread like discharge**, redness and watering in both eyes.

There are two types –

1. Palpebral
2. Limbal

The **palpebral form** is more common than the limbal. The upper tarsal conjunctiva is more involved than the lower. The tarsal conjunctiva develops large papillae which are almost square with smooth surface. They vary in size and number. They become smaller with treatment and may disappear either with treatment or without treatment.

The **limbal form**, the similar papillae develop in the limbus. The upper limbus and temporal (towards the ear) are more involved. Rarely the papillae may involve the cornea.

Rarely both the types may be present in the same eye.

Management

The condition is **nonblinding** in spite of its long course. It requires prolonged treatment over years. The aim of the treatment is to give maximum comfort to the children with minimum medicine without side effects of the medicine.

Weak corticosteroid drops give prompt relief. They should always be prescribed under supervision of ophthalmologist.

Giant Papillary Conjunctivitis

This is less common than other types of allergic conjunctivitis. It is seen in persons using **contact lens, artificial eye** or have **nylon sutures left** in the eye following surgery. The symptoms are itching, mucoid discharge, and recurrent redness. The itching is less severe than in spring catarrh but the papillae are larger than in spring catarrh. It can be unilateral. The management is removing the cause and mild steroid drops.

Growth of the Conjunctiva

The growth of the conjunctiva can be:

1. Infective
2. Neoplastic

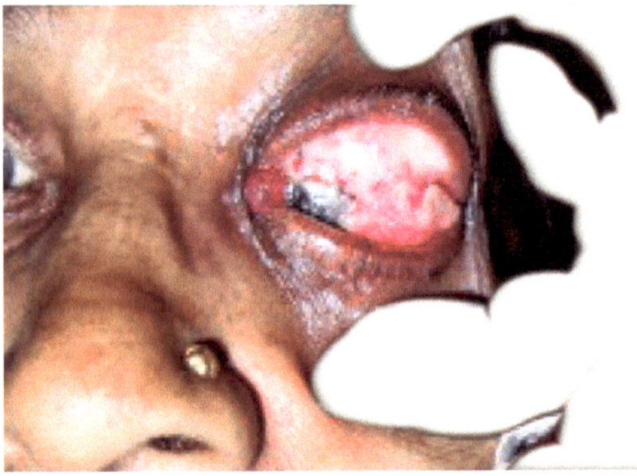

Fig. 8.9: Epidermoid (squamous cell) carcinoma arising from conjunctiva (*Courtesy:* Dr Santosh Patel)

Infective growth of conjunctiva are:

1. Burst chalazion
2. Foreign body granuloma
3. Rhinosporidiosis

The neoplastic growths of the conjunctiva can be:

- Benign (noncancer)
- Malignant (cancer)

The benign tumors of conjunctiva are:

- Nevus
- Limbal dermoids
- Dermolipoma
- Papilloma
- Hemangioma
- Neurofibroma

The malignant tumors of the conjunctiva are:

1. Epidermoid carcinoma (Fig. 8.9)
2. Basal cell carcinoma
3. Malignant melanoma

CHAPTER

9

Disorders of the Cornea

The **cornea** is the transparent anterior 1/6th (front) of the globe. The remaining 5/6 part of the globe is opaque (can not see through), white in color and called the **sclera**.

The average diameter of adult cornea is 11.7 mm. This is measured by **corneal caliper**. A cornea with diameter less than 10 mm is called **microcornea** and a cornea larger than 13 mm is called **megalocornea**.

The cornea is more curved than the sclera. The average corneal curvature is 7.5 mm. Cornea is thicker on the periphery and thin in the center. Corneal curvature is increased in **keratoconus** and is reduced in **microcornea** and **phthisis** (soft eye). The junction of cornea and sclera is **limbus**.

The main function of the cornea is visual (to see). The total power of the eye is **+60 D sphere**. Out of this power of the cornea is **+43 D**, rest **+17 D** is due to lens. To focus, the cornea should be transparent. Loss of transparency causes diminished vision when in front of the pupil.

The anterior surface (front surface) of the cornea is shinning and smooth. It is kept wet and bright by tear. The anterior surface of the cornea acts as a **convex mirror** and forms a **small, erect, virtual image** called **Purkinje image**. (Fig. 9.1).

In disease of the cornea these two properties, i.e. transparency and mirror effect are lost. Loss of these two properties result in diminished vision.

Common Features of Corneal Diseases

1. **Loss of transparency:** This results in formation **corneal opacity**. Any disease that involves the cornea results in corneal opacity. It may be temporary or permanent. The permanent opacities are the end result of diseases.

   The opacities cause diminished vision when central (in front of the pupil). The peripheral (away from the pupil) opacities do not cause diminished vision. The opacities may be single or multiple. Opacities do not stain with fluorescein. Staining of any opacity means keratitis. The opacities of cornea have been graded according to their density (Figs 9.2 to 9.5).

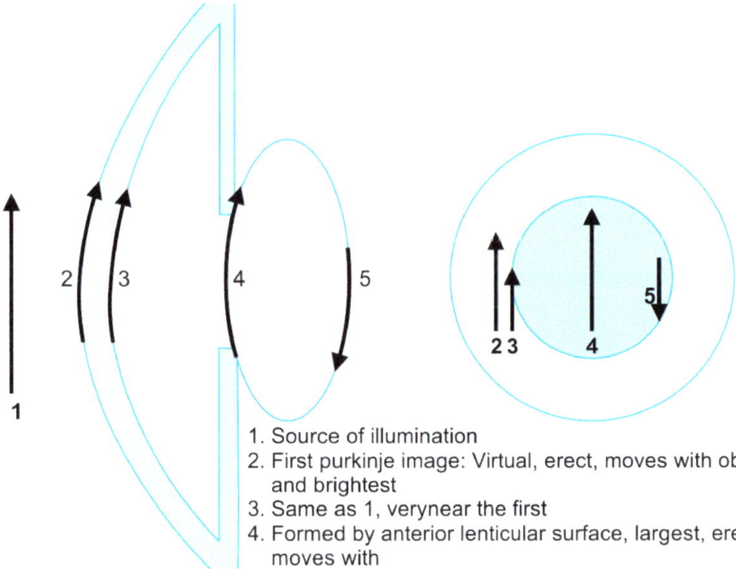

Fig. 9.1: Purkinje images

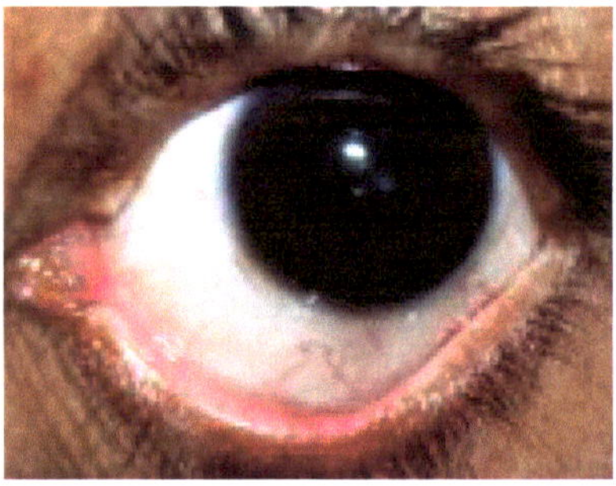

Fig. 9.2: Macular corneal opacity

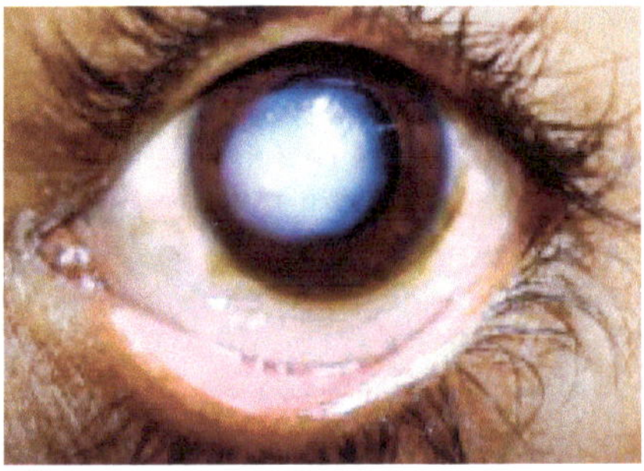

Fig. 9.3: Leukomatous corneal opacity

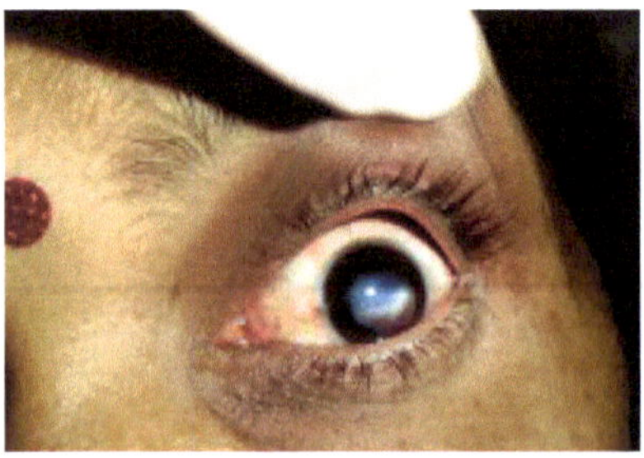

Fig. 9.4: Vascularized corneal opacity

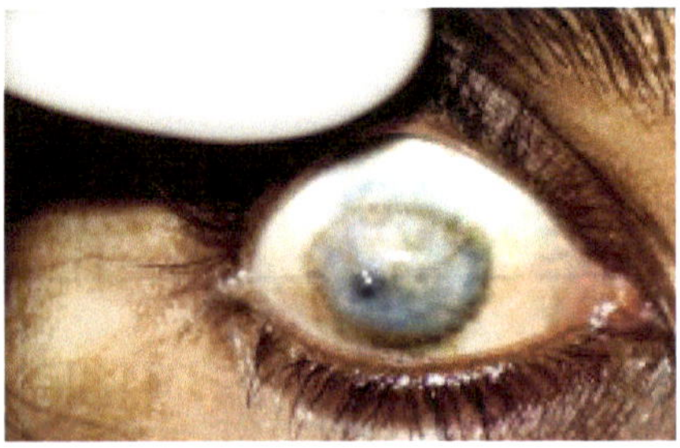

Fig. 9.5: Total corneal opacity

They are:

Nebula: Very faint, visible only on slit lamp.
Macula: Denser than nebula, visible with torch light.
Leukoma: Densest, visible in natural light.
If iris is attached to any of the opacities, it is called **leukoma adherans** (Fig. 9.6).

Corneal opacities on long run, may get vascularized (Fig. 9.4).

2. **Keratitis:** Inflammation of cornea is called keratitis. It can be infective (microorganism) or noninfective. The superficial infective keratitis is called **corneal ulcer**. The shape, size and position of corneal ulcer vary. Central ulcer cause diminished vision. The corneal ulcer stain with **fluorescein**. They are associated with pain, watering, photophobia. Severe form of corneal ulcers are associated with **hypopyon** (Fig. 9.7) (pus in the anterior chamber) (Figs 9.8 and 9.9). When corneal ulcers heal, they leave corneal opacities. Most of the corneal ulcers are associated with circumciliary congestion. This is also called circumcorneal congestion. The circumciliary congestion starts at the limbus and fades away from the limbus. Presence of circumcorneal

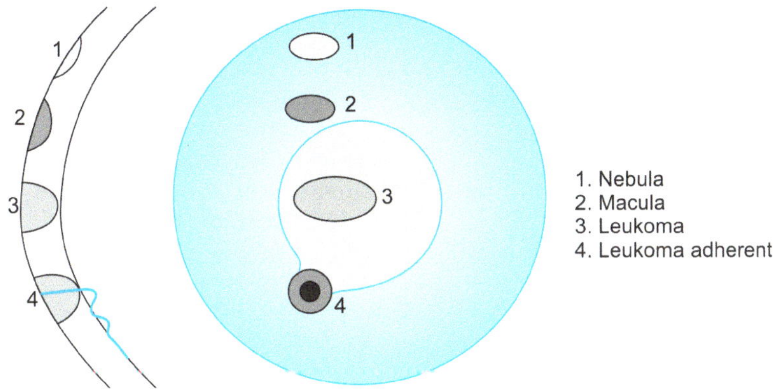

Fig. 9.6: Various grades of corneal opacities

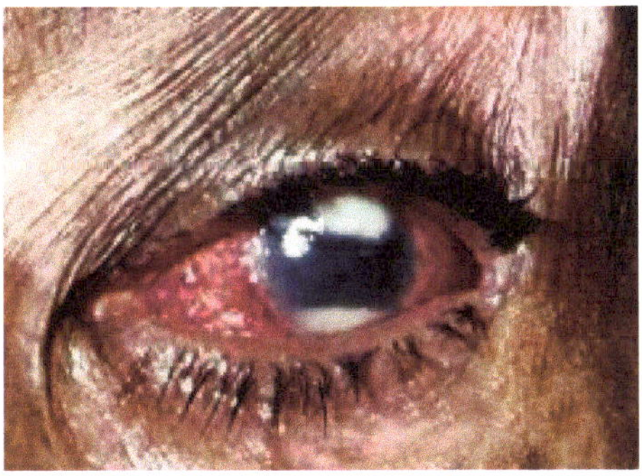

Fig. 9.7: Hypopyon corneal ulcer (*Courtesy:* Dr Santosh Patel)

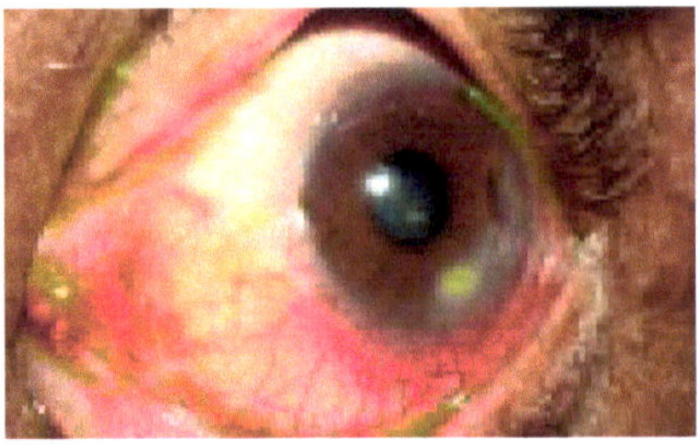

Fig. 9.8: Positive stain of corneal ulcer (*Courtesy:* Dr Santosh Patel)

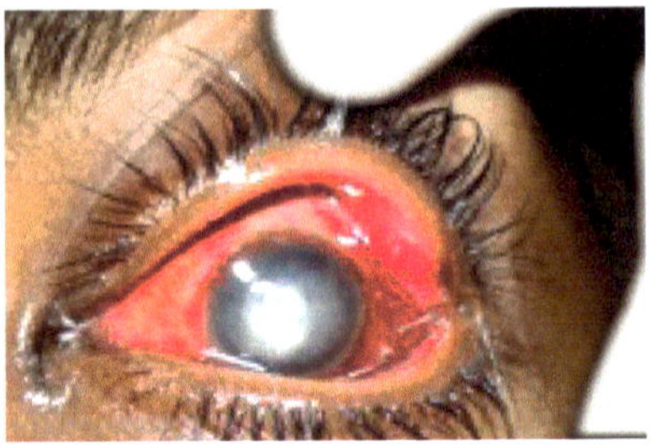

Fig. 9.9: Large corneal ulcer (*Courtesy:* Dr Santosh Patel)

congestion always does not mean corneal ulcer. Other causes of circumciliary congestion are:
- Acute iridocyclitis
- Acute congestive glaucoma
- Noninfective deep keratitis (interstitial keratitis)

Circumcorneal congestion should be differentiated from conjunctival congestion. It is common to have both the types of congestion at the same time in the same eye.

Differentiating features are given in the following chart.

Conjunctival congestion	**Circumciliary congestion**
Start in periphery	Start round the cornea
Spread towards cornea	Spread away from cornea
Large irregular branching join each other	Small regular straight, do not join each other
Move with conjunctiva	Do not move
Associated with conjunctiva discharge	Watery discharge
May extend over the cornea	Do not invade cornea

3. **Vascularization of cornea**

Cornea is avascular (no blood vessels are present). Presence of blood vessels always means corneal disease. The vascularization can be **superficial** or **deep**. Superficial vascularization is seen in kerato-conjunctivitis. Deep vascularization is seen in deep keratitis. They can be differentiated from each other by following features: (Figs. 9.10 and 9.11)

Superficial corneal vascularization	**Deep corneal vascularization**
Start in the conjunctiva and cross the limbus in the epithelium	Start in the sclera, are not visible at the limbus, grow in the corneal structure
Bright red in color, branching irregular, join each other. Seen in trachoma, phlycten, chronic corneal ulcer	Pink in color, do not join seen in deep keratitis

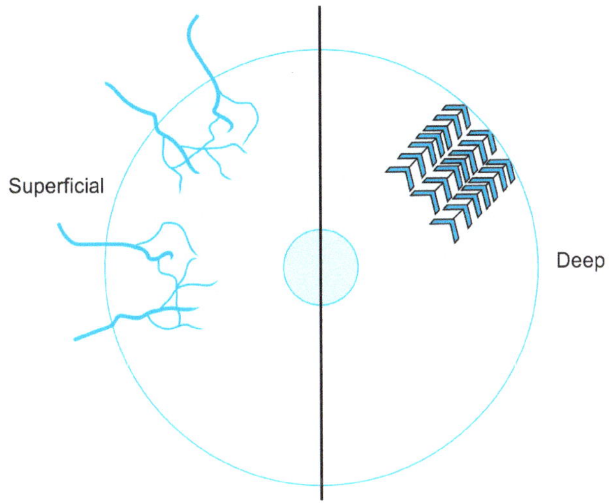

Fig. 9.10: Vascularization of the cornea

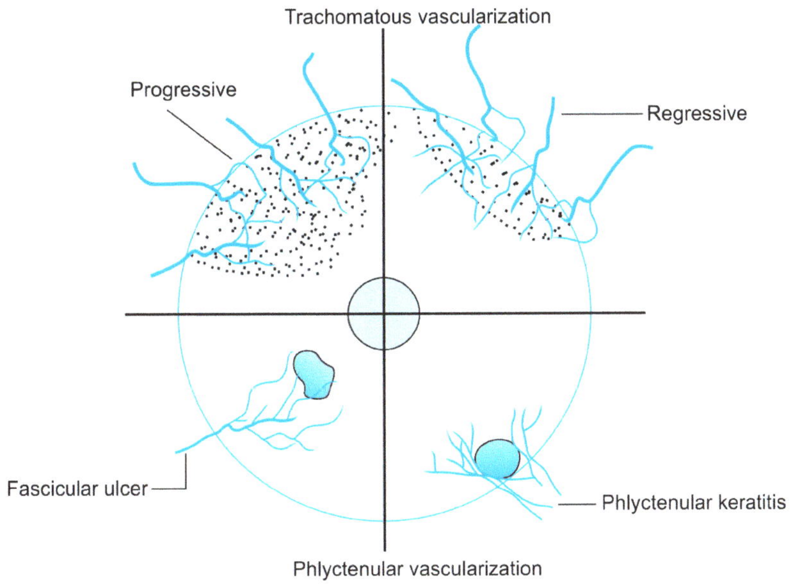

Fig. 9.11: Types of superficial vascularization of cornea

4. **Change in size and shape of the cornea**
   Corneal size is **reduced** in **microcornea** and **microphthalmos** (where whole size is smaller than normal) and **phthisis** (soft and shrunken eye). Corneal size is **increased** in **buphthalmos** and **keratoglobus**.
   Curvature is increased in keratoconus and keratoglobus.
   Curvature is irregular in corneal staphyloma.
   Corneal disorders can be:

- Congenital (present from birth)
- Acquired (developing after birth)

CONGENITAL DISORDERS OF THE CORNEA

Microcornea

The cornea is smaller than 9 mm in diameter. It is flat. It may be unilateral or bilateral. The anterior chamber is shallow. The pupil may be circular or key hole shaped. The eye has poor vision. The error of refraction is generally hypermetropic. Treatment consists of improving vision by glasses as far as possible.

Buphthalmos

The corneal diameter is more than 13 mm, may be as much as 17 mm. The corneal curvature is increased. The anterior chamber is deep. The commonest cause is **congenital glaucoma**. It may be unilateral or bilateral. Treatment is management of glaucoma by surgery.

Keratoglobus: This is similar to buphthalmos but the tension is not raised, does not require any treatment except correction of error of refraction when present.

Acquired disorders of cornea can be:

- Trauma
- Infection
- Inflammation
- Allergy
- Nutritional

Commonest Acquired Disorders of the Cornea

The term **keratitis** is used for both superficial and deep infection of the cornea. The superficial infective keratitis is called corneal ulcer. There is breach in epithelium in corneal ulcer.

Corneal ulcer: There are two types of corneal ulcers; **central** and **peripheral (Fig. 9.12)**. The corneal ulcer can be caused by any of the following : Bacteria, virus, fungus and parasites.

Bacterial Corneal Ulcer

Many pus forming bacteria cause corneal ulcer. Bacterial ulcers are very common. They are generally **central** (in front of the pupil). Bacterial corneal ulcers generally develop **after injury** to the epithelium. The injury may be very mild like a fine scratch in the epithelium which should normally heal in two to three days if it is not contaminated by microorganisms. In case of contamination a corneal ulcer develops.

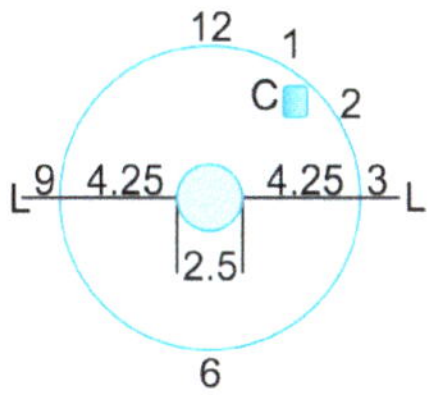

Corneal ulcer 'C' is situated 1 mm inside the limbus, 3.25 mm away from the pupillary margin, between 1 O'clock and 2 O'clock

Fig. 9.12: Recording of the position of corneal ulcer

> There are few bacteria that can cause corneal ulcer without injury. They are gonococcus and diphtheria.

A bacterial ulcer develops within 24 to 48 hours after injury. It sometimes develops within hours of injury.

Following conditions cause corneal ulcers more frequently:

Chronic dacryocystitis, trichiasis, corneal foreign bodies, entropion, ectropion, lagophthalmos, loss of sensation and diabetes.

Bacterial corneal ulcers are generally unilateral. They can be central (in front of the pupil) or peripheral (away from the pupil).

A bacterial corneal ulcer has acute onset with foreign body sensation, pain, watering, redness, diminished vision. Some corneal ulcers are very painful.

On examination, the conjunctiva is congested. There is circumciliary congestion. The ulcer looks gray in color and stains with fluorescein. Central corneal ulcers cause more loss of vision than peripheral. In severe infection hypopyon (pus in anterior chamber) may be present.

A simple corneal ulcer with mild infection should heal within seven to ten days with treatment without complication or may leave faint corneal opacity.

If the corneal ulcer does not heal, it not only spreads on the surface of the cornea but also becomes deep reaching the Descemet's membrane. This causes the Descemet's membrane to bulge through the corneal ulcer. This is called **Descemetocele** or **keratocele**. If the Descemet's membrane perforates, a small hole develops in the cornea, this is called **perforation of corneal ulcer**.

As soon as the corneal ulcer perforates, the aqueous leaks from the anterior chamber and the iris moves to close the perforation resulting in **leukoma adherent**.

If the perforation is large, the corneal cells from periphery shift towards the center and a **pseudocornea develops**. The pseudocornea is thin, irregular and white. Due to its thinness, it bulges forward and the condition is called **anterior staphyloma**. This can involve whole or part of the cornea.

On many cases the lens and vitreous may come out of the large perforation and a **phthisis** results (Flow chart 9.1).

Flow chart 9.1: Fate of a corneal ulcer

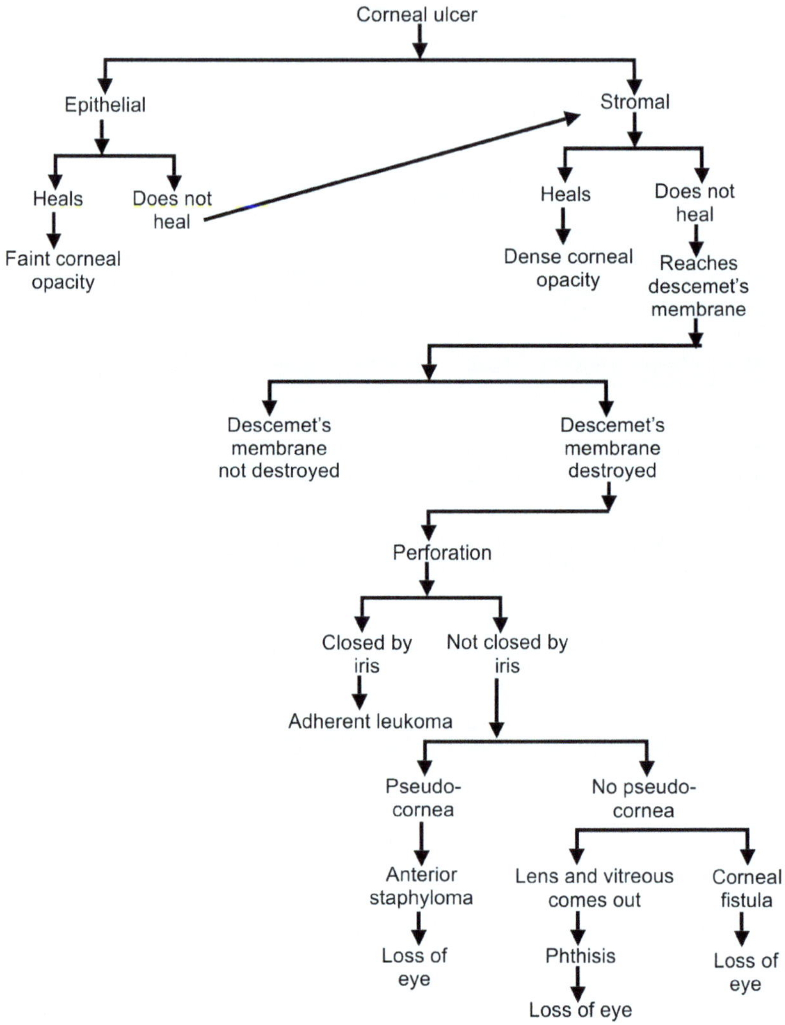

Hypopyon Corneal Ulcer

Corneal ulcer with pus in anterior chamber is called **hypopyon corneal ulcer**. It is a serious condition. The pus is sterile (does not contain micro-organism). However, hypopyon may develop without corneal ulcer in case of severe iridocyclitis (Fig. 9.13).

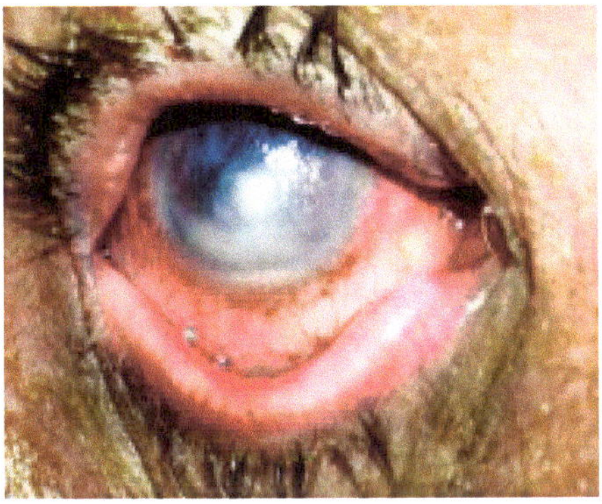

Fig. 9.13: Hypopyon corneal ulcer (*Courtesy:* Dr Santosh Patel)

Causes of bilateral corneal ulcers are:
1. Keratomalacia
2. Ophthalmia neonatorum
3. Measles
4. Leprosy
5. Herpes simplex
6. Blast injury

There are many causes that result in corneal opacities that can be bilateral or unilateral.

Causes of Bilateral Corneal Opacity

1. Congenital (Present at birth)	– Rare
2. Trauma	– Blast injury
	– Chemical injury
3. Infection	– Ophthalmia neonatorum
	– Smallpox (fresh cases are not seen now a days)
	– Leprosy
	– Trachoma
	– Interstitial keratitis
4. Allergy	– Phlyctenular keratitis
5. Nutritional	– Keratomalacia
6. Degeneration	– Arcus senilis (old age)
	– Arcus juvenilis (young age)
	– Band keratopathy
7. Dystrophy	– Epithelial
	– Stromal
	– Endothelial
	– Combined

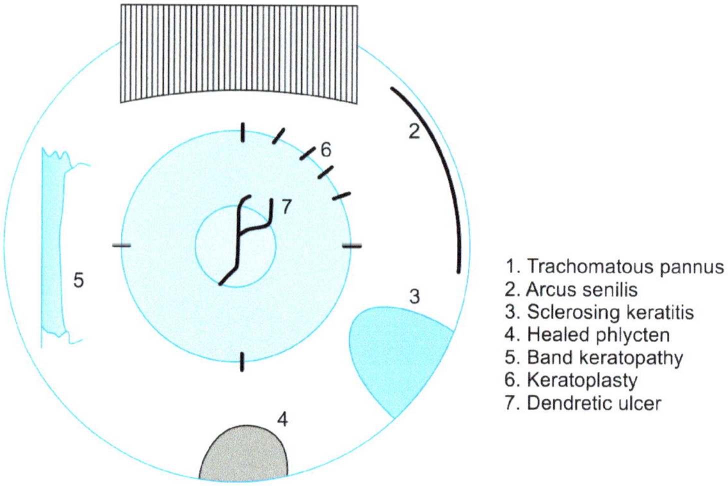

Fig. 9.14: Position of various common corneal opacities

8. Miscellaneous
   - Pterygium
   - Blood staining of cornea
   - Keratoplasty
   - Radial keratotomy
   - Keratoconus
   - Limbal dermoid

Management of Bacterial Corneal Ulcer

Bacterial ulcers are ocular emergencies. All central ulcers even of short duration that stain with fluorescein should be treated without delay.

The treatment of simple bacterial corneal ulcers consists of:

1. Cleaning of the lid margin, and remove discharge. There is no need to wash the conjunctival sac.
2. Instillation of any broad spectrum antibiotic hourly during the day and eye ointment of the same antibiotic by night.
3. One drop of one percent atropine sulfate once a day in children and two times a day in adults for two to three days.
4. Systemic antibiotics are not needed.
5. If there is no discharge from the eye, the eye may be bandaged with pad at night. Other wise left open.

Treatment of Hypopyon Corneal Ulcer

Presence of hypopyon (pus in AC) is more serious than simple corneal ulcer. It requires more frequent instillation of antibiotic.

The treatment consists of

1. Cleaning the lid margin.
2. Removal of discharge.
3. Instillation of atropine sulfate one percent in the morning and at night.
4. Instillation of fortified drop of gentamycin or cephazoline:
   - Every five minutes for six times.
   - Every ten minutes for six times.
   - Then every hourly by day.
   - Every two hourly by night.
   - Tablet acetazolamide 250 mg two times a day.
5. If the above method does not improve in 24 hours, then **subconjunctival gentamycin 20 mg** is recommended in addition to local fortified antibiotic drop.

How to Prepare Fortified Solution of Gentamycin

Drops of gentamycin are available as 0.3% solution in bottle and injection is available as 20 mg per mm in ampoule. To prepare fortified drop of gentamycin, 40 mg of injectable gentamycin is added to 5 ml bottle of gentamycin eye drop. This drop should be used within ten days of preparation and kept in refrigerator in between the use.

Management of Corneal Opacity

1. Best management is to prevent formation of opacity in keratitis and corneal ulcer by prompt and proper treatment.
2. Once corneal opacities have developed, there **is no medical** method to remove them.
3. Only method of removing them is by **keratoplasty**.

All opacities do not require keratoplasty, only central opacities require keratoplasty.

Keratoplasty

Keratoplasty is a surgical procedure by which the opaque cornea is replaced by a clear cornea. **Keratoplasty is not replacement of whole eye**. Keratoplasty will not improve vision unless the cause is in the cornea. In keratoplasty cornea from a dead body is grafted in place of opaque cornea. The cornea has to be removed from the dead body within four hours of death. The unused cornea can be stored in eye bank. There are two types of keratoplasty, **full thickness keratoplasty** also known as **penetrating keratoplasty** and **lamellar keratoplasty** or **partial thickness keratoplasty** (Fig. 9.15).

Viral Keratitis

1. All viruses that involve conjunctiva can infect the cornea.
2. The common viruses that infect the cornea are:

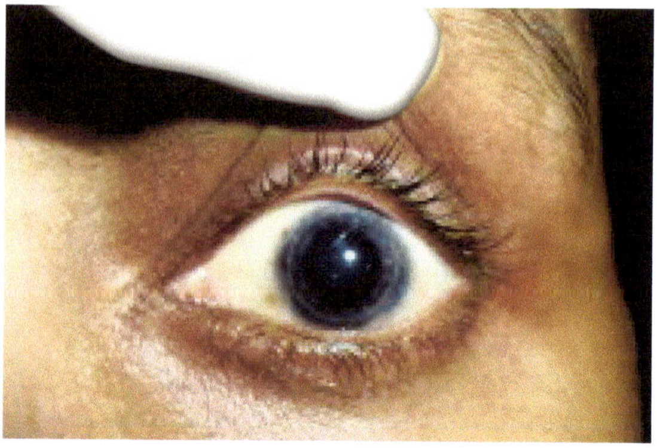

Fig. 9.15: Keratoplasty (*Courtesy: Dr Santosh Patel*)

i. Adenoviruses
ii. Epidemic keratoconjunctivitis virus
iii. Pharyngo conjunctival fever virus
iv. Acute hemorrhagic conjunctivitis virus
v. Measles virus
vi. Herpes simplex virus
vii. Herpes zoster virus

Out of the two herpes viruses, i.e. the herpes simplex and herpes zoster, the former is more common.

Herpes Simplex Keratitis

The herpes simplex keratitis is seen in all ages from neonate to old age. Fortunately in neonates it is mild and self-limiting. In adults, it is troublesome and recurrent, may cause permanent diminished vision. There are two types of corneal involvement in herpes simples, i.e. the primary and recurrent.

The **primary herpes simplex keratitis** is commonly seen between six months to ten years of age. It develops due to transfer of infection from an infected person to a nonimmune child. The features of primary herpes simplex keratitis are **unilateral blepharitis**, may have **vesicles** on the lid skin, follicular conjunctivitis and keratitis that is generally in the form of **superficial punctate keratitis**. It does not develop usual dendretic form seen in adults. The disease may pass into recurrent stage. Treatment consists of local antiviral drops for few days.

Recurrent Herpes Simplex Keratitis

This is more common than the former. It may be localized to epithelium only or may involved deep layers.

The progress of the epithelial lesions are:
Superficial punctate keratitis→Dendretic ulcer→Geographic ulcer→ Keratitis meta herpetica

The deep keratitis are:
- Stromal keratitis
- Disciform keratitis
- Trophic keratitis

Epithelial lesions are seen in adults. This is due to reactivation of primary lesion of childhood. The lesions start as small lesions in the epithelium that stain with fluorescein. **The corneal sensation is reduced**. This may heal or may pass into stage of dendretic ulcer.

Dendretic ulcers develop when punctate (pin point) join to form branch like epithelial defects. The bed of the ulcer stains with fluorescein and the margin and tips of the ulcer stain with Rose Bengal. The corneal sensation is reduced, hence, the patient does not complain of pain. Only reduced vision with watering are the two common complaints. The dendretic ulcer may heal with treatment or may pass into next stage of **geographic ulcers**. These are also called **ameboid ulcers**. They are larger than the dendretic ulcer. When these ulcers fail the condition passes into stage of **keratitis meta herpetica**.

Treatment

Punctate keratitis, dendretic ulcer and geographic ulcers require frequent antiviral drops or ointment for five days. No steroids should be used in herpetic keratitis. If it fails than the ulcer should be cauterized (burnt by carbolic acid). The meta herpetic keratitis does not heal by antiviral therapy alone, requires soft contact lens to heal in addition to antiviral drops.

Deep herpetic keratitis may either be caused by the virus or hypersensitivity (allergy) to the virus. The invasion by virus may lead to perforation. The disciform keratitis and trophic ulcers require specialized treatment under trained ophthalmologist.

Fungal Keratitis (Myotic Keratitis)

Fungal keratitis is one of the most serious forms of keratitis. It was commonly seen in villages following injury by plants or animals but now-a-days it is seen in urban (town) people as well in persons who are:
1. On corticosteroid drugs both local or oral
2. Long-term broad spectrum antibiotics
3. Cancer drugs
4. Suffering from
   - AIDS
   - Diabetes
   - Leprosy
5. Contact lens user

Typical ulcer develops seven to fifteen days after injury by organic matter (plant or animal) in the stroma as yellowish raised area with irregular margins. There may be small areas of keratitis around the main ulcer. The eye is much congested. Vision is diminished, soon develops a thick hypopyon. The ulcer does not respond to usual antibiotic and atropine.

The treatment consists of –

1. Atropine sulfate one percent two times a day
2. Anti fungal drops and ointment
3. Systemic anti fungal
4. Oral diamox

If the ulcer does not heal, a penetrating keratoplasty may help.

Marginal Corneal Ulcers

Marginal corneal ulcers are noninfective except herpes simplex. They are hypersensitive (allergic) in nature.

The common marginal ulcers are

- Phlyctenular ulcer
- Marginal infiltrates
- Mooren's ulcer

Out of the three, the phlyctenular ulcer is the commonest and Mooren's ulcer is the least common. The marginal ulcers are generally nonvision threatening. They do not perforate. They are self-limiting but very painful.

Phlyctenular Corneal Ulcer (Figs 9.16 and 9.17)

This is seen in children between one to ten years in both sexes. It may be unilateral or bilateral. Ulcers are part of phlyctenular keratitis and follow a phlycten that is partly on the conjunctiva and partly on the cornea. The number of phlycten may be one or more. When more than one they may develop all-round on the periphery of the cornea. Once phlycten develops at the limbus, it is very painful associated with redness, watering,

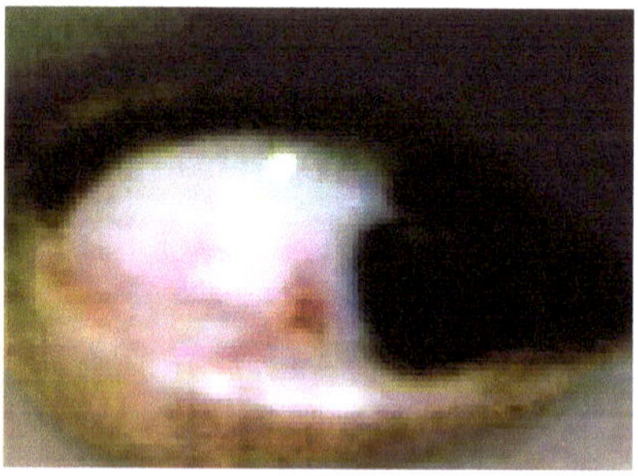

Fig. 9.16: Conjunctiva phlycten not likely to involve cornea (*Courtesy*: Dr Nidhi Pandey)

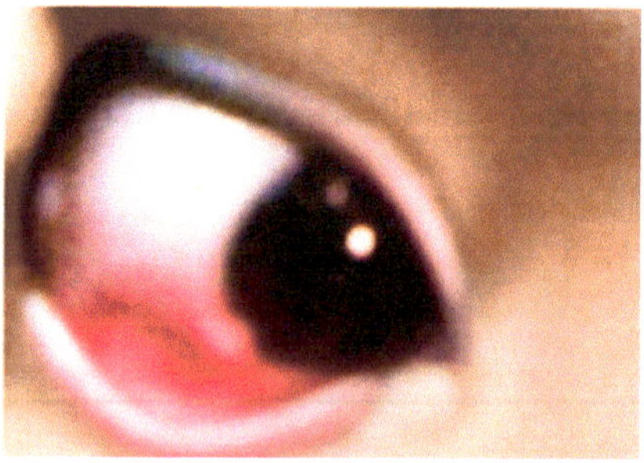

Fig. 9.17: Limbal phlycten likely to involve cornea (*Courtesy*: Dr Nidhi Pandey)

photophobia and blepharospasm (forceful closure of lid). Phlyctenular keratoconjunctivitis is the commonest cause of photophobia and blepharospasm in children. The phlycten generally ulcerates before healing. A phlyctenular ulcer may heal even without treatment or may shift over the cornea. When the phlyctenular corneal ulcer moves towards the pupil, the ulcer is accompanied by a bunch of blood vessels. Such a phlyctenular corneal ulcer is called **fascicular ulcer**. The vision is greatly reduced when the fascicular ulcer is on the pupil (Fig. 9.18).

The anterior chamber and pupil are not effected by phlyctenular keratitis. Management of phlyctenular keratoconjunctivitis is local steroid drops under supervision of ophthalmologist.

Marginal Corneal Infiltrates

These are less common than phlyctenular keratitis, seen in adults. They are self-limiting (heal without treatment) but recurrent. They are very painful. They respond well to mild steroid drops.

Mooren's ulcer rare degenerative deep ulcers seen in elderly persons. They generally do not perforate unless infected. They require specialized treatment in specialized hospital.

Trachoma

Trachoma is a chronic keratoconjunctivitis that has acute (sudden) onset in childhood. It is an important cause of treatable and preventable blindness. Involvement of the cornea is the cause of blindness. The cornea is involved in acute as well as chronic stage. The corneal changes can be divided into following groups:

1. Early
2. Late
3. Delayed

The early corneal changes consists of:

i. Superficial punctate keratitis in the upper part. The keratitis is visible after fluorescein with cobalt blue filter under high magnification.
ii. Micropannus—Small areas of superficial vascularization that does not extending more than one millimeter towards the pupil.

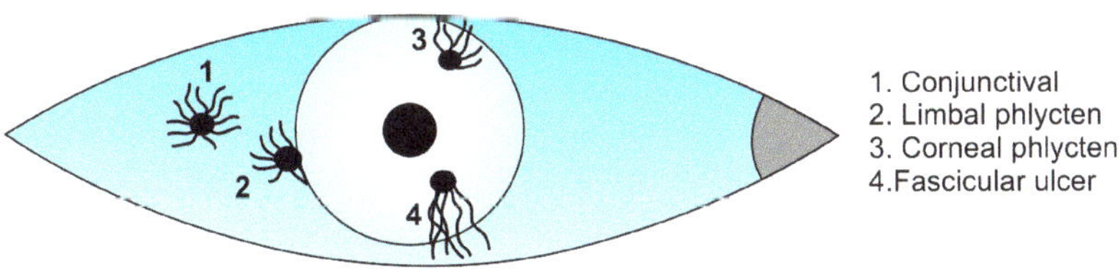

Fig. 9.18: Various stages of phlycten

Late changes consists of:

i. Gross pannus
ii. Herbert's follicles—Follicles similar to those seen in tarsal conjunctiva are seen at the upper part of the cornea.
iii. Herber's pits—The Herbert's follicles mature and burst to form small pits at the limbus. They are signs of established trachoma.
iv. Superficial vascularisation of the cornea—This is called **pannus** formation. There are two types pannus—**progressive pannus** and **regressive pannus**. They may develop anywhere on the corneal periphery but the most common site is upper part of the cornea. The blood vessels grow from the conjunctiva between the epithelium and the Bowman's membrane towards the pupil and may cover the pupil reducing vision. If treated before they destroy the Bowman's membrane. They may disappear fully otherwise they leave a permanent scars.

The delayed corneal changes are due to:

1. Secondary bacterial infection—Secondary bacterial infection in trachoma results in **blinding trachoma**.
2. Constant rubbing of the cornea by trichiasis or entropion.

Management of corneal involvement in trachoma

The early changes are treatable by usual antitrachoma antibiotics and do not require any surgery.

The late changes are partly treatable by antitrachoma antibiotic, do not require any surgery.

The delayed changes are not treatable medically but require surgery.

The surgery is divided into two parts:

i. Correction of trichiasis and entropion
ii. Keratoplasty. No keratoplasty should be done without correcting trichiasis, entropion and vascularization.

Deep Keratitis

This group of diseases is also known as **parenchymatous keratitis** or **interstitial keratitis**.

Common causes of interstitial keratitis are:

1. Congenital syphilis
2. Acquired syphilis
3. Tuberculosis
4. Herpes simplex (disciform keratitis)
5. Herpes zoster (disciform keratitis)

Interstitial keratitis is inflammation of corneal stroma due to allergic reaction of the cornea to the microorganisms. It is seen in two forms: (1) Children, (2) Adults.

Interstitial keratitis in children is more common than in adults. It is seen between one year to fifteen years of age. It is bilateral. It is caused by inherited syphilis. The mother passes the infection to the fetus via placenta. It is caused due to sensitization of cornea by a organism of syphilis known as *Treponema pallidum*. Associated iridocyclitis is always present with the condition. It has an acute onset and a long course.

It starts as watering, photophobia and blepharospasm. On examination there is circumciliary congestion. Deep vessels encroach from the periphery all-round in sectors to meet in front of the pupil. The vessels are straight and have a look of bottle brush. They do not join each other as in case of superficial vascularization. The vascularization gives a ground glass (hazy) appearance to the cornea and the blood in the vessels give the cornea a dull pink color. Once the vessels meet in front of the pupil, vascularization stops and the vessels start disappearing from the periphery. The acute stage last for weeks. The chronic stages lasts for months and the stage of recovery lasts for years.

It is generally associated with diminished hearing and flat nose bridge. The condition is self-limiting. It is relieved over the months. Instillation of steroid drops one hourly along with one percent atropine sulfate give prompt relief but steroid has to be used for years. Treatment of syphilis by antibiotics does not cure interstitial keratitis but is essential to treat congenital syphilis to prevent damage to the heart and brain.

Adult form of Interstitial Keratitis

The adult form develops years after the person has been infected by *Treponema pallidum*. It is unilateral, less severe and starts in the upper limbus. It is also associated with iridocyclitis. The treatment is systemic penicillin, local atropine and strong steroidal drops. The steroid has to be administered for months to years with usual precautions.

Tubercular interstitial keratitis is seen less commonly than syphilitic interstitial keratitis, is unilateral and sectorial. The lower sector is more involved than upper. The symptoms and signs are similar to interstitial keratitis due to acquired syphilis. The treatment is local atropine and steroid. The patient should get complete antitubercular treatment.

Disciform Keratitis

This is a localized form of deep keratitis. The common causes are herpes simplex and herpes zoster virus. Many a times no cause can be found out. It may also be seen in acquired syphilis, tuberculosis and injury. It is an unilateral condition seen in adults generally in front of the pupil causing diminished vision. The cause of the disease is allergy to the virus in case of herpes simplex and zoster and hypersensitivity to tubercular or treponema protein. Treatment is local weak solution of steroids.

Corneal Degenerations

Degenerations are a group of diseases that develop in cornea secondary to some primary diseases like iridocyclitis, glaucoma or injury. They are generally unilateral and nonhereditary.

The two common corneal degeneration are **band keratopathy** and **nodular keratopathy**.

Band Keratopathy

The degeneration is seen exclusively in the inter palpebral aperture (between the lids) in front of the pupil as a horizontal band of white rough opacity. A fully developed band keratopathy is visible in ordinary torch light. The color is due to deposition of calcium in the anterior corneal stroma, Bowman's membrane and epithelium. Its starts on the periphery of the cornea from both sides leaving a clear zone between the opacity and the limbus, gradually growing to meet the other end in the center. The band has circular clear areas in the white deposits. So long it does not cover the pupil, the vision remains good. Once the pupil is covered, the vision drops. It takes months to years for the band to develop fully. It is not painful because it develops when the iridocyclitis or glaucoma has subsided.

It requires specialized treatment that includes keratoplasty.

Nodular Degeneration of Cornea

This is less common than band keratopathy, seen in adults, who have suffered from phlyctenular keratitis and fascicular ulcer in childhood. This consists of white nodules in anterior stroma and Bowman's membrane. This nodule may bulge under the epithelium. They generally do not reduce vision and do not require treatment.

Corneal Dystrophies

Corneal dystrophies are rare in Indians. They are often hereditary, bilateral, may start in childhood and progress over years and then stop increasing. They are not related to any ocular disease or trauma. The loss of vision due to dystrophies is not marked. They are bilateral and equal in both eyes. They may involve any of the layer of the cornea or may involve more than one layer.

Keratoconus (Conical Cornea)

This is a bilateral condition. The age of onset is between ten to twenty years. It is supposed to be a dystrophy. It involves all the layers of the cornea in the central part. The cornea bulges in the center. It progresses slowly up to forty years of age but may stop at any age as well. In some cases it progresses very fast and ruptures the Descemet's membrane. In such case the aqueous enters the cornea. The cornea becomes cloudy and painful and the vision suddenly falls to hand movement.

Otherwise the only symptom is fall of distant vision due to irregular myopic astigmatism which is confirmed by retinoscopy, keratoscopy, keratometer and video keratograph.

Retinoscopy shows:

1. Myopic refraction with scissor movement. The axes are always oblique.
2. The central part shows a black spot.
3. A black circle at the base of the cone.

   The keratoscope placido disc shows irregularity in the rings.

   In advance cases the corneal bulge is visible when seen from the side.

Miscellaneous Condition of Cornea

Arcus senilis: This is a very common bilateral symptomless condition seen in persons after 40 years of age. It is hereditary. It is due to deposition of lipid (fat) in the cornea. It starts as grey line 1mm inside the limbus on the upper and lower part of the cornea and spread on each side till the ends meet. Sometimes it is so prominent that it is visible in natural light. It does not require any treatment. only importance of the condition is that many persons with arcus have raised cholesterol in their blood which requires treatment.

When the arcus develops under 40 years, it is called **arcus juvenilis**. It also does not require any treatment.

Neurotrophic Keratitis

This happens whenever the corneal sensation is lost permanently or for long time due to **lesion of fifth cranial nerve**. Normal corneal sensation is essential to protect the cornea from injury by blinking and Bell's phenomenon.

Bell's phenomenon is upward rotation of the eyeball when the lids are closed. This movement of the globe up is not present in absence of corneal sensation. In absence of corneal sensation, the blinking are lost and the cornea is exposed to outward injury. This causes corneal ulcer. The commonest cause of permanent loss of corneal sensation is **leprosy**. This may be bilateral. Others causes are **herpes zoster ophthalmicus** and destruction of trigeminal ganglion by surgery or injection of alcohol or tumor. The condition is unilateral. As there is no corneal sensation, the patient is not aware of corneal ulcer but circumciliary congestion is always present. The ulcer stains with fluorescein. Hypopyon is common. Perforation is common.

Treatment consists of early diagnosis, soft contact lens and tarsorrhaphy. In tarsorrhaphy the skin of the lid margins is removed and the two raw surfaces are stitched. This protects the cornea from injury and allows the ulcer to heal.

In all cases of corneal ulcer the corneal sensation must be tested not to miss the diagnosis.

Neuroparalytic Keratitis

In this case, the corneal sensation and the Bell's phenomenon are present but the patient is unable to close the lids due to paralysis of the seventh cranial nerve. This is called **lagophthalmos**. Here corneal ulcer develops in the lower part. The commonest cause is **leprosy** where sensation is also abolished. The other cause is Bell's palsy. As the **corneal sensation is present**, the patient can feel the pain of corneal ulcer. The ulcer starts in the lower part and spreads towards the pupil. Hypopyon is common.

Treatment is protection of cornea by tarsorrhaphy along with usual treatment of corneal ulcer. Thus in all cases of corneal ulcer, specially of lower part, the action of orbicularis should be examined and if it is found to be absent or poor, all steps should be taken to protect the cornea.

Bullous Keratitis

Normal corneal epithelium is loosely attached to the Bowman's membrane. It is flat and smooth. Though it is sensitive to touch, the normal movement of lids do not cause discomfort. Once fluid gathers under the epithelium, it is separated from the Bowman's membrane, the surface of epithelium is converted into fluid filled nodule called bullae, which is very painful even to normal movement of the lids. The source of fluid is not from the epithelial surface (the front surface) but the endothelial (back surface). Presence of bullae on the anterior surface always means damage to the endothelium.

The common causes of bullus keratitis are **aphakia**, **pseudophakia** specially with AC, IOL, long standing **glaucoma** and **uveitis**, **disciform keratitis**, some corneal dystrophies, vitreous in anterior chamber.

The condition is painful. There is lot of watering, vision is reduced. If the bullae bursts and gets infected, a corneal ulcer develops.

The usual treatment consists of instillation of hypertonic saline five percent two to three times a day, therapeutic contact lens, penetrating keratoplasty. If all fail, a tarsorrhaphy may give relief to the pain.

Exposure Keratitis

Exposure keratitis is a corneal ulcer that develops when the lids fail to cover the cornea. It happens in proptosis, exophthalmos, lagophthalmos, coloboma of lids, ectropion of lower lid.

Management is correction of the defect, i.e. reduction of proptosis and exophthalmos, correction of coloboma and ectropion and tarsorrhaphy.

Welding Arc Injury

If a person watches welding procedure from very short distance for a few minutes without protective glasses he develops acute severe pain, photophobia, blepharospasm and watering. These symptoms do not take place immediately after exposure, it takes six to eight hours to develop the symptoms. It is a bilateral condition. On examination, there is severe blepharospasm. The cornea is bright in most of the cases or may develop scattered staining by fluorescein. The anterior chamber and pupil are normal.

The management consists of instillation of four percent xylocaine in each eye. This initially causes intense burning but in a few minutes give relief. This is followed by instillation of broad spectrum antibiotic and non steroidal antiinflammatory drugs three to four times. Pain killers by mouth may be required.

Keratomalacia

Keratomalacia is a serious bilateral condition. It is an important cause of blindness in children. It is fully preventable. Once it has happened, it is difficult to treat. It is due to lack of vitamin A in child's diet. A child may complain of diminished night vision before the onset of keratomalacia but it may develop without night blindness as well. The keratomalacia is always associated with xerosis (dryness) of conjunctiva.

On examination the child is malnourished. The conjunctiva is dry. The cornea is hazy and dull. The ulcer when present is central and fast growing without circumciliary congestion and perforates soon.

Management

The condition is fully preventable by administering 100000 units of oral vitamin A to every child from six months to six years every six months.

CONTACT LENSES

Contact lenses are optical devices that are put on the cornea to improve vision and some corneal disorders in stead of spectacles. They are made of special plastic material. They remain in place in front of the cornea by surface tension of the tear film. The optics of contact lens differs from optics of the spectacles. When a contact lens is put on the cornea, a thin film of tear enters in between the back surface of contact lens and front surface of the cornea. This abolishes the corneal curvature. Thus, cornea, tear film and contact lens forms an optical unit. The power of the contact lens is given on the front surface of the contact lens by changing its curvature. A curvature more than normal corneal curvature produces minus effect and a curvature less than normal corneal curvature gives plus effect. The corneal curvature is called **K reading** that is measured by an instrument called **keratometer**. Power of the contact lens and spectacle lenses are not equal. Power of the minus contact lens is always less than the minus power in the spectacle and power of plus contact lens is more than plus power in spectacle. The low degree of astigmatism is corrected by ordinary contact lenses. For high astigmatism, special contact lenses are required. Contact lenses are given for distant correction. They do not correct presbyopia which requires spectacle in addition to contact lens, unless special bifocal contact lenses are used. The size and material by which the contact lenses are made differ from lens to lens. As per material used, contact lenses can be hard, soft or gas permeable hard (rigid lenses). Each has its own merits and demerits Table 9.1.

Table 9.1: Comparison between hard, soft and gas permeable hard lenses

	Hard lenses	Soft lenses	Gas permeable rigid lenses
Material	PMMA	HEMA	Silicone with PMMA
Size	Smaller than cornea 8.5 mm to 10.0 mm	Larger than cornea 13.5–14.5 mm	Larger than hard contact lens
Water content	3% of weight	40% of weight	In between
Oxygen supply to cornea	Nil	Good	Fair
Wear	Daily 8 hourly	Extended—more than 24 hours.	Between 8 hours to 24 hours
Vision correction	Very good	Fair	Moderate
Correction of astigmatism	Best	Poor	Moderate
Tolerance	Poor	Best	Moderate
Maintenance	Easy	Difficult	Difficult
Complication	Least	Most	Intermediate
Cost	Cheap	Most expensive	Expensive

Contact lenses are made of special nontoxic plastics called polymers. Commonly used materials are—Polymethyl methacrylate (PMMA) and hydroxyethyl methacrylate (HEMA). The first is used for hard contact lenses and the second for soft contact lenses. The PMMA lenses are rigid (hard). They contain only three percent water and do not contain oxygen or allow oxygen to pass through them. They are small, 8.5 mm to 10 mm diameter. The HEMA lenses are soft. They contain 40% water and allow oxygen to pass through them. They are larger than hard lenses, i.e. 13.5 mm to 14.5 mm in diameter. There is a third type that has more water content than hard but less than soft lenses and allow a large amount of oxygen to pass through them. They are called gas permeable hard lenses. They contain silicone as well as PMMA.

Indications for Contact Lens (Why Contact Lenses are Prescribed)

1. Optical
   - i. High error of refraction
     - Myopia
     - Hypermetropia
   - ii. Aphakia
     - Unilateral aphakic to avoid diplopia
     - Bilateral aphakia
       - a. Cosmetics
       - b. Avoid difficulties of aphakic

	correction, i.e. magnification, ring scotoma, poor peripheral vision, face turn
iii. Anisometropia	– Difference of power in two eyes more than three diopter
iv. Astigmatism	
v. Keratoconus	
2. Cosmetic	– To hide corneal opacity
	– To change color if iris
	– Albinism
3. Therapeutic	– Drug delivery
4. Occupational	– Sports
5. Low vision aid	

Methods of Contact Lens Fitting

1. Contact lenses are generally not given if the error of refraction is less than two diopter.
2. Children under ten years of age can not manage contact lenses, hence, they are not given hard lenses.
3. Soft lenses can be given if the parents are capable to handle the contact lenses.

To prescribe contact lenses the following protocol is followed:

1. Record distant vision and near vision.
   Inform presbyopes that to correct near vision, they will require specially designed lenses that are costly or may have to near correction in spectacle in addition to contact lenses.
2. Find out if the diminished vision is due to error of refraction or not. This is done by pinhole. If the vision improves with pinhole, the person has error of refraction that will benefit by contact lens.
3. Do refraction under cycloplegic and find out exact error of refraction and amount of astigmatism. High astigmatism is not fully corrected by soft contact lenses. Hard contact lens can neutralize some astigmatism. Soft contact lenses do not correct astigmatism well. The patient may either use specially designed contact lenses that are costly toric lenses or have to use spectacle over contact lens.
4. Do keratometry—This gives correct corneal curvature and axis of astigmatism.

With above information available, contact lenses can be fitted by any of the following methods:

1. By trial lenses only
2. By keratometry only
3. By keratometry followed by trial frame

Table 9.2: Complications of contact lens

Complication	Symptoms	Management
1. Difficulty in inserting and removal	–	Go back to the contact lens practitioner, he will demonstrate the correct method
2. Slipping of contact lens	Diplopia Blurring of vision Foreign body sensation	Consult contact lens practitioner
3. Infection	Foreign body sensation, watering, redness, pain	Immediately remove the contact lens. Stop using till the contact lens practitioner has been consulted. Use broad spectrum antibiotic

Contraindications of Contact Lenses

(Conditions when contact lenses are not prescribed)

1. Lagophthalmos
2. Proptosis
3. Loss of corneal sensation
4. Dry eyes
5. Presence of chronic dacryocystitis
6. Pterygium
7. Limbal dermoid

Contact lenses are not free from complications. They may be as mild as difficulty to insert or as serious as infection Table 9.2.

CONTACT LENS CARE

Contact lens need proper handling, storing, cleaning and disinfecting, a poorly stored lens is damaged. Each contact lens is provided with a storing case (box) and storing fluid. The contact lenses should be cleaned by especially prepared solution. They should not be washed with drinking water or disinfected by home made disinfectant.

Corneal Surgeries

Corneal surgeries to improve vision are **keratoplasty** and **refractive keratotomy**.

Keratoplasty is replacing diseased opaque cornea of the recipient by healthy transparent cornea of a donor.

There are two types of keratoplasty, i.e. full thickness keratoplasty (penetrating) and partial thickness keratoplasty (lamellar). In full thickness keratoplasty, a circular button of cornea from the center of the cornea of a donor eye is removed. It includes all the layers of the cornea from epithelium to endothelium. It is essential that there should be no opacity or active disease in donor eye. The endothelium should be healthy.

The donor eye is removed from a donor within six hours of death in winter and two hours in summer. No eyes are removed from any living person.

The two methods of collecting donor cornea are:

1. Whole of the eyeball is removed by enucleation.
2. Only cornea with a rim of sclera is removed.

The donated tissue is transported to eye bank in a special bottle kept in ice box and used within twenty four hours of removal.

The corneo scleral disc can be kept in special nutrient fluid for five to six days.

Cornea can be frozen and dehydrated in special refrigerators in nutritional media for three weeks. Such cornea is useful for lamellar graft only.

To do a penetrating keratoplasty, a circular disc which contains all the diseased part of cornea with all the layers is removed from the recipient eye and a full thickness donor cornea of same size is stitched in the gap created by removal of diseased cornea. A keratoplasty needs sixteen to twenty stitches by very fine thread under microscope. It takes about three to four weeks for the donor cornea to be incorporated in the recipient eye. It is not alway possible for the donor cornea to get accepted and remain clear in the recipient eye. It may be well united but becomes opaque. This is called **graft rejection** and may require regrafting.

In case of lamellar graft, only a partial thickness diseased cornea is removed and a donor cornea of same size and thickness is stitched to the recipient eye.

Refractive Corneal Surgeries

In keratoplasty an opaque cornea is replaced by a transparent (clear) cornea. In case of refractive corneal surgery, the surgery is done on clear cornea to change the curvature of the cornea without removing any part of the cornea.

The commonly used refractive surgeries are:

1. Radial keratotomy (RK)
2. Photorefractive keratectomy (PRK)
3. Lasik

In the first, multiple partial thickness incision (cuts) are given on the anterior (front) surface of the cornea leaving the pupil clear. No stitches are required. It is most useful in myopia of moderate degree, i.e. between -2 D to -10 D. Its results in hypermetropia are not so good. The surgery is done only after the error of refraction has stabilized (no more increasing) after 20 years of age. Higher errors may require repeat surgery. The surgery is no more preferred because the other surgeries PRK and Lasik give better results. All the refractory corneal surgeries are done under local anesthesia.

Both PRK and LASIK require special type of excimer laser to perform them.

In Lasik, a thin circular flap of cornea is formed but not removed by a special instrument called microkeratome and the underlying stroma is treated by excimer laser. Then the flap is put back. It does not need any stitching. The method gives best results when used between -12 D and +6 D.

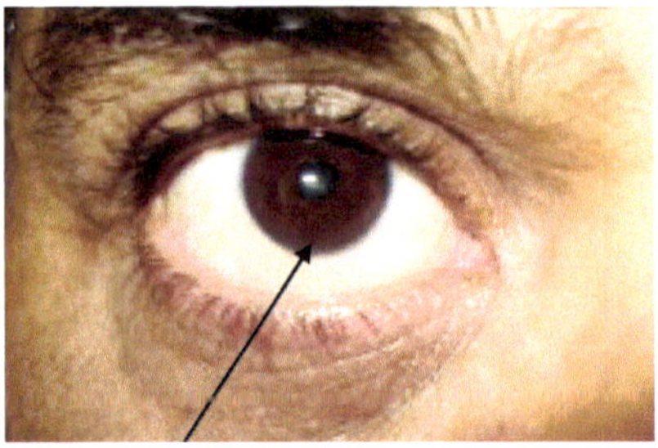

Fig. 9.19: Small superficial corneal body (*Courtesy*: Dr Nidhi Pandey)

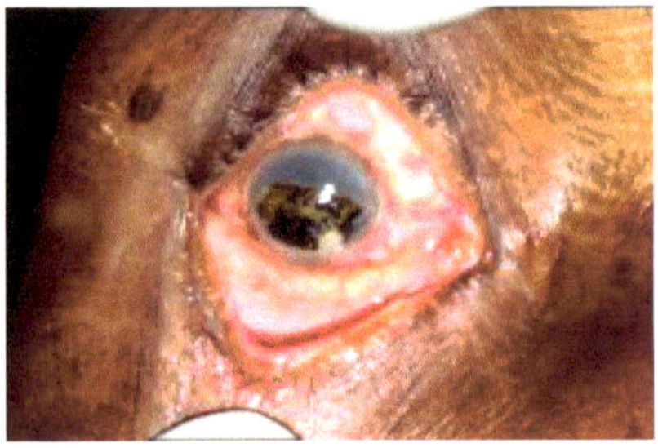

Fig. 9.20: Large corneal foreign body covering half of the cornea causing severe keratitis (*Courtesy*: Dr Santosh Patel)

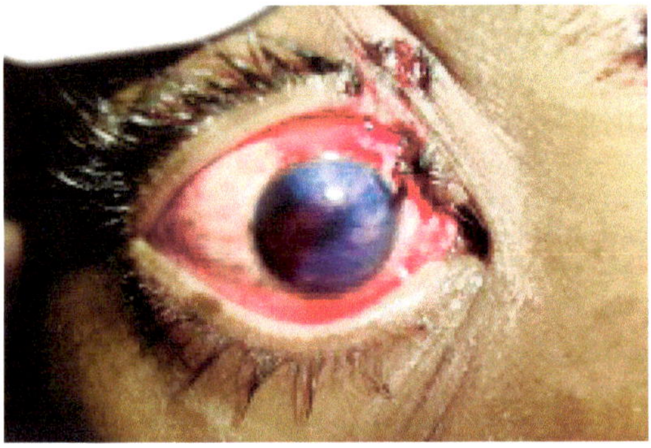

Fig. 9.21: Rupture of cornea with iris prolapse following blast injury (*Courtesy*: Dr Nidhi Pandey)

It can correct very high astigmatism also. It is done under local anesthesia and not painful. The improvement of vision is noticed next day.

In photorefractive keratectomy no flap is raised, only the corneal epithelium is removed and the cornea is treated by excimer laser. It gives good result between -6 D to +3 D. It takes few days to notice improvement of vision. It is done under local anesthesia but the eye remains painful for few days.

Corneal Trauma

Corneal trauma are common causes of unilateral or bilateral diminished vision that may range between loss of a few lines on Snellen's chart to loss of perception of light. The commonest trauma is corneal abrasion. Cornea is a common site for foreign body to be lodged (Fig. 9.19 to 9.21).

CHAPTER

10

Disorders of the Globe and Sclera

The globe (eyeball) is a spherical shape. It consists of two structures, a larger opaque (through which light does not pass) called **sclera** and a smaller transparent part called cornea. The **cornea** is more curved than sclera. The junction of the two is called **limbus** (Fig. 10.1). The cornea plays an important part in vision. The sclera does not have any role in vision. Its main function is to contain and protect intraocular structure. Besides these two functions, it acts as attachment of extraocular muscles. The blood vessels and nerves passes through it. It is white in color. Its anterior part is covered by **bulbar conjunctiva**. The posterior part is not visible. It is surrounded by orbital fat in the posterior part. The eyeball can freely move in the orbit by action of extraocular muscles. The average diameter of the sclera is 24 mm.

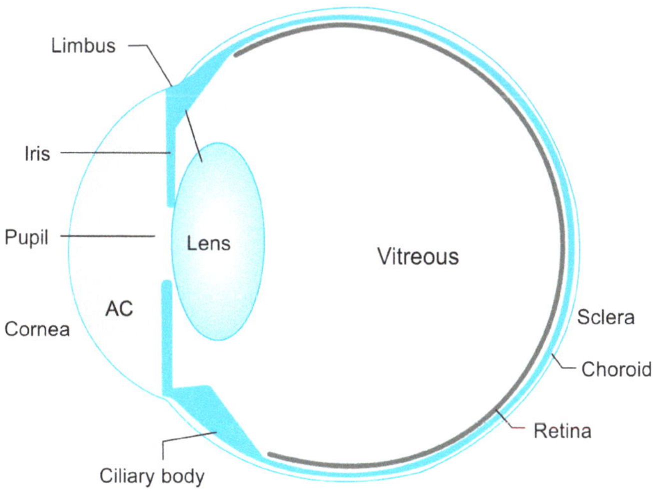

Fig. 10.1: Diagram of globe

The common disorders of the sclera are:
1. Congenital
2. Inflammation
3. Ectasia (bulging) of the sclera
   The commonest congenital anomalies of the globe is microphthalmos.

Microphthalmos

In microphthalmos, the diameter of the globe is **less than 20 mm**. It may be as low as few millimeters. The condition can be **unilateral** or **bilateral**. The cornea is also small in size and called **microcornea**. The curvature of cornea is flatter than normal. The anterior chamber is shallow. The pupil is small. The pupil is generally associated with coloboma of the iris below the pupil. The lens is spherical. The other intraocular structures are under developed. The movements are normal. As the eyeball is small, the inter palpebral aperture is narrow. The vision is less than normal. The error of refraction is generally hypermetropic (Fig. 10.2).

There is no way to increase the size of the globe. All that can be done is to improve vision as far as possible by glasses.

The conditions that should be differentiated from microphthalmos are **enophthalmos** and **phthisis bulbi**. Both are acquired conditions.

ENOPHTHALMOS

In enophthalmos, the shape, curvature and size of the eyeball including the cornea are normal. The movements are normal. The vision is generally good. The only feature common with microphthalmos is narrowing of the interpalpebral aperture. The commonest cause of enophthalmos is **fracture floor of the orbit**. The other cause is **Horner's syndrome** due to paralysis of sympathetic supply to the eye.

No specific treatment is required. A prompt repair of fracture floor of orbit may prevent development of enophthalmos.

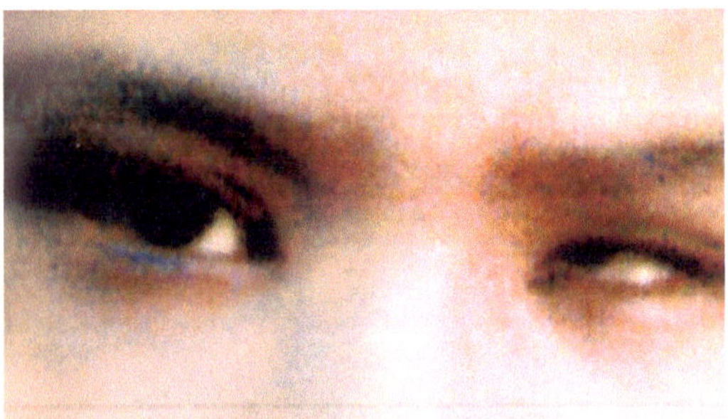

Fig. 10.2: Microphthalmos

PHTHISIS BULBI

Phthisis bulbi is irregular shrinkage of the globe due to destruction of ciliary body. Destruction of ciliary body either stops or diminishes production of aqueous so the intraocular tension falls under 5 mm of Hg. The causes of destruction of ciliary body are severe intra ocular inflammation like endophthalmitis or penetrating injury (Fig. 10.3).

In phthisis, the size of globe is reduced in all direction. It looses its circular shape and becomes cubical. The eyeball shrinks and goes back in the orbit. The corneal curvature is lost and the shape becomes quadrilateral. The anterior chamber is generally shallow but can be deep if the eye is aphakic. The movements are normal. The interpalpebral aperture is narrow. The vision is either poor or absent.

Once the eye has gone in phthisis, there is no treatment available to correct it. An artificial eye may be worn over the phthisis (to make it look normal). A proper treatment of endophthalmitis and management of penetrating wound of the globe may prevent phthisis formation.

> One point must be remembered that a phthisis bulbi may contain a retinoblastoma, which is a cancer of the eye in children.

Inflammation of Sclera

Sclera is an **avascular structure**, so it is rarely infected by microorganisms. Only on rare occasions it may develop a scleral abscess (pocket of pus) if an infected foreign body is lodged in it.

More common are inflammations of sclera proper and episclera. Episclera is an ill defined vascular loose tissue between the conjunctiva and sclera.

Inflammation of episclera is called **episcleritis** while inflammation of sclera is called **scleritis**. The first is more common than the second. The second is more serious, requires longer period of treatment and is more likely to develop complications.

> Sclera is never involved in simple episcleritis but episclera is almost always involved in scleritis.

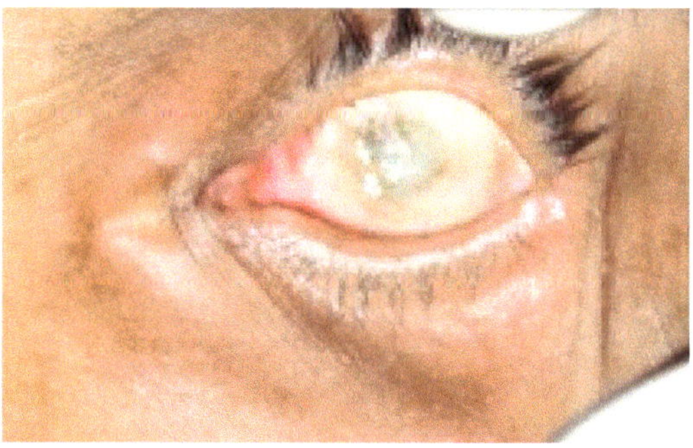

Fig. 10.3: Phthisis bulbae

EPISCLERITIS

Episcleritis is inflammation of episcleral tissue. The exact cause of which is not known, but it is more common in persons who suffer from **diabetes** and painful inflammation of joints (**arthritis**). It is seen between 20 years to 40 years, more commonly in **females**. It can be unilateral or bilateral. There are two types—**simple episcleritis** (diffuse) or **nodular episcleritis** (localized). The simple episcleritis is almost symptomless except localized congestion over the white portion of the eye. The congested area moves with the conjunctiva. It is a self-limiting disease that disappears in a few days only to reappear after few months. Weak steroid solution or Nonsteroidal anti-intrammatory drug drops once a day for months are required to prevent recurrence. It should be differentiated from phlycten. The difference between the two is even in table 10.1

In nodular form, a well formed subconjunctival nodule similar to conjunctival phlycten generally on the temporal sclera (towards the ear) is seen. It is not painful but may be tender (pain on pressure). It requires treatment by steroid eye drops.

Scleritis

Scleritis is inflammation of scleral tissue. It is more serious but rare than episcleritis. It is seen after 25 years of age in both males and females, more commonly in females. It is generally unilateral but can be bilateral. It mostly develops on temporal side, however can be seen at other places as well. There may be more than one lesion at the same time. It develops over many days as localized congestion that is converted as a nodule away from the limbus. The nodule is fixed to the sclera. It is painful on pressure. There may be dull pain without pressure on the nodule. If the nodule is near the limbus, the lesion may extend in the cornea causing a form of deep keratitis called **sclerosing keratitis**. The sclerosing keratitis is a tongue shaped white opacity at the level of stroma of cornea. It is associated with some degree of uveitis. On a long run it causes thinning of the sclera that bulges out as staphyloma. Scleritis is called **anterior scleritis** when it is visible by torch light and **posterior scleritis** when it develops on the back surface of sclera and not visible. Posterior scleritis causes mild to moderate proptosis. The posterior scleritis is best diagnosed by B-scan ultrasound.

Table 10.1: Difference between phlycten and episcleritis

Features	Episcleritis	Phlycten
Age	Adults	Children
Location	Away from limbus	Mostly at limbus
Blepharospasm	Nil	Severe when on the cornea
Tenderness	±	Non tender
Conjunctiva	Moves over the nodule	Nodule moves with conjunctiva
Conjunctivitis	Nil	Common
Corneal involvement	Rare	Keratoconjunctivitis ++

Scleritis requires prolonged treatment by oral steroids with usual precautions.

STAPHYLOMA

A bulging of the outer coat of the eyeball, i.e. cornea or sclera which are lined by uvea is called staphyloma. The outer coat is thin at the spot of the bulge (Fig. 10.4).

According to location, the staphyloma of the eyeball can be –

1. Corneal
2. Scleral

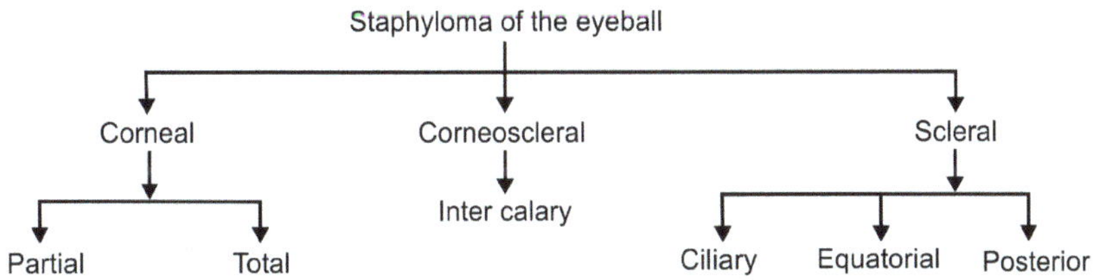

Corneal Staphyloma (Anterior Staphyloma) due to Sloughing of Corneal Ulcer

The ulcer bed is replaced by scar tissue in which iris gets attached. The scar tissue along with iris is called **pseudocornea**. When it involves only a part of cornea, it is called partial corneal staphyloma. When whole of the cornea is involved, it is called total corneal or **total anterior staphyloma**. The scar is weaker than normal cornea; hence it bulges with normal intraocular tension as well. The color of corneal staphyloma is a mixture of black and white. Generally eyes with total anterior staphyloma are blind due to associated secondary glaucoma.

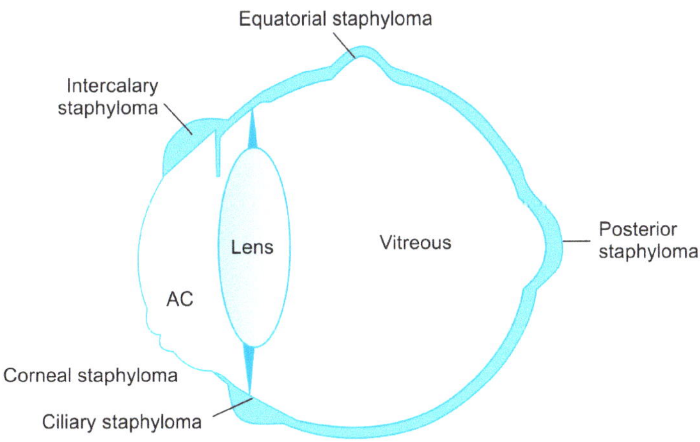

Fig. 10.4: Diagram showing various types of staphyloma and intraocular structures lining them

Smallpox used to be the commonest cause of bilateral anterior staphyloma before smallpox was eradicated. Other causes of bilateral anterior staphyloma are **keratomalacia** and **blast injury**. Once a staphyloma has developed, there is no treatment except enucleation for cosmetic reasons. Partial staphyloma may have some vision which can be improved by low vision aids.

Scleral staphyloma develops at anatomically weak spots in the sclera. More after injury, scleritis and long standing glaucoma that cause thinning of sclera which bulges out under the conjunctiva. The thin sclera is lined by uvea, hence the color of the staphyloma is black. According to position of the staphyloma and the part of the uvea lining at the staphylomas are called **intercalary**, **ciliary**, **equatorial** and **posterior**.

Intercalary Staphyloma

This is situated at the limbus and lined by root of the iris. This happens following penetrating injury at the limbus. It is a visible staphyloma.

Ciliary Staphyloma

This is situated between the limbus and the equator. It is lined by ciliary body. This is the commonest type of staphyloma. The common causes are absolute glaucoma and long standing scleritis. It is a visible staphyloma (Fig. 10.5).

Equatorial Staphyloma

This type of staphyloma develops under the recti muscle, hence are generally not visible. The causes are long standing scleritis. It can be congenital.

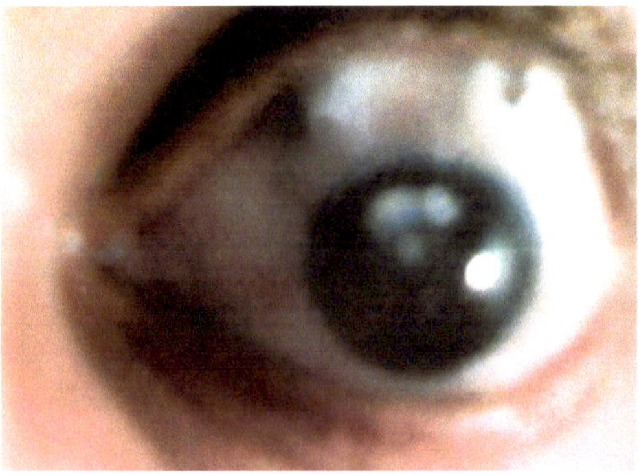

Fig. 10.5: Ciliary staphyloma

Posterior Staphyloma

These are congenital staphylomas. Commonest cause is **high myopia**. These are also not visible. They are seen either by **indirect ophthalmoscopy** or **ultrasound**.

Staphylomas are untreatable condition that may perforted by sharp or blunt injury, hence patient must be careful and avoid injury.

There are no known malignancies of sclera.

CHAPTER

11

Disorders of the Lens

Lens is a transparent circular disc like structure that is thick at the center. (Figs 11.1A, B and 11.2). The thickness gradually diminishes on the periphery. The edge of the disc is rounded and is called the **equator** of the lens. The central part on the front surface is called the **anterior pole** and the corresponding point on the back surface is called the posterior pole of the lens. The lens is situated behind the iris. The pupil lies in front of the centre of the lens. The lens is suspended from the ciliary body by **zonule** of the lens. The ciliary body, the zonule and the lens divides the inner part of the globe into two unequal parts (chambers):

1. A large **vitreous chamber** that is filled by vitreous. The back of the lens lies on the front surface of the vitreous.
2. A smaller **aqueous chamber** that is filled by a clear fluid called **aqueous humor**. The aqueous chamber is again divided in two unequal chambers:
    a. A large **anterior chamber**
    b. A small **posterior chamber**
    The two chambers communicate with eachother through the pupil.

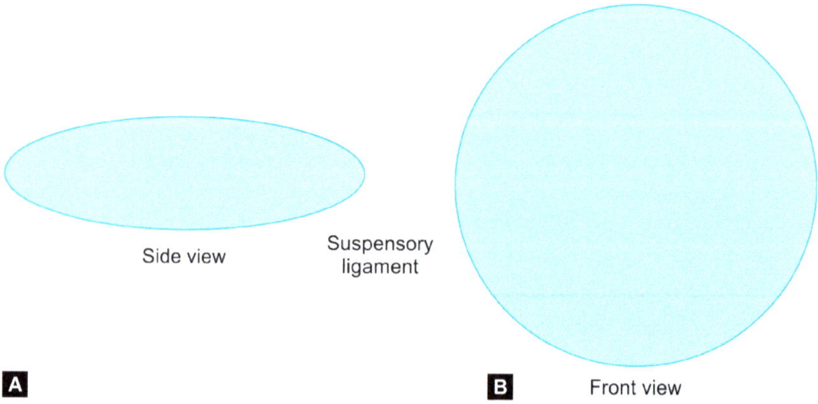

Figs 11.1A and B: Side and front view of normal lens

The lens has following parts (Fig. 11.3):
1. The capsule
2. The epithelium
3. The lens fibers are again divided into two parts, i.e. the lens cortex and the nucleus of the lens.

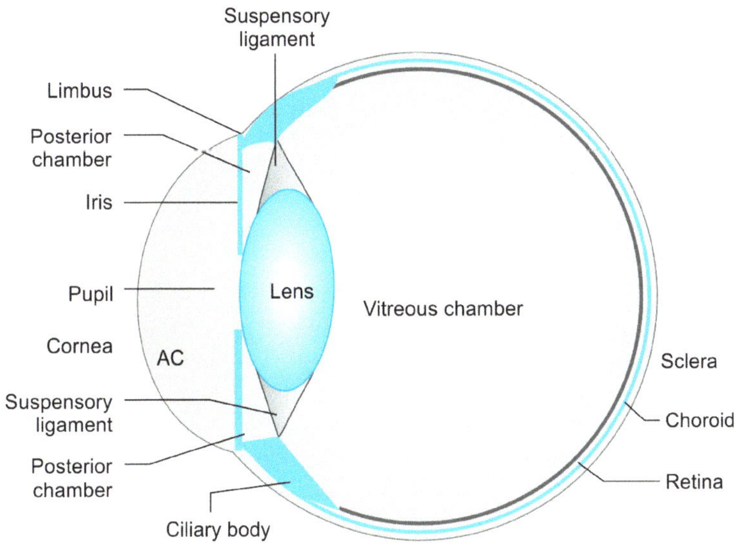

Fig. 11.2: Lens suspended by suspensory ligament and position of various chambers

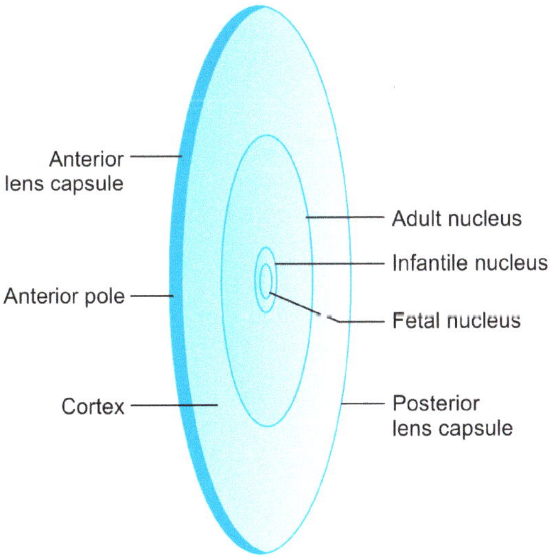

Fig. 11.3: Side view of the normal lens showing various parts

4. The **capsule** is an ill defined structure that surrounds the contents of the lens all-round. It is thicker in front and thin at the back. The zonules get attached to the lens capsule all-round at the equtor.
5. The **epithelium** is present on the front surface only under the capsule.
6. The **lens fibers**—The lens fibers form the main bulk of the lens. They can be divided into two groups, the peripheral fibers which form the **cortex**. The fibers are formed constantly and pushed towards the center. The central fibers form the **nucleus** of the lens.
7. The nucleus starts forming very early. As the lens grows, more and more cortical fibers are compressed and converted into nucleus. The nucleus keeps on enlarging throughout life.
8. In children, it is not possible to separate the nucleus from the cortex. As age advances the nucleus becomes hard and can be seen separately on slit lamp.
9. The zonules are strong under 40 years of age but become weak as age advances and can be broken with ease.
10. The lens in children is also attached to the vitreous firmly and can not be pulled out without injury to the vitreous.

The main function of the lens is to focus:
1. Parallel rays from infinity and
2. Diverging rays from near point on the retina

The second function is brought about by increasing the power of the lens. This process is called **accommodation**. This is brought about by contraction of the ciliary muscle and increasing the curvature of the lens. A child has maximum accommodation. The power of accommodation gradually decreases with age and by the age of sixty it is almost lost. This is called **presbyopia** that sets in at about forty years of age. The other cause of loss of accommodation is **paralysis of ciliary muscle**. This is called **cycloplegia**. This can be produced by putting drugs like atropine in the eye. The drugs that abolish accommodation are called cycloplegics. The other causes of cycloplegia is **paralysis of third nerve**.

The diseases of the lens can be broadly put in three groups:
1. Loss of transparency called **cataract**
2. Displacement of lens called **ectopia lentis**.
3. Change in shape and size of the lens

The first two can be:
- Congenital
- Acquired

Absence of lens totally or partially is called **aphakia**. An eye with intact lens is called phakic eye.

CATARACT

Loss of transparency of the lens is called cataract. Cataract can be localized or generalized. The opacity can be in the cortex or the nucleus. Sometimes

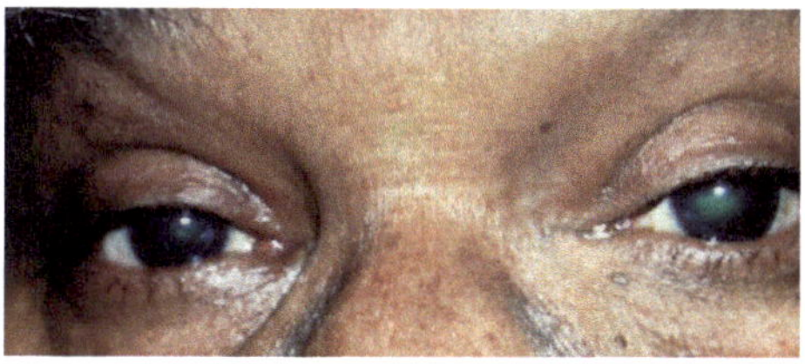

Fig. 11.4: Immature cataract

both the structures are involved and the eye develops a **total cataract**. This is called **mature cataract**. If the cataract does not extend from the anterior capsule to the posterior capsule, it is called **immature cataract** (Fig. 11.4).

The cataract can be present at birth, and called **congenital cataract**. It may develop after birth but before thirty years of age, it is called **developmental cataract**. Cataracts that develop round about fifty years of age are called **senile cataract** or age related cataract. These are the commonest type of cataract.

From the above description it is clear that cataract can be divided into two groups –

- In aged (past 40 years of age)
- In children

The type of cataract seen in adults are:

- Senile cataract (commonest)
- Traumatic cataract
- Cataract in systemic disease
- Cataract due to drugs
- Cataract due to injury

Cataract seen in children are:

- Congenital (present at birth)
- Developmental
- Traumatic
- Drug induced
- Secondary to intraocular inflammation

CATARACT IN ADULTS

Senile Cataract

This is a slow growing opacity in the lens after fifty years of age in both the sexes. It is generally bilateral (both eyes). One eye has more advanced opacity (cataract) than the other. Only symptom of senile cataract is **gradual painless diminished vision**. Cataract does not cause any pain or redness of the eye. If pain and redness are present in the eye, causes other than cataract should be looked for.

According to position of the opacity, the cataract can be nuclear cataract, cortical cataract or posterior subcapsular cataract (Figs 11.5A to D).

Nuclear cataract is the commonest type of cataract. The nucleus become translucent and allows less light to pass through. This results in diminished distant vision. Hardening of the nucleus causes scattering of rays that leads to glare. In nuclear cataract the vision is greatly diminished in bright light as well. One of the advantages of nuclear cataract is that the near vision improves. A person who required plus glasses for near work can see near things without glasses with nuclear cataract. This is due to myopia introduced by the hard nucleus. This improvement of near vision is called **second sight**.

The nuclear cataract rarely becomes total. As time passes, the nucleus becomes harder and changes color from white to brown. The whole of the cortex is converted to opaque nucleus and vision is reduced greatly.

Symptoms

Symptoms of nuclear cataract can be divided into two groups:
1. Without pain or redness
2. With pain and redness

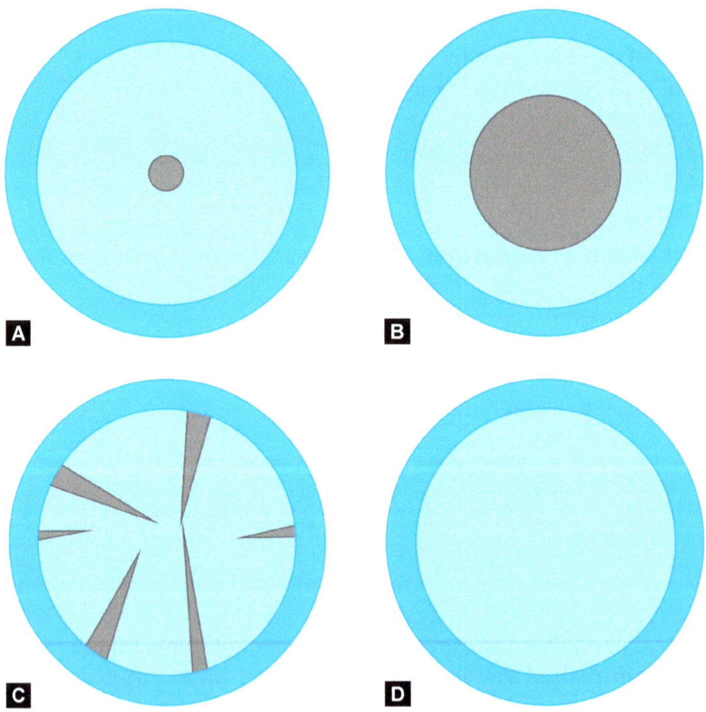

Figs 11.5A to D: Retinoscopic figures of (A) Posterior polar; (B) Central nuclear; (C) Cortical; (D) Complete cataract

The first group are very common and almost all patient have them. The second group develops over the symptoms of the first group and are rare. They are ocular emergency.

Symptoms of cataract without pain or redness consists of:

1. Gradual fall of distant vision
2. Glare—Intolerance to light
3. Poor vision in bright light (noon)
4. Better vision in dim light (evening)
5. Polyopia (one thing looks more than two or three)
6. Improvement of near vision (patient can read without glasses)

The painful symptoms are:

1. Gross loss of distant and near vision
2. Redness
3. Severe pain in eyes
4. Headache

These symptoms are rare and develop only if the protein leaks from the capsule.

Progress of Nuclear Cataract

Nuclear haze →Nuclear scerosis →Brown cataract →Black cataract →Total nuclear cataract

Signs of Nuclear Cataract

- The eye is normal externally except visible whiteness in the cornea.
- The cornea, anterior chamber are normal.
- The pupil is circular, central and brisk to light both direct and indirect.
- The pupil has a grey reflex that look like dull pink spot in bright pink reflex on retinoscopy.
- Intraocular tension is within normal limits.
- **The iris shadow** is present. Iris shadow is the shadow of iris on partially opaque lens when light is thrown obliquely. The iris shadow is not visible if the lens is clear or is totally opaque.

Treatment

- There is no medical treatment for any cataract.
- The definite treatment is removal of lens and replacing it by a posterior chamber intraocular lens.

Some nonsurgical procedures may give good vision till the patient agrees to get operated. They are:

1. Increasing the minus power for distances.
2. Asking the patient to do near work without glasses.
3. Use umbrella or hooded cap while going out.

Cortical Cataract (Flow chart 11.1)

In contrast to nuclear cataract, in this condition opacity starts in the cortex in spoke like manner and spread towards the center as well as on either side. Thus, converting the whole of the cortex into grey opaque mass. Sometimes the cortex between the nucleus and posterior capsule becomes opaque in the shape of a disc. The above two changes are called **incipient stage** of cortical cataract. On retinoscopy the opaque areas stand out as black cones (Fig. 11.5C) that are broad towards the limbus and pointed towards the pupil. As days pass the cortex gathers fluid and the whole of the lens increases in size. This is called **intumescent stage of cortical cataract**. The increased size of the lens pushes the iris towards the cornea. This narrows the angle of anterior chamber and the intraocular tension rises (Fig. 11.5C).

The incipient stage and intumescent stage together are called immature cataract.

Flow chart 11.1: Progress of cortical cataract

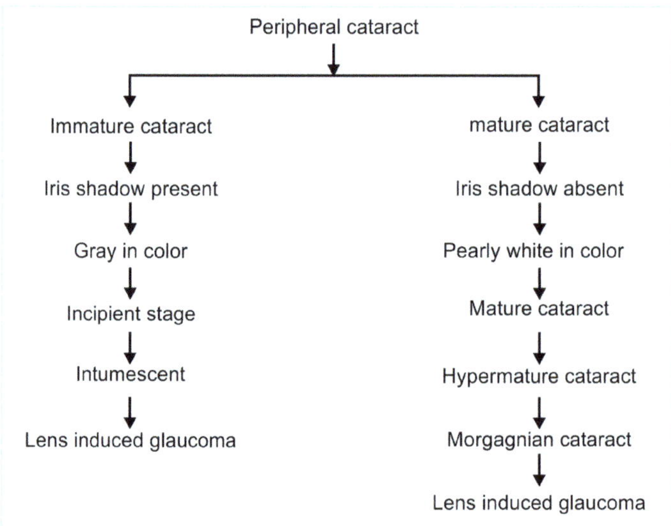

Symptoms of Cortical Cataract

The symptoms are same as in nuclear cataract except that a person with cortical cataract has fairly good vision in bright light and poor vision in dim light. The fall of vision in cortical cataract is faster than in nuclear cataract. Chances of lens induced glaucoma and uveitis are more in cortical cataract than in nuclear cataract.

Treatment

There is no treatment except lens extraction with intraocular lens implant.

Posterior Subcapsular Cataract (Fig. 11.5A)

Posterior subcapsular cataract is a slow growing cortical cataract that develops as a layer of opacity behind the nucleus and in front of the posterior capsule. The central part of the opacity becomes denser and is visible as a small black dot in the center of the pink glow on retinoscope. It develops early than nuclear or cortical cataract. The exact cause is not known. It may be hereditary. Other causes are chronic uveitis and prolonged use of steroid. Loss of vision is disproportionate to opacity. As the opacity is near the posterior pole, hence vision becomes less, as the pupil constricts as is seen in bright light.

Treatment is lens extraction, posterior capsule polished and posterior chamber intraocular lens implants. These patients are more likely to develop posterior capsular opacification after intraocular lens implant.

Congenital Cataract (Figs 11.6A and B)

Congenital cataracts are those opacities in the lens that develop in the nucleus during early weeks of development. The exact cause of congenital cataracts is not known but they have a strong hereditary tendency. About one-third congenital and developmental cataracts are hereditary. In about one-third no cause can be found out. Remaining are due to **maternal rubella** (mother suffers from a virus infection called rubella during first three months of pregnancy), and a type of diabetes seen in children called **galactosemia**. In diabetes there is rise of glucose in blood which is passed in urine. In galactosemia there is rise of galactose in blood which is passed in urine.

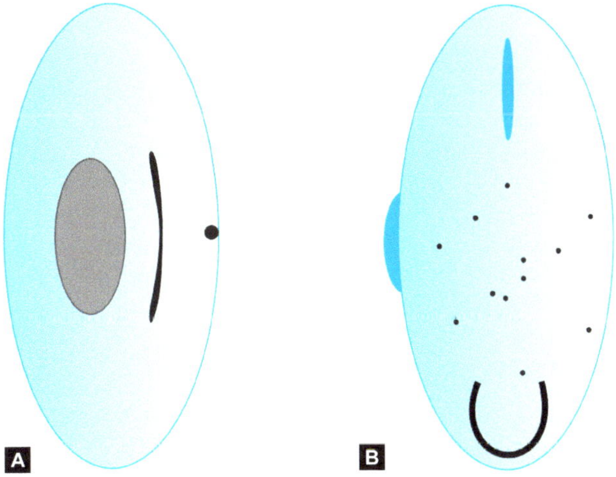

Figs 11.6A and B: Types of congenital cataract (A) that cause dliminished vision; (B) that do not cause much loss of vision

The congenital cataracts can be unilateral or bilateral.

The symptoms of congenital cataracts depend upon the position and size of opacity. They can be divided into two groups:

1. Those that cause diminished vision.
2. Those that do not cause diminished vision.

To the first group belong the opacities in the visual axis. An opacity near the posterior pole (back of center of the lens) causes severe loss of vision while an opacity on the anterior pole causes least diminished vision. A total cataract causes maximum loss of vision. In the second group are the opacities which are not on the visual axis except anterior polar cataract which is situated in the visual axis but does not cause loss of vision.

Though the commonest symptom of congenital cataract is diminished vision, other symptoms are:

1. Visible white opacity in the pupillary area. The child does not complain of this but the parents become aware of this soon.
2. Effect of diminished vision
   a. Amblyopia
   b. Squint
   c. Nystagmus.

Generally the child is brought with squint or squint and nystagmus and after examination under mydriasis is found to have lenticular opacity and amblyopia.

An unilateral dense opacity is more likely to develop squint and amblyopia.

Commonest type of congenital cataract is soft central cataract. This requires early surgery and visual rehabilitation.

The next common congenital cataract is lamellar or zonular cataract.

Zonular Cataract

This type of cataract account for about 50% of all congenital cataracts. They are generally bilateral. They can develop before birth or after birth. They are central, circular disc shaped opacities that show layers. The opacity does not reach the periphery. There is a clear zone in the surrounding cortex which is visible when the pupil is dilated. The central opacity send radial spoke like opacities in the clear cortex. These are called **riders**. If the opacity is larger than the normal pupil, the vision falls very much but improves when the pupil is dilated (Figs 11.7 to 11.9).

Traumatic Cataract

It is equally seen in children as well as adults. They are more common in males than in females. Generally traumatic cataract is unilateral except in blast injuries where multiple foreign bodies may injure the lens.

The two common types of traumatic cataracts are:

1. Due to penetrating injury (needle, knife, thorn)
2. Due to blunt injury

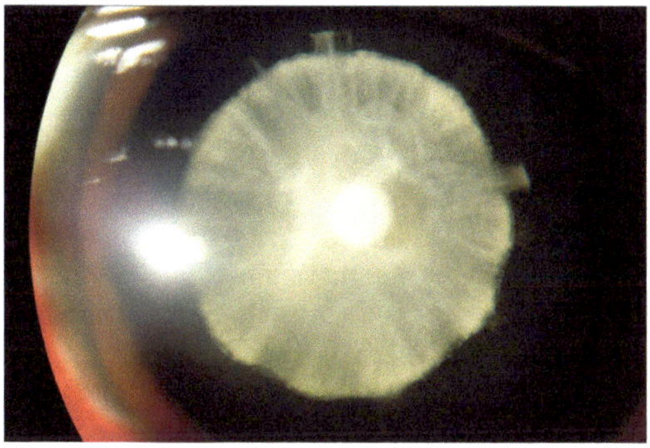

Fig. 11.7: Lamellar cataract (*Courtesy*: Dr Santosh Patel)

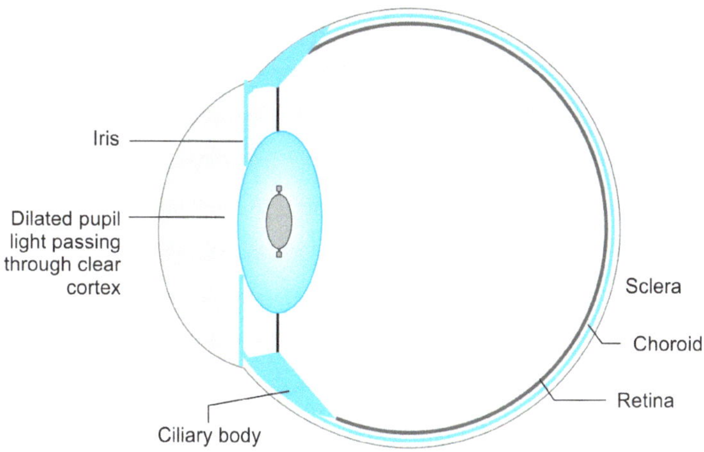

Fig. 11.8: Lamellar cataract—side view dilated pupil, fairly good vision

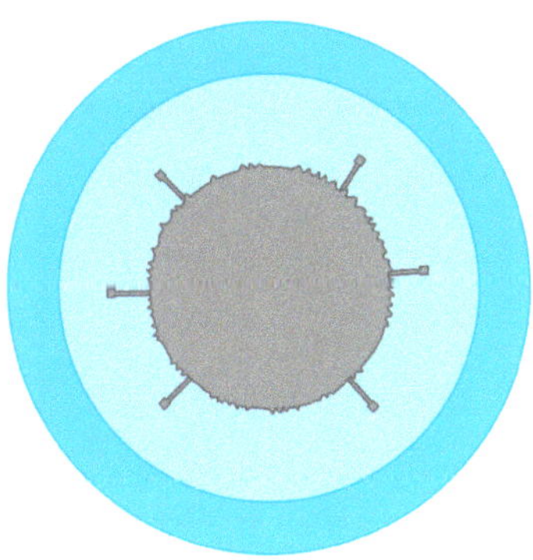

Fig. 11.9: Lamellar cataract as seen in retinoscope with riders from periphery

Cataract Due to Penetrating Injury

The sharp object penetrates the cornea and then passes through the anterior lens capsule. If the injury in the lens is pin-point, it allows little aqueous to enter the lens that turns the cortex opaque. The wound heals and a localized opacity develops in the cortex which most of the time remains stationary. But if the wound is large a large, opacity develops that spreads to cover whole of the cortex and nucleus. A large wound does not close automatically, it remains open. As more and more cortex get opaque the total volume of the cortex increases and the lens swells up. A swollen lens causes secondary glaucoma. If the swelling is too much, the opaque cortical matters leaks through the opening and pours in the anterior chamber again causing secondary glaucoma. The vision falls to just perception of light. Most of the time the iris prolapses through the corneal wound.

After few weeks the cortical matter starts absorbing and only strands of opacity are left and a dense **after cataract** results. If the nucleus is formed before the injury, it is not absorbed and requires removal surgically.

Cataract Due to Blunt Injury

Cataract due to blunt injury differs from that caused by penetrating injury in the sense that there is no visible opening in the capsule.

The changes brought about blunt injury to lens are –

1. Vossius ring
2. Concussion cataract
3. Anterior subcapsular opacity
4. Posterior subcapsular opacity
4. Subluxation or dislocation of lens.
5. Changes in the macula in the form of commotio retinae or **Berlins edema**.
6. There may be associated changes in iris like dialysis (Fig. 11.10).

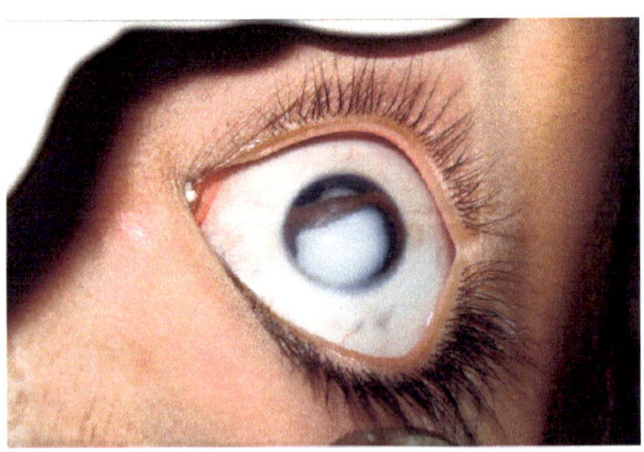

Fig. 11.10: Traumatic cataract with iridodialysis (*Caurtesy:* Professor AK Chandrakar)

Vossius Ring

This is deposition of iris pigment on the anterior lens capsule when the posterior surface of iris is forced against the anterior lens capsule. The iris pigment is deposited in a circular fashion. The diameter of the circle is equal to the size of the pupil at the time of injury. As the iris pigment deposition in away from the center of the lens, it does not cause any loss of vision. The Vossius ring does not require any treatment, it passes off in weeks to months.

Concussion Cataract (Fig. 11.11)

Concussion cataract develops few days after the blunt injury. It is more common in posterior cortex than anterior cortex. This is due to entry of very small amount of aqueous through micro tear in the capsule. It develops as **flower petal like opacity** arising from a central point as prominent opaque lines. From each opaque line develop branches of opacity like bottle brush which causes diminished vision. Opacity is best visible on slit lamp and as black start like opacity on retinoscopy.

A small concussion opacity may remain stationary, a large opacity enlarges and may involve whole of the cortex.

Rubella Cataract

Rubella is a virus that causes cataract in unborn child if the mother gets infected by the virus during first three months of pregnancy. It causes congenital changes in many organs of the unborn child like heart, lung, brain, ear and eyes.

The changes in eyes are **bilateral** cataract, **microophthalmos** (small eye) and **glaucoma**. The rubella cataract is generally large and contains live virus in them. The disease in mother is fully preventable by rubella vaccine given at the age of nine months. Every girl should get a shot of rubella vaccine compulsorily.

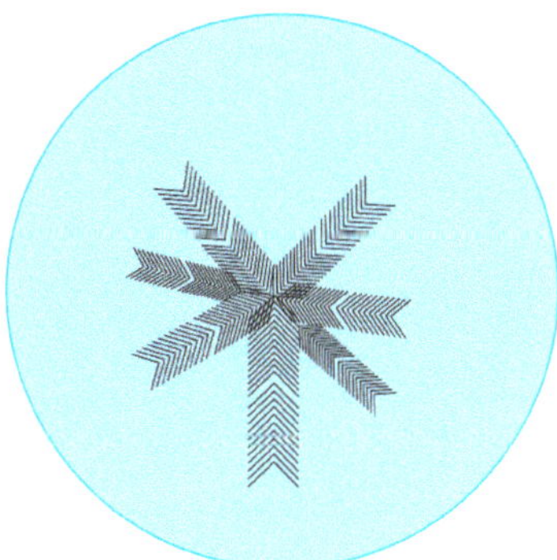

Fig. 11.11: Concussion cataract

Once rubella has developed, there is no treatment either for the mother or the child.

The only treatment of rubella cataract is surgery in a specialized hospital.

Treatment of Congenital Cataract

1. There is no medical treatment for congenital cataract.
2. All girls should be immunized against rubella at the age of nine months.
3. All congenital cataracts do not require treatment. The opacities away from the optical axis does not require treatment. Central opacities with clear cortex after dilatation of pupil, may be operated late. Uniocular cataracts have poor results even after successful surgery. Complete bilateral cataracts should be operated as soon as the child can be given general anesthesia for at least half an hour.

The best results are obtained by putting intraocular lens after lens extraction.

Congenital cataracts should be operated only in specialized hospital.

Treatment of Cataract in Adults

Mere presence of opacity in the lens does not require any treatment. A cataract requires treatment only when it causes diminished vision.

> There is no medical treatment for cataract.

A patient may benefit from change in power of glasses for sometime but will have to be operated ultimately. A patient with nuclear cataract may postpone surgery for sometime by increasing minus power.

Similarly keeping the pupil dilated may improve vision for sometime but the eye has to be operated ultimately.

> The definite treatment of cataract is surgery with IOL.

- **Maturity of cataract is not important for surgery**. It is the visual requirement of the patient that decides if an eye should be operated or not. A professional like doctor, engineer, lawyer, teacher may have to be operated even with vision of 6/36 to 6/24 but a farmer or a labor may postpone his surgery till his vision has come down to less than 6/60.

> Only one eye is operated at a time even when both eyes have operable cataracts.

Evaluation of Patient for Lens Surgery

1. First, find out that loss of vision is due to cataract.
2. When due to cataract, find out if the loss of vision is due to cataract only

or there are other causes also present in the same eye. Such common causes are—**Central corneal opacity, high error of refraction, squint, amblyopia, glaucoma, macular lesion, retinopathy, optic atrophy** because all of them will result in poor vision even after perfect surgery.

3. Once it has been decided that the person requires lens extraction, following conditions should be excluded:
   a. Ocular
   b. Systemic

Ocular causes that are contraindicated in lens extraction (The eye should not be operated) –

1. Acute infection – Conjunctivitis, corneal ulcer
2. Chronic infection – Chronic dacryocystitis
3. Deformity of lid – Trichiasis, entropion, ectropion, lagophthalmos
4. Dry eye
5. Raised intraocular tension (glaucoma)

Before operation following should be checked

1. There is minimum perception of light and accurate projection of light. Patient with vision less than this will not benefit from surgery.
2. The eye should be white (not congested = red).
3. The cornea should be bright.
   AC normal
   Pupil central, circular and brisk to light in both eyes.
4. Intraocular tension should be less than 20 mm Hg.
5. Regurgitation test should be negative.
6. Diabetes, blood pressure are not contraindicated. They should be under control before surgery and remain controlled after surgery.

The surgical principle behind the lens extraction is to:

1. Remove the lens fully—Intracapsular lens extraction (ICCE)
2. Remove the opaque part of the lens leaving the posterior capsule and part of the anterior capsule intact—Extracapsular lens extraction (ECCE)

> Both the methods leave the eye aphakic. The aphakic eye is highly hypermetropic. There is no accommodation left after removal of lens totally or partially. This causes diminished near vision. The vision is generally less than 6/60 and no near vision.

These two are corrected by:

High plus lenses for distance and addition of plus three to distant correction for near. This generally means plus 10 lens for distance and plus thirteen lens for near. These powers are given in spectacle.

Persons with spectacle correction for aphakia have many difficulties:

1. The most common disadvantage is 33% magnification which means that an object one meter tall looks 1.33 meter high.

2. To have best vision, the patient has to look through the center of the lens. Hence, he has to elevate the chin.
3. The vision becomes less when seen through the periphery of the lens, hence the patient has to move his head to see side rays instead of moving the eye.

These difficulties can be reduced or eliminated by using **contact lens** or putting an **artificial lens** in place of opaque lens. The second gives best results for distant vision. In both the condition additional near correction is required in the spectacle.

Putting an artificial lens in place of opaque lens is called **intraocular lens implant** (IOL) and an eye with IOL is called **pseudophakia** in contrast to aphakia where no artificial lens is put inside the eye.

APHAKIA

When a lens is partly or completely absent from the pupillary area, the condition is called aphakia. Examples of total absence of lens from pupillary lens is surgical total removal of lens (ICCE) and dislocation of lens in the vitreous (Figs 11.12A to D).

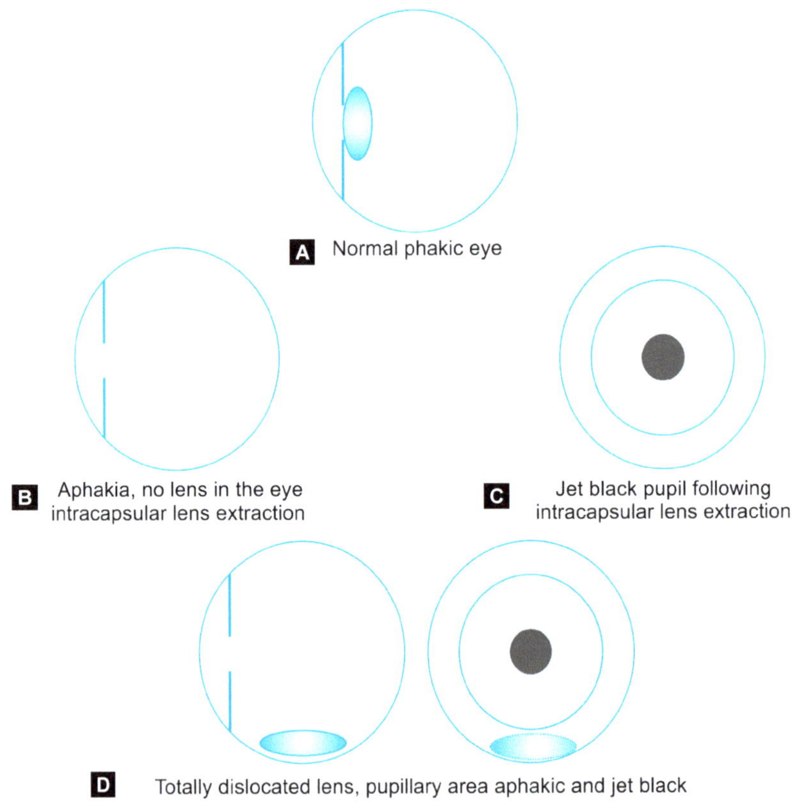

Figs 11.12A to D: Total absence of the lens from the pupillary area

Examples of partial absence of lens from pupillary area are—Partial removal of lens matter by ECCE and subluxation of lens. (Figs 11.13A to C)

The commonest cause of aphakia is surgical removal of lens. Other causes are dislocation of lens and absorption of lens after traumatic cataract.

The symptoms of aphakia are:

- Diminished distant vision—Vision less than 6/60
- Absence of near vision

Signs of aphakia are:

1. Scar of surgery at limbus.
2. Scar of injury in the cornea.

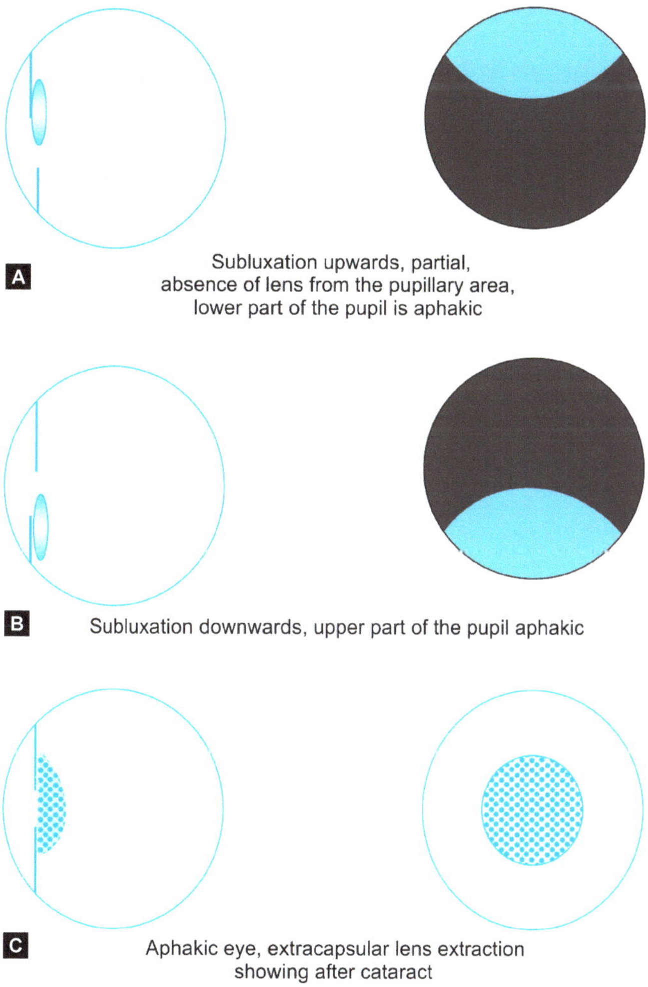

Figs 11.13A to C: Diagram showing partial aphakia

3. Deep anterior chamber.
4. Tremulousness of iris. The iris moves with movement of the eyes.
5. Changes in color of pupil
   i. Jet black, when the lens has been removed completely (ICCE).
   ii. Grey white pupil if ECCE has been done or traumatic cataract.
6. High hypermetropia with high astigmatism, i.e. +10 Dspl with +1.5 to 2.0 Dcyl.
7. Total loss of accommodation.
8. On fundus examination the disc looks small.

Treatment of Aphakia (Figs 11.14A to I)

Any of the following:
1. Spectacle correction for distance and near.
2. Contact lens with near correction in spectacle.
3. Intraocular lens with near correction in spectacle.

PSEUDOPHAKIA

In pseudophakia the lens is either removed by ECCE or ICCE. The second method is now-a-days used rarely and an artificial lens of suitable power made of special plastic matter is placed in place of the nucleus and cortex.

The lens can be removed by following methods:
1. Small incision extracapsular cataract extraction (SICE). The nucleus and cortex are removed. The capsule is left intact. This may require a stitch to close the wound.
2. No stitch ECCE—Where a small puncture is made to remove the nucleus and the cortex. As the cortex is too large to come out of such a small puncture it is crushed and the crushed material is washed out along with cortex leaving the capsule intact. No suture is required but it takes few days to heal.
3. Phacoemulsification—Here through a small hole, a special probe is introduced that emulsifies the lens and cortex into fluid, which is drained leaving the capsule intact. This is most preferred method now-a-days.

Once the lens has been cleared, an artificial lens of suitable size and power is put in the capsule. The power of the lens required by a particular is calculated by an instrument called biometer.

> No cataract surgery is done by laser. All the procedures are done under operative microscope.

Complications of Lens Surgery

1. Modern lens extraction with intraocular lens implant done under operating microscope with all possible precautions, do not have any complications.
2. In spite of best surgery without any complication, sometimes the vision does not improve to expected level.

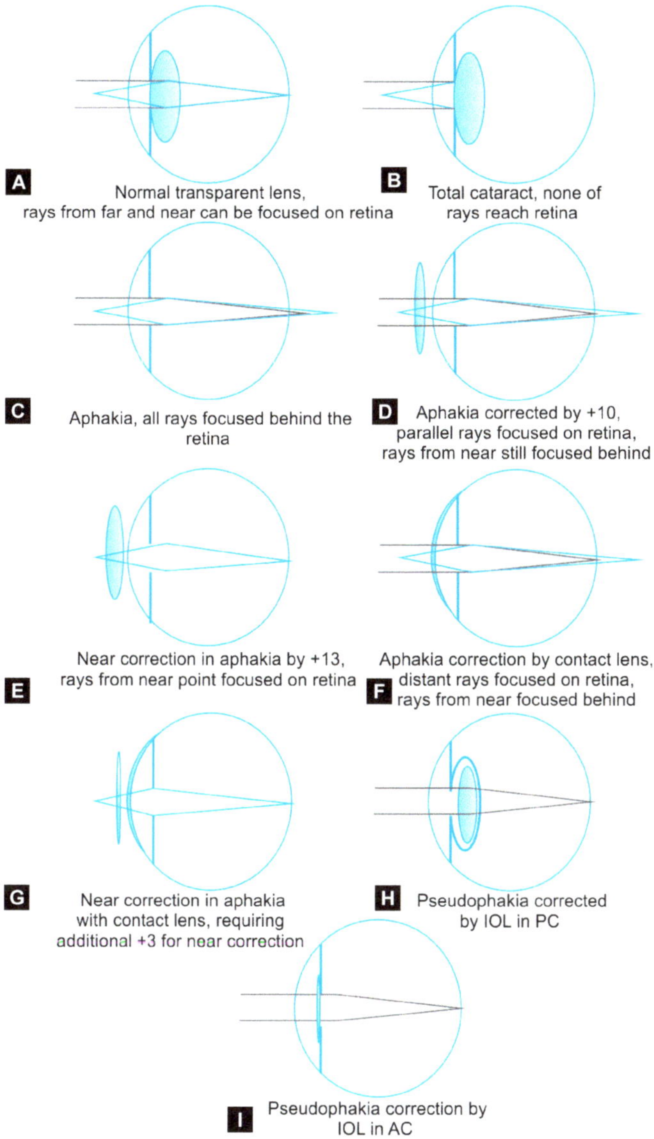

Figs 11.14A to I: Optical correction of aphakia and pseudophakia

3. The causes of nonimprovement of vision following lens surgery can be divided into two groups. They are:
   i. Preexisting causes
   ii. Causes related to surgery

Preexisting causes of nonimprovement of vision following lens surgery are:

1. Those that are visible before surgery:
   a. Corneal opacity
   b. Squint
   c. Amblyopia
   d. Chronic uveitis
   e. Advanced glaucoma
2. Those that are discovered after surgery:
   a. Macular lesion
   b. Retinal dystrophy
   c. Retinopathy
   d. Partial optic atrophy
   e. Pre-existing retinal detachment
3. Those that develop after surgery
   a. Endophthalmitis
   b. Damage to the cornea
   c. Posterior capsular opacification (PCO)
   d. Fresh retinal detachment
   e. Glaucoma in aphakia

Out of these, two require mention. They are:

1. Postoperative endophthalmitis
2. Posterior capsular opacification

The first is an emergency and can cause permanent loss of vision in the operated eye. The second is not an emergency developing slowly and treatable by laser capsulotomy.

Postoperative Endophthalmitis

This is an avoidable and preventable condition if proper antiseptic and aseptic methods are used before and during surgery. It is partially treatable if diagnosed and treated well in time.

Endophthalmitis is infection of all intraocular structures, i.e. uvea, vitreous and retina.

There are two types of postoperative endophthalmitis:

1. Acute
2. Chronic

Acute endophthalmitis develops within two days of surgery due to infection by pus forming bacteria. The eye is painful, red with discharge. The vision is greatly reduced.

On examination:

1. The lids are swollen.
2. The conjunctiva is swollen and red.
3. The cornea is hazy.
4. There may be pus in the anterior chamber.
5. The pink retinal glow is dull on retinoscopy.

6. The fundus is not visible.
7. The movements of the eye are present.

If not treated in time, the eye passes into next stage called **panophthalmitis** where all the intraocular structures and periocular structures are involved with total loss of vision. The movements of the eye are lost. There is no treatment once panophthalmitis develops. The patient gets relief from pain only after the contents of the eyeball have been removed surgically. The surgery is called **evisceration**.

Chronic Endophthalmitis

Develops weeks after the surgery. There is gradual loss of vision. The eye is red and painful. It is caused due to fungus infection.

Posterior Capsular Opacification

This happens due to development of a translucent membrane between the back surface of posterior chamber IOL and posterior lens capsule. About 33% cases of PCIOL develop PCO. Younger the patient, more are the chances of developing PCO. All patients under ten years develop PCO. The main complaint is gradual reduction of vision even after very good surgery.

The treatment is simple. The membrane is cut by NdYAG laser. The procedure is called **laser capsulotomy**.

After Cataract

This is more severe form of PCO. If the lens develops dense white opacity following extracapsular lens extraction, the condition is called after cataract. In after cataract, the vision is poor from the day after surgery. The pupillary area develops a white opacity that is as white as or more than original cataract. The best treatment is to avoid formation of after cataract by fully washing all the cortical matter during extracapsular lens extraction. The only treatment available for after cataract is to cut the newly formed opacity by knife. Laser is ineffective in after cataract.

Congenital Anomalies of the Lens

The common congenital anomalies of lens are:
1. Loss of transparency—Congenital cataract
2. Abnormal position of lens—Subluxation of lens
3. Abnormal shape and size of the lens
   Microphakia—Lens smaller than normal
   Spherophakia—Lens more spherical than normal

ABNORMAL POSITION OF LENS

Ectopia Lentis

The normal lens hangs behind the iris, in front of the vitreous by zonules that are attached to the ciliary body. The center of the lens lies just behind the pupil.

If the lens shifts from this position, the lens is called **subluxation** of lens and the condition is called **ectopia lentis**. If the lens is totally absent from the pupillary area, it is called **dislocation** of lens (Figs 11.15 and 11.16).

Commonest cause of sub luxation of lens is congenital absence of zonule. The lens moves away form the site of absent zonule. If the lower zonule are absent, the lens will shift upwards and if the zonules are absent at upper part, the lens will move down. Similarly the lens may move on either side.

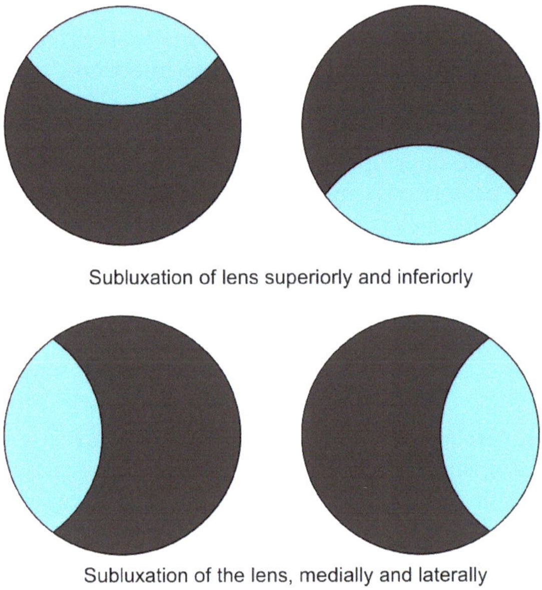

Fig. 11.15: Ectopia lentis

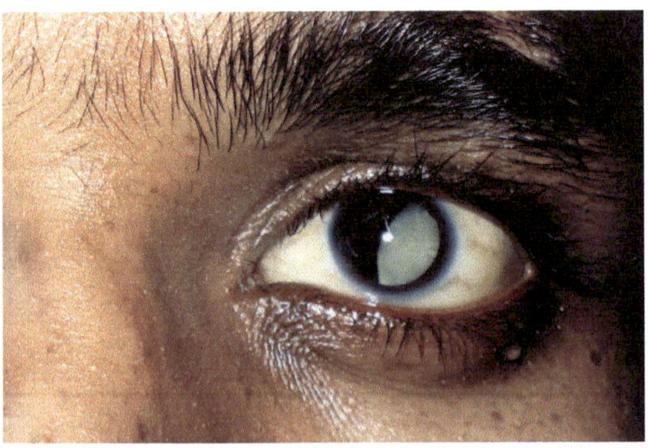

Fig. 11.16: Mature ectopic cataract (*Courtesy*: Professor AK Chandrakar)

The congenital ectopia lentis is generally bilateral and similar. It may be so mild that the child has no symptom or may be gross enough to cause diminished vision and uniocular diplopia. The pupil has two types of error of refraction, i.e. myopia through the subluxated lens and hypermetropia through aphakic lens.

On examination

- The iris is tremulous at the site of aphakia.
- The AC is deep over the aphakia.
- The AC is shallow over the subluxated lens.

In oblique illumination, the phakic and aphakic areas are seen clearly in the pupillary area. The ectopia lens may be the only defect in the body or may have many abnormalities in the body other than eyes. They are long hands, feet and fingers and changes in heart.

CHAPTER

12

Disorders of the Uvea

Uvea is the middle layer of the eyeball. It is rich in blood supply and is pigmented. It has three parts: The **iris**, **ciliary** body and **choroid**. Each has its own function. The iris lies parallel to the cornea and forms the posterior (back) surface of anterior chamber. It has a hole in the center called **pupil**. The function of iris is to regulate the size of the pupil on which depends the amount of light that can enter the eye. It also regulates the flow of aqueous from posterior chamber to anterior chamber. Normal iris does not bleed when cut. (Fig. 12.1).

The ciliary body and the choroid line the sclera. The ciliary body bulges into the vitreous chamber. It is highly vascular and bleeds freely due to injury. It has plain muscles in its substance. It has two functions, i.e. accommodation and formation of aqueous. The lens is attached to the ciliary body by **zonules**. The inflammation of iris and ciliary body cause redness of the eye, pain in the eye and pain on pressing the eye (tenderness).

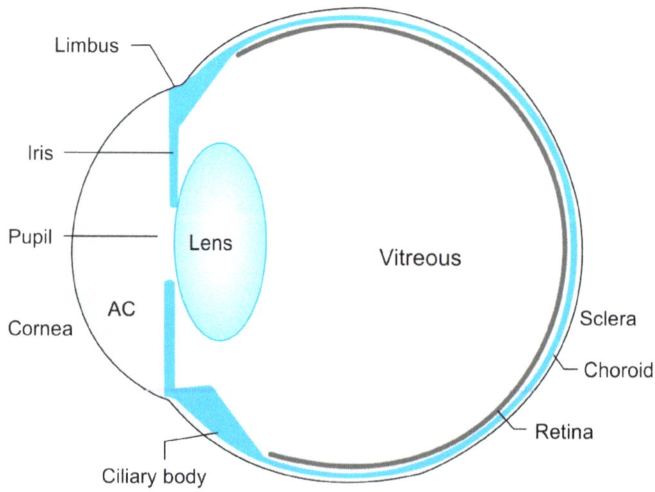

Fig. 12.1: Diagram showing uvea

The choroid lies between the retina and the sclera. It is firmly attached to the retina but loosely attached to sclera. Its function is to supply nutrition to the retina specially to the macula. It also keeps the inside of the eye dark. It is highly vascular. It does not have any muscles. Its disorders do not cause any pain or redness of the eye.

The disorders of the uvea can be divided into:
1. Congenital and
2. Acquired

The acquired disorders can be:
- Trauma
- Inflammations
- Degenerations
- Neoplasm

The congenital disorders of the uvea are –
- Total or portial absence of uvea (coloboma) and absence of pigment in the iris (albinism) (Fig. 12.2).
- Absence of uvea limited to iris only is called **aniridia**. In fact the iris is not totally absent, it is present in small pieces which are not visible on ordinary illumination and seen on slit lamp examination and gonioscope.
- It is a hereditary condition seen equally in both sexes.
- It is generally present in both the eyes.

The child is brought to eye specialist for any of the following symptoms:
1. Intolerance to light
2. Diminished distant vision
3. Nystagmus

On examination the pupil is widely dilated and no iris is visible. The lens generally has some opacity. The edge of the lens is visible on retinoscopy.

These eyes have raised intraocular tension which is difficult to treat.

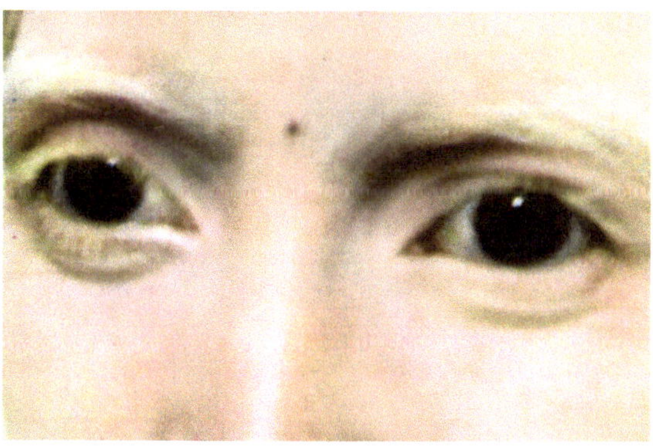

Fig. 12.2: Albinism light pigmented iris

Management consists of prescribing colored glass for glare. Correction of any error of refraction, keeping intraocular pressure under control by medicine and rehabilitation of child.

Coloboma of Uvea

These are more common than aniridia. The coloboma means absence of uvea in a localized area. Colobomas are generally situated at the lower part of the iris. It can be limited to iris only or may extend into choroid. In such a case the ciliary body is also absent at the site of coloboma.

The iris coloboma are situated at six o'clock position. It extends from pupil up to the limbus. The coloboma looks like a key hole. (Figs 12.3 to 12.5). The edge of the lens can be seen through the coloboma. Generally the eyes with coloboma are microphthalmic. The cornea is small, anterior chamber shallow, the pupil reacts to light. The vision varies from normal to hand movement.

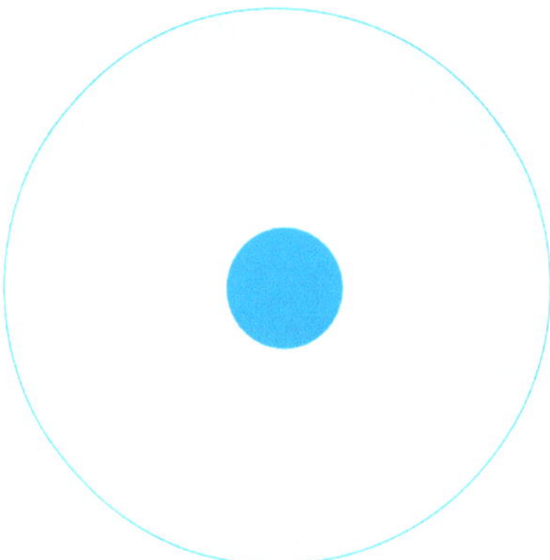

Fig. 12.3: Normal iris pupil and lens (blue)

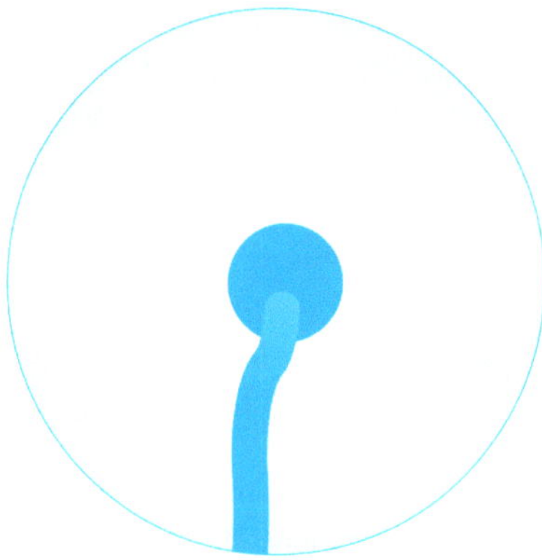

Fig. 12.4: Typical coloboma of iris with normal lens

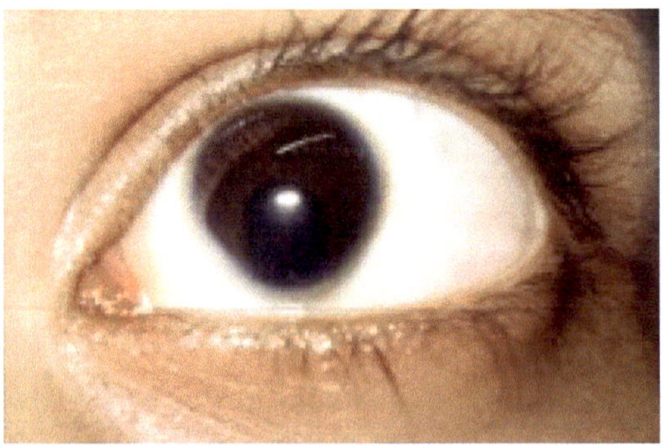

Fig. 12.5: Typical coloboma of the iris extending into the choroid

The choroidal coloboma may be extension of iris coloboma in the lower part. (Fig. 12.6) Sometimes the coloboma may invlove the choroid only. Such colobomas lie between the optic disc and the ciliary body in the lower part. Extensive coloboma may reach up to optic disc. Generally these eyes have poor vision. On retinoscopy the coloboma shines as white reflex. The details of the coloboma are best seen by direct and indirect ophthalmoscopy.

There is no treatment. Generally the vision does not improve with glasses.

Coloboma of Macula (Fig. 12.6)

Unlike coloboma of iris and choroid which are situated at 6 o'/clock position below the optic disc, the coloboma of the macula, is situated 2 ½ disc away from the disc on the temporal side, the usual place of macula as a punched out area oval in shape. The choroid and retina are absent in the coloboma. The white floor is formed by sclera. The size of coloboma form 1 mm to 10 mm. As there is no retina in the coloboma there is no vision in the area. The vision is very poor. It can be unilateral or bilateral. Coloboma of the macula are cause of profound visual loss, squint and nystagmus. There is no treatment. It must be differentiated from congenital toxoplasmosis (a parasitic disease).

Persistent Pupillary Membrane

The colobomas are due to deficient uveal tissue. Persistent pupillary membrane may be called excess of uveal tissues in the eye.

Till few weeks before birth there is no formed pupil. The area where the pupil should be present is covered by uveal tissue and vascular sheath of the lens. By birth these tissues disappear fully and a clear pupil becomes visible. In some cases these tissues do not disappear completely but stays as fine strands of tissue. These strands are called **persistent pupillary membrane**. This fine strands may be seen as bands across the pupil, may be attached to the lens capsule or float freely in the aqueous (Fig. 12.7).

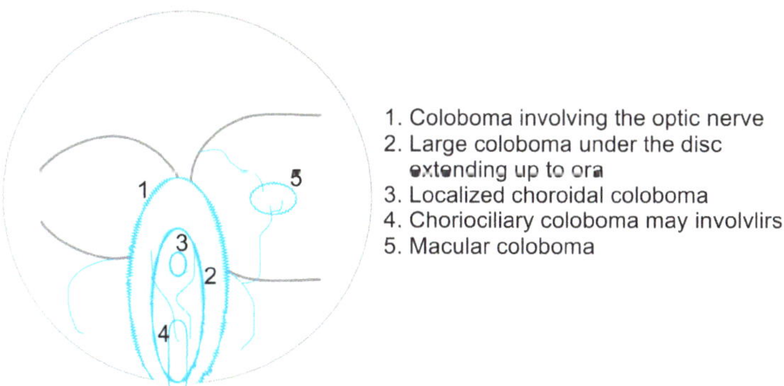

Fig. 12.6: Diagram showing various types of congenital choroidal coloboma and macular coloboma

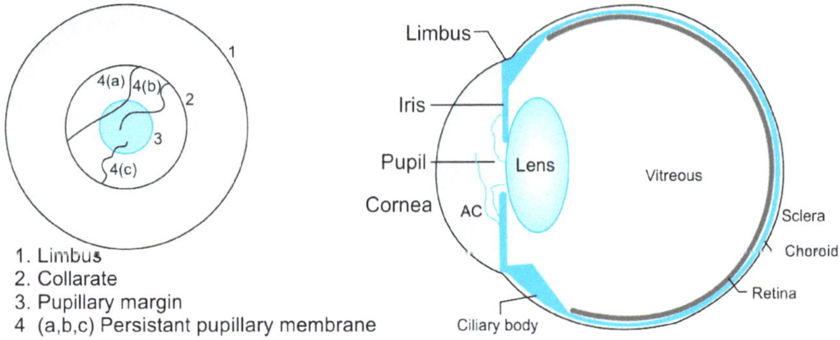

Fig. 12.7: Diagram showing persistant pupillary membrane

They are very common. Large strands are visible with torch light, the small strands are visible on slit lamp examination. The patient has no knowledge of them. They do not cause any symptoms. They do not require any treatment. Most of them disappear with age.

Albinism

The dark color of the uvea is due to pigment melanin. More is the pigment, darker is the iris. In case of albinism there is no or very little melanin in the body. The albinism can be generalized or may be restricted only to the eye. The latter is called **ocular albinism** which is less common than generalized albinism. (Fig. 12.8)

In albinism the skin is very pale. The hair, eyebrows and lashes are golden brown. The iris is bluish white, the pupil is pink. The patient have severe photophobia, diminished vision and nystagmus. There is no treatment. Correction of error of refraction by dark colored glasses give some relief to the child.

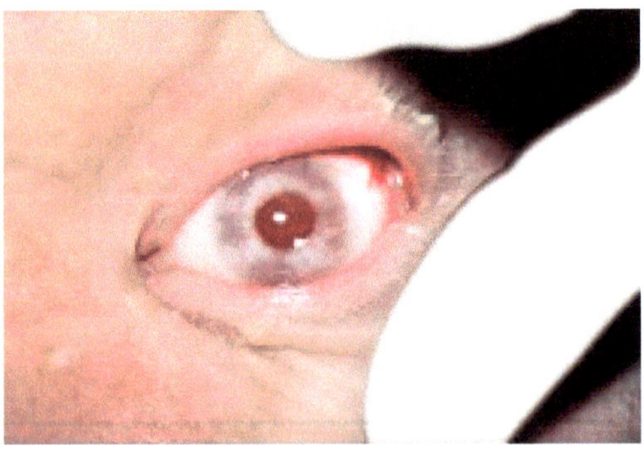

Fig. 12.8: Albinism showing absence of pigment in the iris and pink pupil (*Courtesy*: Dr Santosh Patel)

Trauma (Injury) to Uvea

Uvea may be injured in two ways:

- Penetration injury
- Blunt injury

Penetrating injury is that injury which cuts either the cornea, sclera or both. Penetrating injury of the cornea is always associated with **prolapse of iris** (iris comes out of the cornea). In severe cases it may involve the ciliary body and choroid as well. Injury to the lens is very common. The penetrating injury may be associated with intraocular foreign body. If the foreign body is light and slow, it gets lodged in iris, a large foreign body with force may penetrate the iris and injury to lens. It may pass through the lens or zonule and reach the retina.

Corneal injury requires stitching. If the iris has prolapsed, it should be cut. The process of cutting the iris is called **iridectomy**. If the lens is injured and opaque, it should also be removed. All cases of penetrating injury to the eye should **be X-rayed** for evidence of **intraocular foreign body** and when found to be so, the foreign body should be removed in specialized hospital. The penetrating injury of the ciliary body and choroid bleed profusely which may not be stopped by any means. In such cases the intra-ocular structures are removed by **evisceration.**

Blunt Injury to the Eye

1. Hyphema—Accumulation of blood in anterior chamber is called hyphema. The blood may be only in traces or may fill whole of the anterior chamber. In blunt injury the blood most of the time comes **from the ciliary body** and not from the iris. The normal iris does not bleed even when it is cut. Iris bleeds only when it is diseased as in chronic uveitis, diabetic retinopathy or neovascular glaucoma. Blood settles down at the bottom of the anterior chamber with a horizontal upper border when the head is erect and spreads all over the iris and pupil and when patient is lying. A large hyphema fills whole of the anterior chamber giving the cornea a red look. (Figs 12.9 to 12.11). It is not the cornea that is red but the red blood is visible through the cornea. If the hyphema covers the pupil, the vision is reduced otherwise it does not change the vision. Small hyphema disappears in a day or two without any trace. A large hyphema may take weeks to months to clear. A large hyphema may close the angle of anterior chamber and cause glaucoma. A large hyphema with glaucoma causes **staining of the cornea by blood**. This is called blood staining of cornea. A **blood stained cornea** is not red but yellowish grey. Blood staining of cornea requires treatment at specialized hospitals.

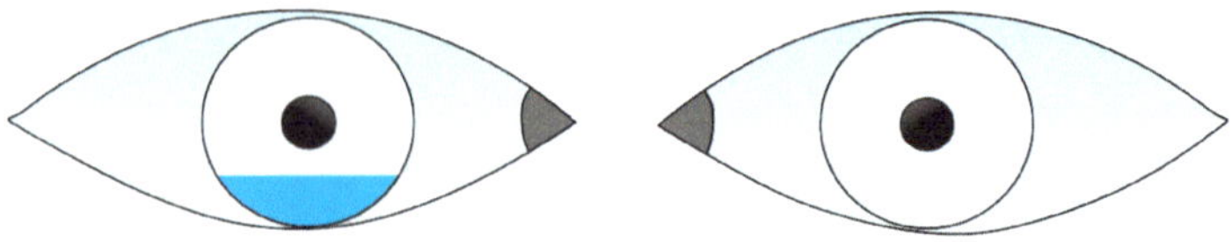

Fig. 12.9: Diagram showing fresh Hyphema at the bottom of AC when the eye is erect

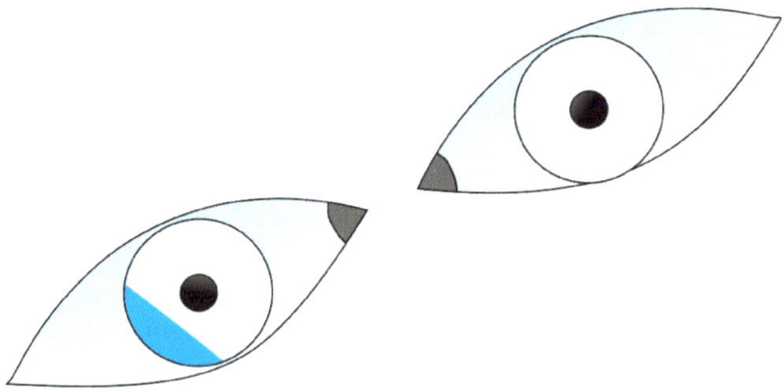

Fig. 12.10: Diagram showing fresh Hyphema when the head is filled right

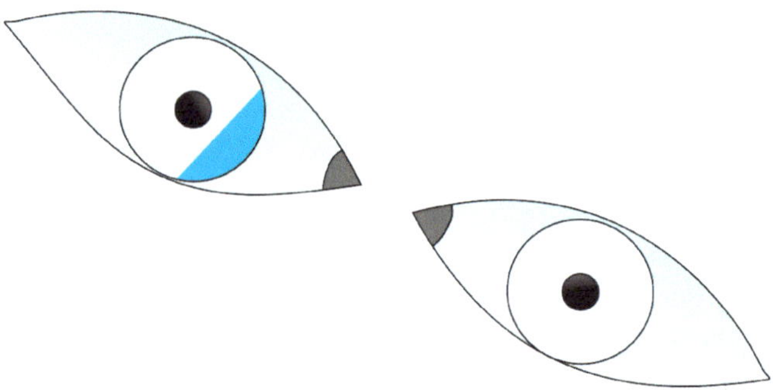

Fig. 12.11: Diagram showing fresh Hyphema when the head is tilted left

2. Changes in the pupil: followin blunt injury
   i. Change in size:
      A blunt injury can cause either constriction or dilatation of the pupil. The first is called **traumatic miosis** (Fig. 12.12C) and the second is called **traumatic mydriasis** (Fig. 12.12B). Traumatic miosis is caused due to paralysis of dilator muscles. The pupil is small and irregular, reacts sluggishly to light. In a few days it returns to normal size. It may cause **Vossius ring** on the anterior surface of lens.

Traumatic Mydriasis

This is due to paralysis of constrictors of pupil. The pupil is larger than normal and sluggish to light and accommodation. The pupil is irregular. It takes longer time for the pupil to come to normal size. In some cases the pupil may remain dilated for rest of the life (Fig. 12.12B).

Change in Shape of Pupil Following Injury

This can be brought about in two ways:

1. Ruptures of pupillary margin – This causes a notch at the pupillary margin (Fig. 12.12D).
2. **Iridodialysis** (Fig. 12.12E)—In this case the iris is detached from the ciliary body. It may be very small and go unnoticed unless searched or may be as large as to involve whole of the iris and the whole of the iris is detached and lies in the anterior chamber as a nodule causing aniridia. Otherwise moderate iridodialysis has following features.

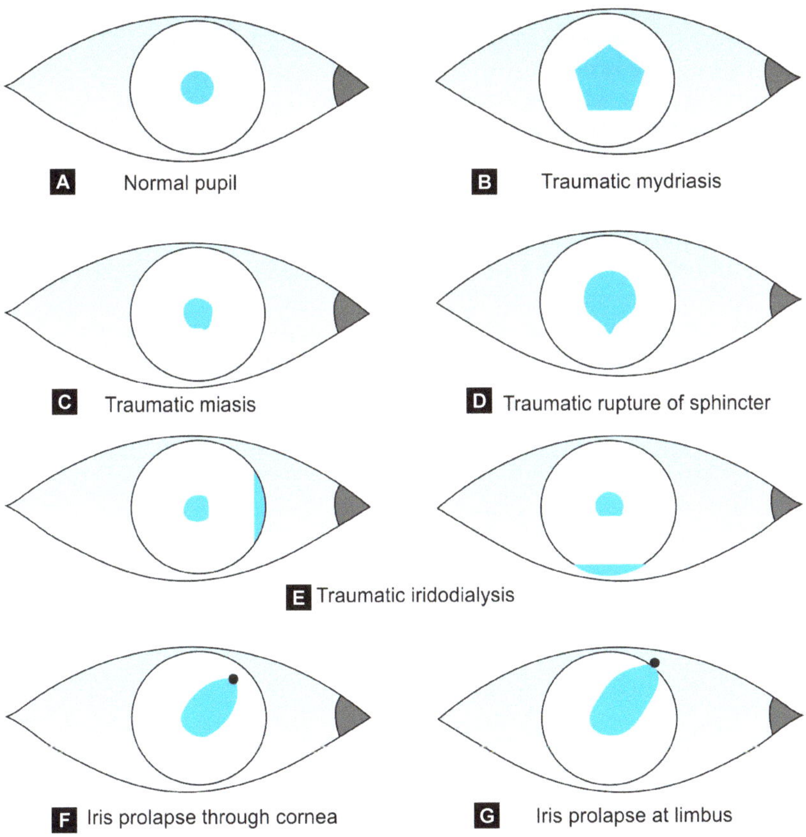

Figs 12.12A to G: Effect of blood trauma on iris and pupil

i. There is hole in the iris at the limbus. The hole is flat towards the pupil.
ii. The pupil is D shaped with flat surface towards the hole.
iii. There may be hyphema in AC.
iv. The lens may be clear and in its normal place or may be dislocated or subluxated. Late cataractous changes are common.

Small dialysis do not require any treatment. Large holes may be required to be closed by stitches.

Blunt injury to ciliary body may rupture the ciliary body causing it to bleed resulting in hyphema or it may be detached from its attachment and a slit develops between the ciliary body and sclera. This is called **traumatic cyclodialysis** and is generally associated with lowering of intra ocular tension. Tear may extends in the substance of the ciliary body and damage the trabecular meshwork. This is called **recession of angle of anterior chamber** resulting to late onset of **wide angle glaucoma**.

Blunt injury to the choroid results in rupture of choroid. Choroids ruptures away from the disc like a crescent of moon with concavity towards the disc. Generally there is only one rupture but there may be two. Initially due to rupture of choroidal vessel there is hemorrhage over the rupture and the rupture is not visible. Ones the blood clears the rupture becomes visible. If it is not between the macula and the disc, there is no loss of vision. No treatment is required (Fig. 12.13).

Inflammation of Uvea

Inflammation of uvea is called **uveitis**. Uveitis is a common disorder of the eye. It can be seen at any age. Both males and females are equally affected. It may be unilateral and remain unilateral or may become bilateral. The course of the disease in the second eye is similar to in the first eye.

Uveitis always does not involve all the parts of the uvea.

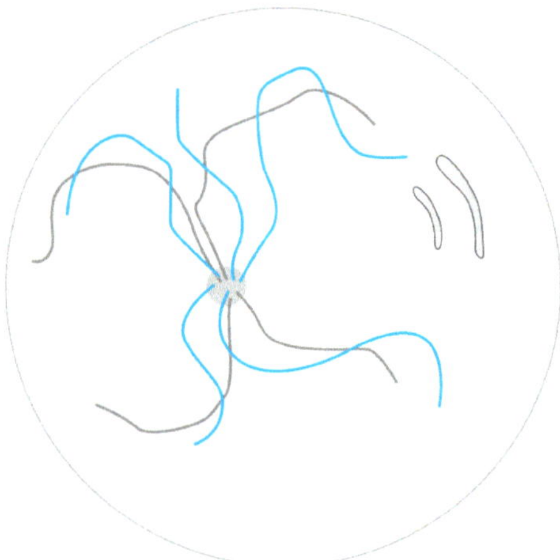

Fig. 12.13: Traumatic choroidal rupture

Flow chart 12.1: Showing anatomical classification of uveitis

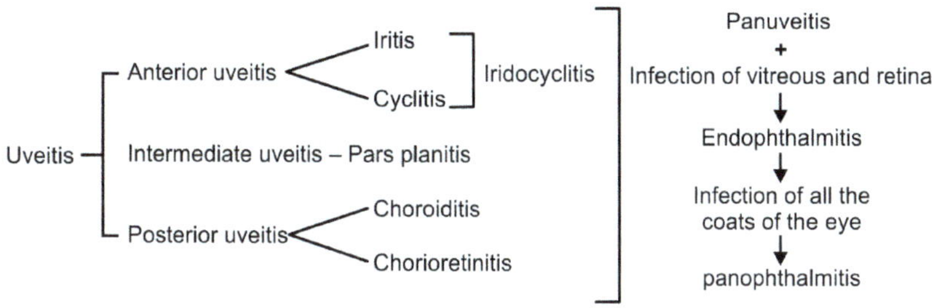

Table 12.1: Shows possible sites of inflammation in uveitis

Name of uveitis	Main part of uvea involved	Other parts of the eye involved
Iritis	Iris	Nil
Cyclitis	Anterior part of ciliary body	Nil
Iridocyclitis	Iris + Ciliary body	Angle of AC
Parsplanitis	Posterior part of ciliary body	Anterior part of choroid, retina, macula and vitreous
Choroiditis	Choroid	Retina, macula, vitreous
Endophthalmitis	All structures inside the globe	Sclera
Panophthalmitis	All intraocular structures	Extraocular muscles

According to the part of uvea invloved it is divided into **anterior** or **posterior** uveitis. When whole of the uvea is involved it is called **panuveitis.** As the retina is very near the choroid and gets its blood supply from the choroid, it is very common for retina to be involved in choroiditis and the condition is called **chorioretinitis**. If the vitreous is affected the condition is called **endophthalmitis.** If the infections spreads outside the coats of the eye, a very serious vision threatening condition called **panophthalmitis** develops Flow chart 12.1 and Table 12.1 showing sites of lesion in uveitis.

Iridocyclitis (Iritis + Cyclitis)

Iritis is inflammation of iris only. Cyclitis is inflammation of ciliary body. It is very rare for one of them to be present, hence they are collectively called iridocyclitis. It is an acute condition seen in children or young adults. It is generally unilateral (one eye). It begins with pain in the eye. The eyeball is tender (painful on pressure). There is headache on the side of the eye to be involved. There is photophobia, lacrimation, redness and diminished vision. Vision ranges from near normal to 6/60 with good projection.

On examination—The lids are moderately by swollen, the eye is red due to **circumciliary congestion**. The discharge is watery, the eyeball is tender, the cornea is bright on epithelial surface (the front surface) but shows small deposits on the endothelial surface (back surface). These deposits are called **keratic precipitates** (KP).

Keratic Precipitates

These are cells that arise from the iris and ciliary body and are deposited on the back surface of the cornea. Their number vary from a few to many. They may be so large as to be seen by torch light or so small as to be seen under high power magnification of slit lamp. The large white KPs are called **mutton fat KPs**. They may be scattered all over the endothelium but the commonest pattern is triangular with apex upwards and base at the limbus. They appear early but may be present when the inflammation has been brought under control (Fig. 12.14).

Flare

The normal aqueous is crystal clear without any suspended particle. In iritis the cells from the inflammed iris, are mixed with the aqueous. Initially they remain suspended in the aqueous and are visible on bright narrow beams of slit lamp under magnification. The suspended particles are heavier than aqueous.

As the number of cells increase, they settle down at the bottom of the anterior chamber as pus and called **hypopyon**.

HYPOPYON

Hypopyon is collection of pus in anterior chamber. The pus gets infected only if the cornea is perforated. The common examples are perforated corneal ulcer and perforating injury of the eye. The hypopyon is heavier than aqueous, so the cells settle at the lowest part of the anterior chamber. Newly formed hypopyon is fluid and moves with position of head. If the head is tilted right it will be seen on lateral side of right eye and if the head is tilted left it will be seen on the medial side of AC of right eye in case of hypopyon of right eye (Fig. 12.15).

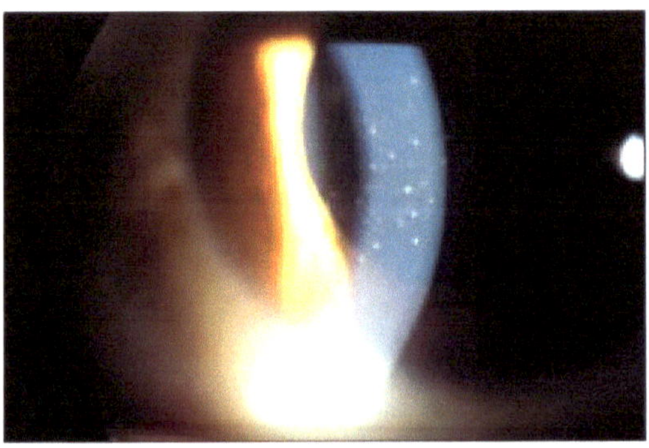

Fig. 12.14: Keratic precipitate (*Courtesy*: Dr Santosh Patel)

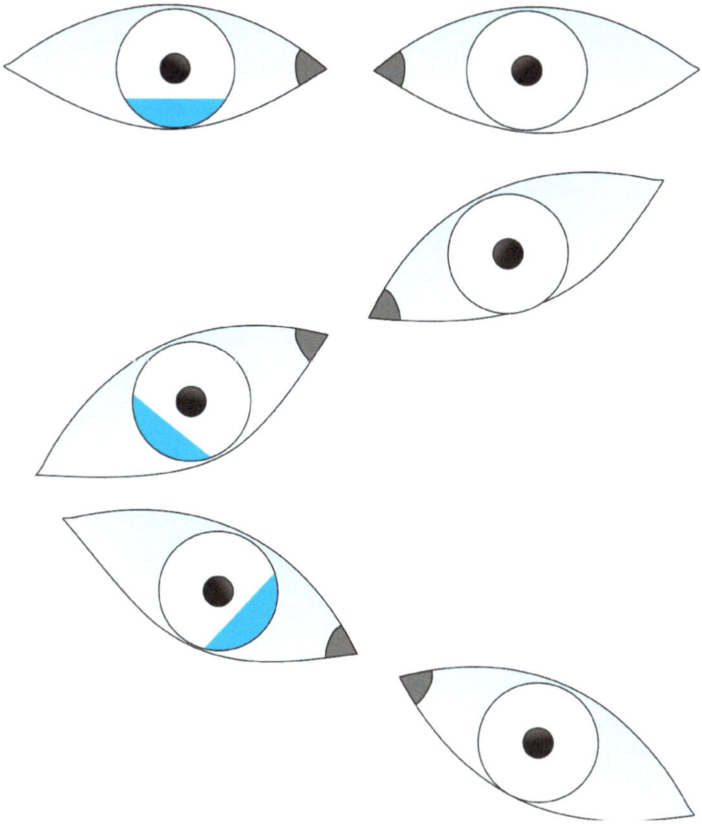

Fig. 12.15: Diagram showing fresh hypopyon at various positions

Hypopyon is **white in color**. In some cases it may become pink when mixed with blood. The uppermost part of the hypopyon is horizontal. The size of hypopyon depends upon seriousness (severity) of the uveitis. It may be very small and not visible unless the patient looks down or it may be large enough to fill the whole of the anterior chamber giving a white color to the cornea. The size of the hypopyon may change many a times during the day even without a treatment. **Hypopyon is always a serious condition** that requires prompt treatment. The conditions that cause hypopyon are iritis, iridocyclitis, cyclitis, panuveitis, endophthalmitis and panophthalmitis. Choroiditis does not cause hypopyon.

Any white matter in anterior chamber should be considered to be hypopyon unless proved otherwise (It turns out not to be pus). Such conditions are called **pseudo (false) hypopyon**. They are: cortical matter in anterior chamber following perforating injury or extracapsular cataract extraction. It could be malignant cells (cells of cancers of the retina or uvea), worm or cyst.

When hypopyon is associated with corneal ulcer it is called **hypopyon corneal ulcer**. In all cases of hypopyon corneal ulcer, the lacrimal sac should be examined for chronic dacryocyctitis because chronic dacryocystitis is an important cause of hypopyon.

Treatment of Hypopyon

Treatment of hypopyon is treatment of the cause, i.e. uveitis/corneal ulcer.

In all cases of hypopyon the pupil should be dilated with **atropine sulfate**. If there is no corneal ulcer patient is put on a combination of steroid and broad spectrum antibiotic four to six times a day or a **subconjunctival injection** of steroid and antibiotic is given.

In case of ulcer corticosteroid is contraindicated (not used). The eye is atropinized and **fortified solution of gentamycine or cephazoline** is put every five minutes for six times, then every 10 minutes for six times, then every hourly. If the condition does not improve subconjunctival gentamycine or subconjunctival cephazoline is given. In all cases of hypopyon urine should be tested for diabetes. If there is rise of intraocular tension it should be brought down by oral diamox.

Pupil in Iridocyclitis

In iritis and iridocyclitis the pupil is small, central, irregular and sluggish. Irregularity becomes more obvious if the pupil is dilated with mild mydriatic cum cycloplegia, i.e. homatropine or cyclopentolate. The cause of irregularity is adhesion (fixing) of posterior surface of iris to the anterior surface of the lens. These adhesions are called **posterior synechia**. The posterior synechia may vary in number. The pupil does not react to light at the place of the posterior synechiae. Irregular pupil following dilatation is called **festooned pupil**. Freshly formed synechiae break with two to three instillation of cycloplegic and leave few pigments on the lens capsule (Fig. 12.16).

Other causes of irregular pupil are: Persistent pupillary membrane (Fig. 12.7), traumatic miosis, traumatic mydriasis, rupture of pupillary margin, iridodialysis, iris prolapse (Figs 12.12 A to F).

In severe cases of iridocyclitis the pupil is covered by exudate and the condition is called **occlusio pupil**. The color of the exudate is white when present in the pupillary area, it may be mistaken as cataract.

If the posterior synechia is extensive, it may be formed all-around the pupil. This is called **ring synechia**. Such synechiae prevent the aqueous to pass from the posterior chamber to anterior chamber through the pupil. As the aqueous can not pass in the anterior chamber it pushes the iris forwards and the condition is called **iris bombe** (Figs 12.17 and 12.18).

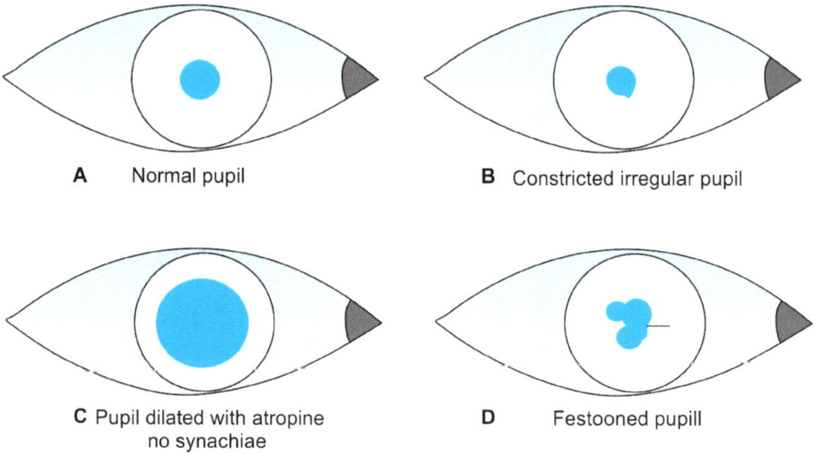

Fig. 12.16: Pupillary changes in iridocyclitis

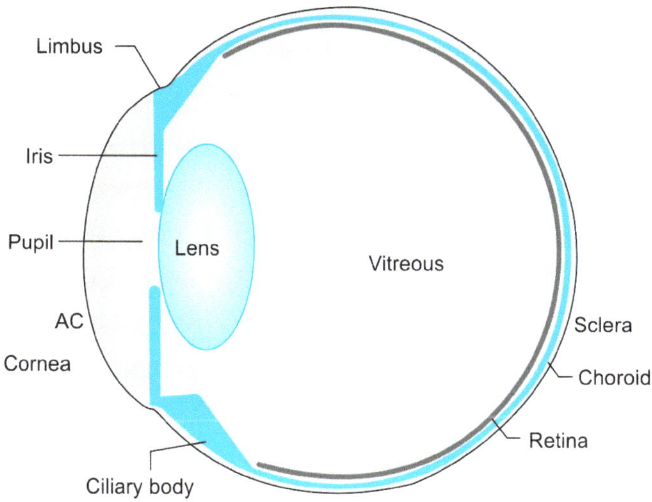

Fig. 12.17: Diagram showing normal depth of AC

Iris Bombe

In iris bombe the anterior chamber is irregular in depth is shallow between the pupillary margin and limbus. There may be exudate in the pupillary area. The angle may be closed due to anterior synechiae resulting in rise of intraocular tension. **Other causes of irregular depth of anterior chamber are** iris prolapse, subluxated lens, adhered leuoma and nodule on the iris.

Peripheral anterior synechiae is an adhesion between the anterior surface of iris and posterior surface of cornea, and blocks the angle of anterior chamber causing rise of intraocular tension (Fig. 12.19).

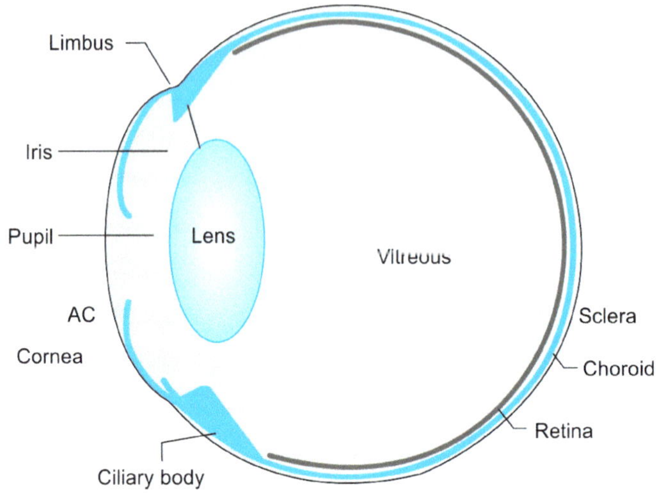

Fig. 12.18: Diagram showing irregular pupil in iris bombee

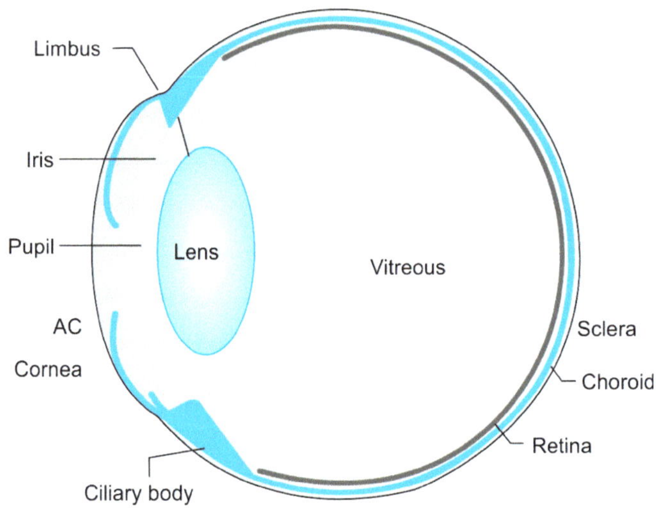

Fig. 12.19: Diagram showing anterior synechiae

Nodule Formation on Iris

In some cases, small nodules develop on the iris. In chronic iridocyclitis they may be anywhere on the iris. Common causes of nodule on iris are **tuberculosis**, **syphilis** and **leprosy**. They disappear with local and systemic treatment (Fig. 12.20).

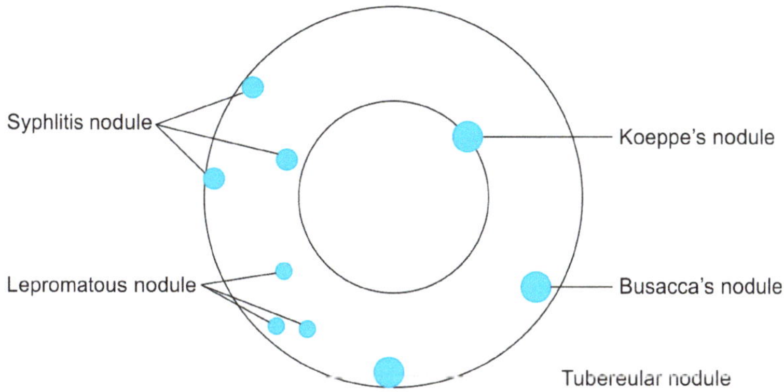

Fig. 12.20: Various types of inflammatory nodules in chronic iridocyclitis with their relative position

Recurrence

Iritis is most of the time a self-limiting disease and responds well to treatment but sometimes there may be recurrence (developing again) in the same eye or the other eye.

Differential Diagnosis of Iridocyclitis

Iritis should be differentiated from corneal foreign body, foreign body in the tarsal plate, acute congestive glaucoma, acute conjunctivitis and phlycten.

Complication of Iridocyclitis

Commonest complication is **secondary glaucoma** (rise of intraocular tension. The second complication is **complicated cataract** (early onset of cataract), **band keratopathy**. On a long run the eye may become soft and a stage of **phthisis bulbi** may develop.

Diagnosis of acute iridocyclitis is easy if the following points are kept in mind—Unilateral, painful, tender eye with redness, no mucopurulent discharge, small pupil, KPs.

Presence of hypopyon is sure sign of iridocyclitis.

Treatment of iridocyclitis consists of instillation of nonsteroidal anti-inflammatory drops three times and cyclopentolate one percent three times a day. If the condition does not improve and cornea does not stain, local steroid should be started and cyclopentolate is replaced by atropine one percent once a day. If hypopyon is present, subconjunctival antibiotic is required.

Posterior Uveitis

This is also called **choroiditis**. It is less common than anterior uveitis. In contrast to anterior uveitis, this is not a painful condition. There is no redness either. Complaints include diminished vision, distorted vision and floaters. It may be unilateral or bilateral.

Posterior uveitis may involve the choroid only or may involve the retina along with. Involvement of macula is cause of loss of vision. Involvement of vitreous is the cause of floaters.

The posterior uveitis may be localized (focal) or scattered. The localized lesion when involves the macula, it is called **central choroiditis** (Figs 12.21A to D).

Rest are called by various names. They are:

1. Diffuse choroiditis—When they are wide spread with little space between two lesions.
2. Disseminated choroiditis—When multiple with some areas of normal choroid in between.

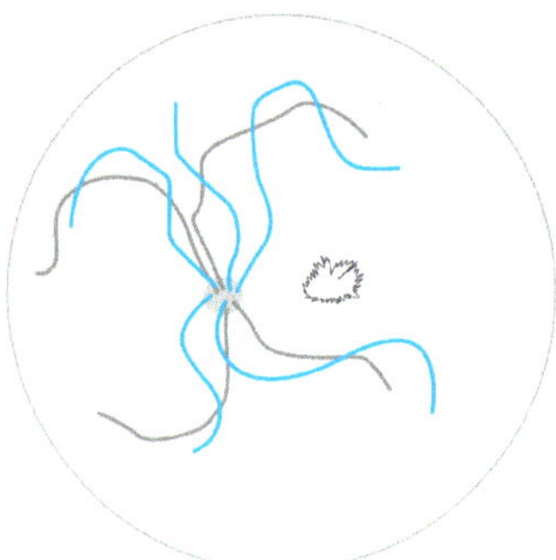

A Central choroIditis

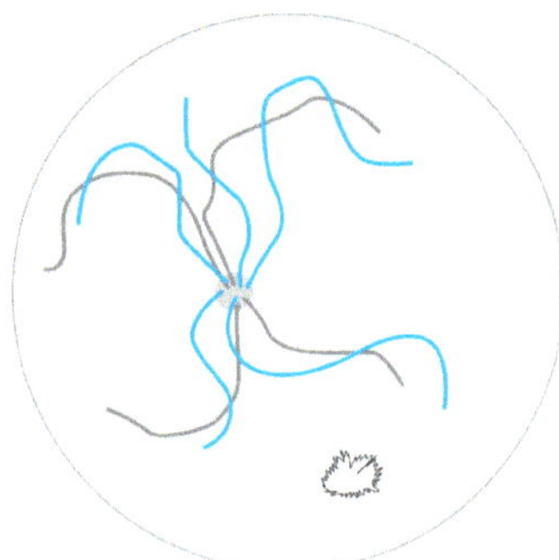

B Isolated peripheral choroiditis

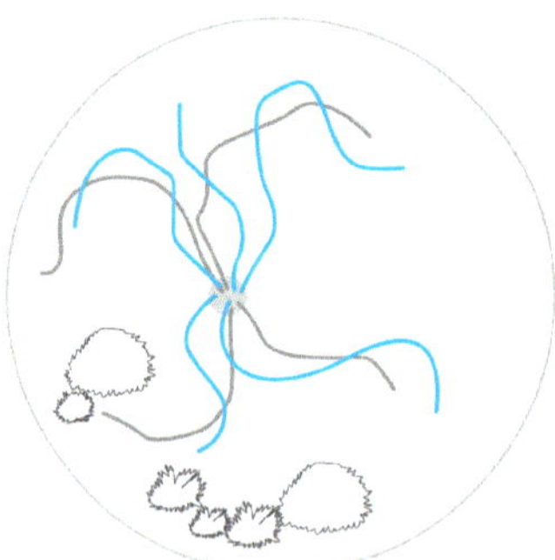

C Diffused choroiditis

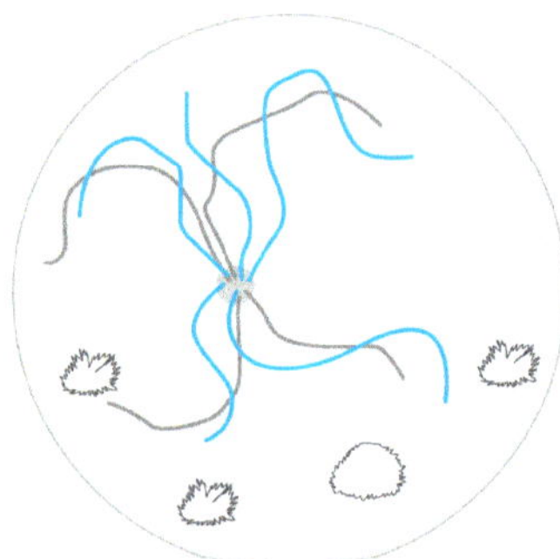

D Disseminated choroiditis

Figs 12.21A to D: Location of various types of choroiditis

These names depend on their ophthalmoscopic picture and location in relation to macula.

The central choroiditis involving macular has poorest vision. Isolated focal choroiditis may not have loss of vision so may be the disseminated choroiditis unless its involves macula also.

The patches of choroiditis produce corresponding field defect.

Management is treatment of cause, i.e. tuberculosis, syphilis, toxoplasmosis, etc. Local antibiotics and steroids do not have any role in posterior uveitis. However systemic steroid may be required. It can be given either by mouth or as sub tenons injection under supervision.

Panuveitis

If all the parts of the uvea, i.e. iris, ciliary body and choroid are involved at the same time, it is called **panuveitis** (Flow chart 12.2). The condition is generally chronic. Most of the infected condition that cause anterior or posterior uveitis can cause panuveitis. The examples are tuberculosis, syphilis, herpes simplex, AIDS. Some of noninfectious conditions can also cause panuveitis. The best example is **sympathetic ophthalmia**. The panuveitis generally involves the retina and optic nerve also.

If the vitreous is involved it is called **endophthalmitis**. In such cases the infection spreads from vitreous to the uvea. It is called **exogenous endophthalmitis**. Spread of infection from uvea to vitreous is less common and called **endogenous endophthalmitis**.

The commonest causes of exogenous endophthalmitis is perforating injury of the globe. It may be surgical or accidental. The other cause is perforating corneal ulcer. The exogenous endophthalmitis can be acute or subacute. The acute exogenous endophthalmitis is caused by pus forming bacteria. The subacute exogenous endophthalmitis is caused by fungus.

The acute endophthalmitis develops within first two to three days of injury. The symptoms are:

1. Pain in the eye
2. Rapid fall of vision
3. Edema of lids
4. Redness of the eye
5. Discharge from the eye

The signs are:

- Edema of the lids
- Swelling of the conjunctiva
- Conjunctival congestion
- Haziness of the cornea
- Wound of entry
- Pus in AC
- Exudate in pupillary area
- Absent retinal glow
- The movements are present

Management

Postsurgical Endophthalmitis

Prevention is the best treatment. Prevention of postoperative endophthalmitis includes:

1. Selection of cases
2. Sterilization of instruments
3. Disinfection of OT
4. Subconjunctival injection of antibiotics after operation

The following cases should not be operated:

1. Case with chronic dacryocystitis
2. Entropion, ectropion
3. Lagophthalmos
4. Loss of corneal sensation
5. Stye, chalazion
6. Uncontrolled diabetes

Once endophthalmitis has developed it is a very serious condition and require urgent treatment that include:

1. Atropine locally.
2. Intravitreal injection of antibiotic.
3. If there is no arrangement of intravitreal injection then subconjunctival injection of broad spectrum antibiotic may be given two times a day.
4. In between the two subconjunctival injection the patient is put on fortified antibiotic drop hourly.

Panophthalmitis

This is an acute condition. In this case all the intraocular structures are involved in infection by pus forming bacteria. It is a severe form of endophthalmitis. The vitreous is full of pus. The sclera and extra-ocular muscles are also involved. There is some degree of proptosis. The movements are absent.

On examination:

1. There is no perception of light.
2. The lids are swollen.
3. Mild to moderate proptosis.
4. The movements are absent.
5. The conjunctiva is chemosed.
6. The cornea is hazy, may be perforated.
7. Anterior chamber is full of pus.
8. Structures beyond the pus are not visible.
9. Generally this is unilateral.
10. The condition does not respond to any medical treatment. The only treatment is removal of all the intraocular contents and cornea. The sclera is left intact. The procedure is called **evisceration**.

Sympathetic Uveitis (Sympathetic Ophthalmia)

This is an example of panuveitis that develops following perforating injury that specially involves ciliary body in the other eye after few days to years. Suppose the right eye is involved in perforation injury, the other eye (left eye) develops panuveitis after 15 to 20 days or may be after years. The injured eye is called **exciting eye** and the other eye that develops panuveitis is called **sympathizing eye**.

It begins as marked photophobia and lacrimation (watering) in the sympathizing eye with blurring of distant and near vision.

On examination there is circumciliary congestion, KPs, flare, signs of iridocyclitis. Iridocyclitis is more marked than choroiditis.

The management of sympathetic uveitis is divided into two parts:

1. **Management of injured eye:**
   i. The wound should be carefully stitched. Any trace of uvea and lens matter in the wound should be removed.
   ii. In the post operative period, the eye is treated by atropine two times a day and local steroid six to eight times a day.
   iii. If there is no perception of light in the injured eye, it should be removed by a procedure called **enucleation**. In enucleation the eyeball is detached from the extraocular muscles and optic nerve and removed.
2. **Management of the sympathizing eye:**
   i. All the patients with penetrating injury in one eye must be told about the danger of developing sympathetic ophthalmia in the un-injured eye.
   ii. They should seek immediate help if they develop any of the following in the un-injured eye
      – Photophobia, lacrimation, redness and blurring of vision.

Once sympathetic ophthalmia has been confirmed, the eye should be treated as severe form of chronic uveitis by

– Atropine two times a day
– Steroid

i. Local drops of strong steroid every hourly
ii. Subconjunctival injection of steroid two times a day
iii. Oral steroid in large doses

The patient requires local steroids and oral steroids for months with all caution.

Tumors of Uvea

Tumors of the uvea can be benign (noncancer) or malignant (cancer).

The common benign tumors of uvea are:

Iris – Nevus hemangioma, neurofibroma, congenital cysts, parasitic cysts, foreign body granuloma.

Ciliary body – Hemangiomas, medullo epithelioma
Choroid – Haemangioma, neurofibroma, benign melanoma (nevus)

Malignant Tumors of the Uvea

The malignant tumors of the uvea may be primary, i.e. arising from the uvea or secondary. In secondary tumor the primary tumor is not in the eye but far away from the eye. They are called **metastatic tumors** of the uvea.

The commonest primary malignant tumor of the uvea is **malignant melanoma of the choroid**. It is less common in ciliarybody and least common in iris.

Malignant melanoma of choroid is seen in persons over fifty years of age. It is unilateral and single. It is more commonly seen on temporal (towards the ear) of the choroid. It may be well defined or diffuse. The tumor is slow growing, may be symptomless or there may be frequent change of near and distant glasses. Initially it is difficult to differentiate from benign melanoma of choroid. The patient may present with loss of field. As the tumor enlarges it may fill a large part of the globe and grow in the angle causing secondary glaucoma. This is a painful stage. It may perforate the globe and pass into the orbit from where it may pass into blood stream causing **distant metastasis**. Commonest site for metastasis **is liver**.

The diagnosis is easy in large tumours otherwise it is confirmed by ultrasonography, CT and MRI.

Treatment

Large intraocular tumours are best treated by enucleation. Small intraocular tumours are treated by radio therapy or laser. If the tumor comes out of the sclera than treatment is exenteration of the orbit followed by chemotherapy.

Exenteration is removal of all the contents of the orbit and lids with periosteom.

Abnormal Contents of Anterior Chamber

1. Hypopyon
2. Pseudohypopyon, any gray substance in AC. It could be:
    i. Lens:
        a. Mature cataract
        b. Cortical matter
        c. Nucleus
    ii. IOL:
        a. AC IOL
        b. Dislocated PCIOL

3. Blood—Hyphema
4. Vitreous in case of intracapsular cataract extraction, subluxated lens or dislocated lens
5. Parasites
   i. Worms—Filaria
   ii. Parasitic cyst—Cysticercosis
6. Foreign body
7. Tumors of iris and ciliary body.

CHAPTER 13

Glaucoma

Glaucoma is a major cause of bilateral blindness world over. Fortunately it is a treatable and unfortunately not preventable.

It is not a single disease. It comprises many disorders. The chief among them is chronic (progressive) damage to the optic nerve that results in diminished vision and loss of field of vision. The commonest factor blamed for damage to the optic nerve is **abnormal rise of intraocular pressure**. As the pressure inside the eye increases, it presses the optic nerve and retinal fibers. Raised intraocular pressure also diminishes blood supply to the optic nerve. All these result in loss of field of vision.

Thus, the four components that comprise glaucoma are:

1. Diminished vision
2. Raised intraocular pressure
3. Field changes (Fig. 13.1) and
4. Optic atrophy

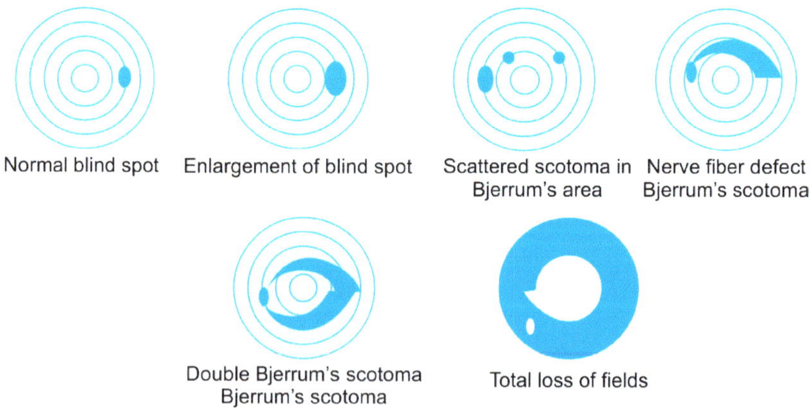

Fig. 13.1: Progressive field changes in glaucoma

Before we proceed to discuss glaucoma, we should understand:

1. The anatomy of the structures related to glaucoma
   The ciliary body, the zonule and the lens form a partition that divides the inner side of the eye in two unequal parts called chambers (Fig. 13.2):
   a. A large **vitreous chamber**—This is not directly related to glaucoma.
   b. A small **aqueous chamber**—This is directly related to glaucoma. The aqueous chamber is divided again in two unequal parts, a small **posterior chamber** and large **anterior chamber**. The two communicate with each other through the **pupil**. The anterior chamber is a plano convex space bound in front by the back surface of the cornea and behind by the iris and lens (in the pupillary area). When the lens is absent the vitreous forms the back surface of the anterior chamber.

      The place where the back surface of cornea and the front surface of the iris meet is called the **angle of the anterior chamber**. This is the most important structure as far as glaucoma is concerned because 95% of the aqueous drains through the angle of anterior chamber. If the angle becomes very narrow or is closed, the aqueous fails to drain and the tension rises.

      The other place where the aqueous may get obstructed is the pupil. If the pupil becomes very small, the flow of aqueous from posterior chamber to anterior chamber is reduced or stopped. This pushes the iris towards the cornea that blocks the angle and tension rises.

      The anterior chamber is not equal in its depth throughout. It is deepest in front of the pupil and gradually decreases in depth on the periphery.

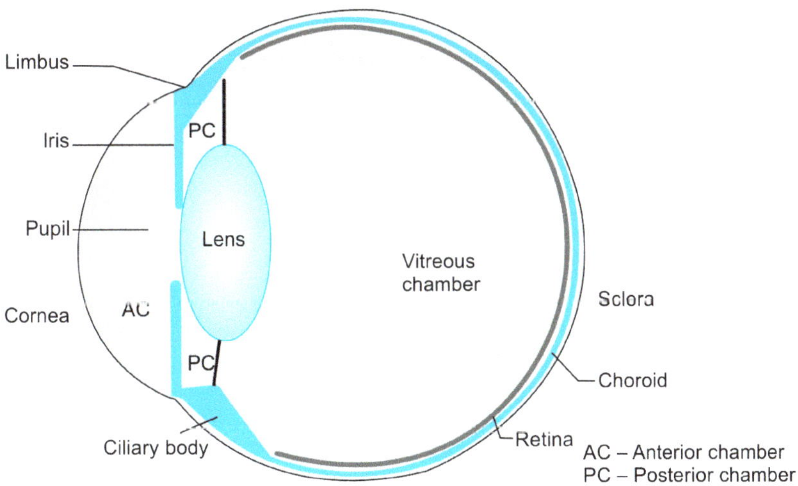

Fig. 13.2: Chambers of eye

2. **Intraocular pressure** is the force (pressure) exerted by intraocular contents on the outer coat of the eye, i.e. sclera and cornea. As the optic nerve passes through the sclera, it is also effected by intraocular pressure.
   The intraocular contents that exert pressure are **aqueous humor, lens, vitreous** and **choroid**. Out of all these, the aqueous humor is the most important factor that produces and maintains intraocular pressure.

FORMATION OF AQUEOUS HUMOR

Aqueous humor is a crystal clear intraocular fluid which is constantly formed in the posterior chamber at a steady rate, in the **ciliary process**. From posterior chamber it passes into anterior chamber through the pupil and circulates in the anterior chamber (Fig. 13.3). It leaves the anterior chamber through the angle of anterior chamber in a steady rate. Thus, there is a balance between formation and drainage of aqueous. This, balance is the cause behind normal intraocular pressure. If the rate of formation falls below normal limit or the drainage is more than normal level, the intraocular pressure will fall and eyeball will become soft. In contrast to this, if the formation is more or drainage is less than normal, the intraocular tension will rise. This rise of tension due to reduced drainage is the main cause of glaucoma.

The aqueous has following functions:

1. **Optical**: Aqueous along with cornea anteriorly and lens posteriorly form a single optical unit of +60 D. Out of which +42 D is due to cornea, +17 D due to lens and rest due to aqueous.
2. **Nutrition**—It supplies nutrition to lens and cornea.
3. **Intraocular pressure**—It creates a pressure higher than outside pressure. Thus, maintain the shape and firmness of the globe.
4. **It removes** waste products from the eye.

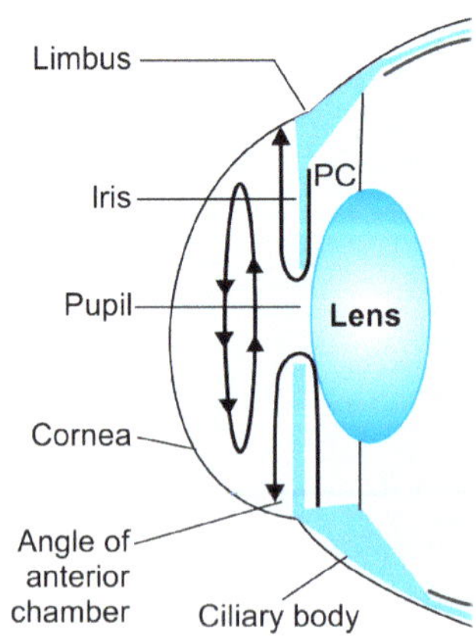

Fig. 13.3: Diagram showing circulation of aqueous

Normal Intraocular Pressure

The normal intraocular tension is between 15 mm Hg to 20 mm Hg. Tension under 10 mm Hg and above 25 mm Hg is abnormal. Tension less than 10 mm Hg is called **hypotony** and above 25 mm is called **glaucoma** and **ocular hypertension**. Ocular hypotony and ocular hypertension both do not cause severe changes that is seen in glaucoma. Generally tension in two eyes is equal but if the difference is more than 6 mm Hg, it is suggestive of glaucoma.

The tension is not constant throughout the day and night. It is highest in the morning and lowest in the evening. In normal eye the change between the two is not more than 5 mm Hg. If it is more than 7 mm Hg it is again suggestive of glaucoma.

There are some drugs that reduce intraocular tension either by reducing production or by increasing the outflow. These drugs can be taken by mouth or as local drops. These drugs are used to treat glaucoma.

The intraocular tension is measured by a group of instruments called **tonometers**. They can be mechanical or optical. The mechanical tonometer commonly used is called Schiötz's tonometer (Fig. 13.4). The optical tonometer is called **applanation tonometer**. Commonest used applanation tonometer is Goldmann tonometer that requires a slit lamp to use it. Other types are hand held applanation tonometer and pneumo (puff) tonometer.

> Tonometers can transfer infection from one eye to the other. Hence, they should be cleaned after each use and sterilized every day.

Optic Nerve

The optic nerve contains about one million fibers that originate in the retina. As the intraocular tension rises, the nerve fibers are compressed, their blood supply is also reduced. This leads to death of the nerve fibers. Death of nerve fibers cause changes in field of vision. The first field of vision to be lost is peripheral field. The central vision remains good. As glaucoma progress

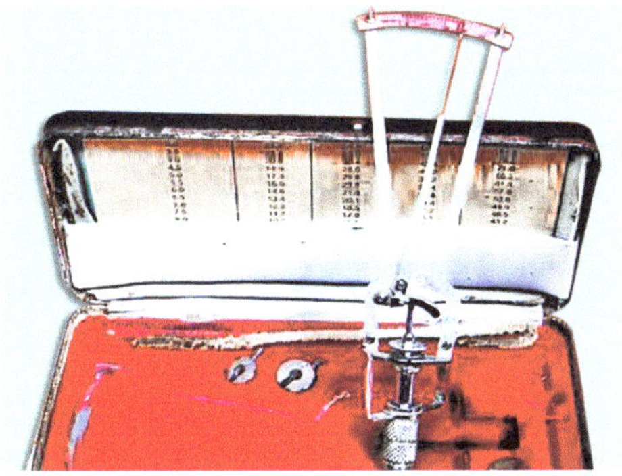

Fig. 13.4: Schiötz's tonometer

more and more retinal fibers get damaged and the field becomes smaller and smaller and at the end the whole of the optic nerve dies with total loss of vision. The change in optic disc is called glaucomatous optic atrophy.

> The vision and field once lost due to glaucoma can not be recovered, hence, glaucoma should be diagnosed and treated as early as possible.

> End result of all untreated glaucoma is **absolute glaucoma**, which results in permanent blindness.

TYPES OF GLAUCOMA (FLOW CHART 13.1)

A child may be born with raised intraocular tension and glaucoma or may develop glaucoma with in first two to three years of age (Fig. 13.5). This is called **congenital glaucoma** (buphthalmos). This is generally bilateral and the tension is generally very high, i.e. more than 40 mm Hg.

Sclera and cornea in children under three years of age are not rigid as in adults. They are stretched under raised tension. This increases the eyeball in size in all direction and the condition is called **buphthalmos**. In buphthalmos the cornea is also large and it becomes hazy. The child gets watering, photophobia and blepharospasm. The child keeps the eyes closed and turns the face away from light.

Flow chart 13.1: Classification of glaucoma

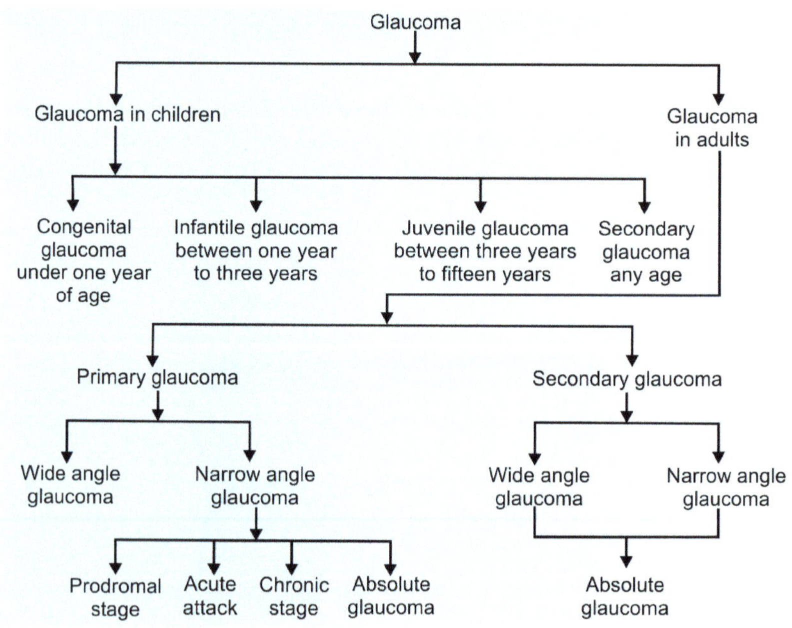

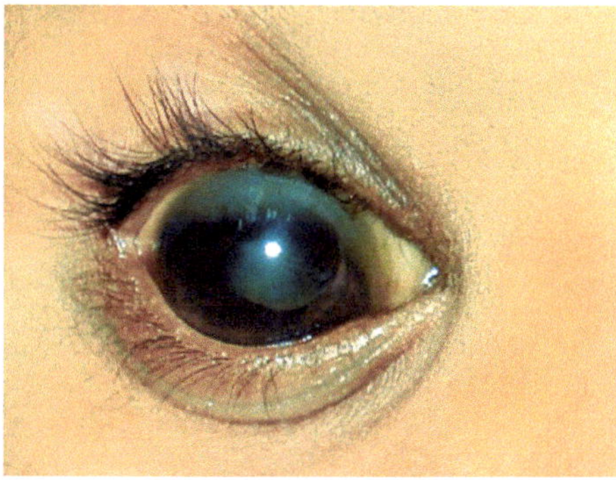

Fig. 13.5: Buphthalmos

The glaucoma developing between one to three years is called **infantile glaucoma**, which is milder than congenital glaucoma.

Glaucoma developing between three years to fifteen years is called **juvenile glaucoma**.

None of these glaucomas respond to medical treatment. They require specialized surgery where an artificial passage is made between the anterior chamber and the subconjunctival space (under the conjunctiva) to drain the aqueous outside the anterior chamber.

Wide Angle Glaucoma

This is also called **chronic simple** or **open angle glaucoma**. This is commonest type of glaucoma seen in adults over forty years and the number increases as age increases, all over the world. It progresses so slowly that its presence is not felt for long time unless the vision is reduced greatly and irreversibly. Due to its presentation it is a **public health problem**. It is equal in males and females. It is generally bilateral, one eye may have more advanced disease than the other. It is also symptomless in the beginning. It does not cause any redness, pain or watering. The only symptom may be diminished vision that is not corrected by glasses. The other symptoms may be loss of peripheral field. The patient says that he has to move the head to see things coming from sides. He has difficulty in diminished light. The loss of vision is so slow that the patient does not pay much attention and thinks that the diminished vision is due to cataract which also develops at the same age. Another difficulty arises because the patient may have both, i.e. cataract and glaucoma in the same eye.

> Vision lost due to cataract can be restored completely following surgery. Vision lost due to chronic simple glaucoma can not be restored either by medicine or surgery. That can only arrest the progress but not cure the disease.

Signs

Chronic simple glaucoma has very few external signs. The signs commonly seen are:

1. Diminished distant vision not corrected by glasses.
2. Faulty projection of light—This is a late feature.
3. Large sluggish pupil
4. Normal anterior chamber
5. Raised intraocular pressure
6. Normal gonioscopy
7. Large disc
8. Glaucomatous optic atrophy
9. Progressive field loss. This is also a late feature.

(Items 7–9: Figs 13.6, 13.7 and 13.8)

Visual Field

When someone looks at an object with normal vision, he not only sees the object of interest but also many things round this. The entire area seen by an eye while looking at a particular spot is the field of vision. This also notes down the dimmest brightness at a given place at a given time.

Field of vision is examined by a group of instruments called **perimeters**. They can be mechanical perimeters or automated computerized perimeters (Figs 13.1 to 13.3).

Gonioscope

In an eye the angle can not be seen by ordinary source of light. Gonioscopes are optical instruments by which the angles can be seen through a reflecting mirror on a slit lamp. It shows if the angle is normal or narrow (Figs 13.9 and 13.10).

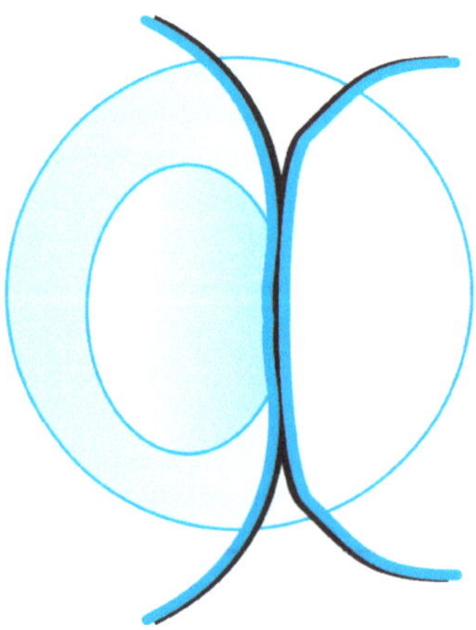

Fig. 13.6: Normal disc, Normal disc cup ratio

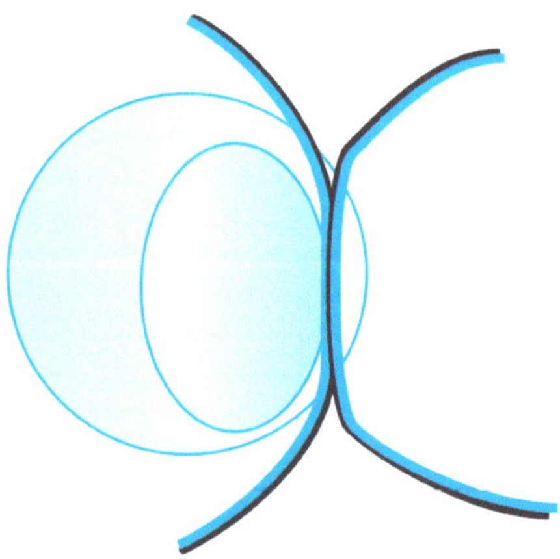

Fig. 13.7: Advanced glaucomatous disc large cup

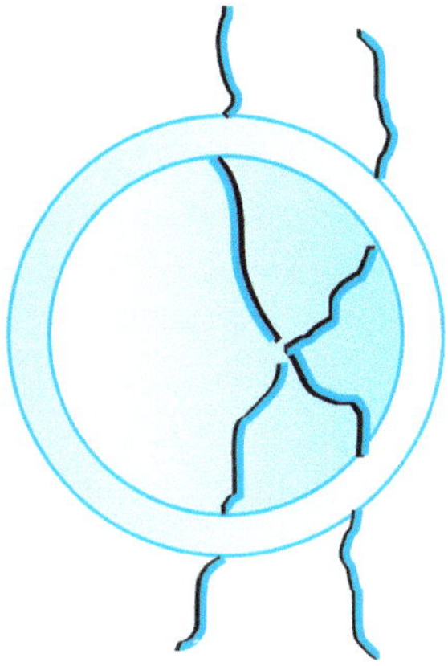

Fig. 13.8: Absolute glaucoma cup filling hole of the disc optic disc atrophied

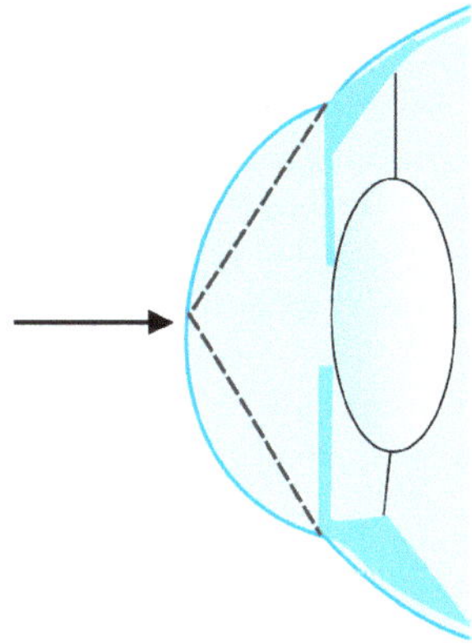

Fig. 13.9: Raise arising from angle are not visible through the cornea

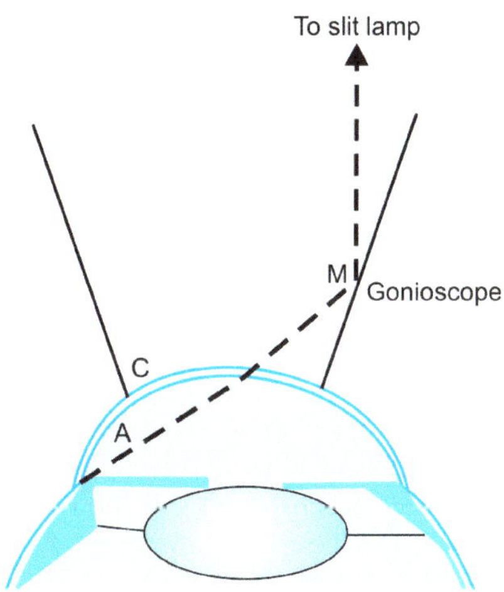

Fig 13.10: Principle of gonioscope light reflected from angle 'A' is refracted by cornea 'C' and reflected by mirror 'M' of gonioscope to be seen by slit lamp

> Persons with narrow angle are likely to develop acute attack of glaucoma when the pupil dilates in darkness or is dilated by drugs.

Ophthalmoscopy

Ophthalmoscopes are optical instruments by which the optic nerve, macula and area round them can be seen magnified. There are two types of ophthalmoscopes—**Direct** and **indirect ophthalmoscope**. The direct ophthalmoscope forms a 15 times magnified erect image of the optic nerve and retina. The indirect ophthalmoscope forms an inverted 3 to 5 times magnified image. Generally it is not used in glaucoma. It is used to see the periphery of the retina.

Most important condition from which chronic simple glaucoma should be differentiated is **immature cataract** by following points:

- Pupillary reaction is brisk, both direct and indirect in cataract.
- IOP—IOP is normal in cataract
- Disc—Disc when visible is normal in cataract.
- Field is normal in cataract.

Treatment

There is no treatment that can cure open angle glaucoma. Treatment only stops progress of the disease by keeping the tension down.

Treatment consists of:

1. **Awareness:** All persons after age of 40 years should get their eye checked by a specialist, who would:
   i. Correct his distant as well as near vision
   ii. Note intraocular pressure
   iii. Examine the optic nerve for early changes for glaucoma. If anything is suggestive of glaucoma, the patient is examined in details for field changes and examination of the angle.
2. **Medial treatment:** There are many drugs that when given locally as drops lower the tension. They are to be continued for rest of life under supervision of ophthalmologist. There are some medicines that work when taken by mouth. They can not be used for long time due to their side effects.
3. **Laser** has limited role in chronic simple glaucoma.
4. **Surgery:** There are many microsurgical methods to keep the intraocular pressure low by creating a passage between the anterior chamber and subconjunctival space (between the sclera and the conjunctiva). The most effective method is **trabeculectomy**.

Narrow Angle Glaucoma

This type of glaucoma has an advantage over wide angle glaucoma in the sense that it is a **symptomatic glaucoma**. The prominent symptom is severe pain, that forces the patient to seek a doctor. The second advantage is that if treated in time, the loss of vision returns to normal and a surgery cures the disease.

The condition is seen over forty years of age, more common in females. It starts in one eye, the other eye may or may not develop similar glaucoma. The disease is more common in hypermetropics and persons with shallow anterior chamber.

It has following stages:

1. *Prodromal stage*: In this the patient sees rainbow like colored circles round light called **colored haloes**, mild headache, slight redness and watering. This happens mostly in the evening or doing near work for few hours. The stage passes off without any treatment but recurs many a times. As time passes the frequency becomes more and one day the patient goes into acute attack. There are two more conditions that also produce rainbow like colored circles (haloes) round the eye but are not due to glaucoma. These are incipient stage of immature cataract and acute mucopurulent conjunctivitis.
2. *Stage of acute attack*: This develops suddenly with rapid fall of vision, redness and watering of the eye and severe pain in the eye, same sided headache and the patient is restless, may vomit.

   On examination the lids are swollen, the eye is red due to circum-ciliary congestion. The cornea is hazy. The anterior chamber is shallow. The pupil is sluggish, dilated and vertically oval, does not react to light. The tension is very high. The fundus is not visible. This stage is so painful that the patient seeks medical help.

   The condition should be differentiated from the two conditions, i.e. acute iritis and acute conjunctivitis. The condition requires immediate treatment.

Table 13.1: Points to differentiate acute congestive glaucoma from acute iritis and acute conjunctivitis

	Acute congestive glaucoma	Acute iritis	Acute conjunctivitis
Age	Generally over 40 years	Any age	Any age
Sex	More common in females	Equal in males and females	Equal in males and females
Onset	Sudden, within one to two hours	Gradual, within eight to ten hours	Gradual, within eight to ten hours
Laterality	Generally unilateral	Generally unilateral	Bilateral mostly
Pain	Severe	Dull	Foreign body sensation
Vision	Very low	Normal or slightly low	Normal
Tenderness	+	++	–
Circum-corneal congestion	+++	++	–
Cornea	Hazy	KP++	Bright
AC	Very shallow	Normal	Normal
Pupil	Semi-dilated, sluggish	Constricted, irregular, sluggish	Normal
Tension	High	Normal or low	Normal

Most of the time the eye responds to medical treatment within 48 hours and the vision improves and pain subsides. If the tension is not lowered by medical treatment, the patient may require an **iridotomy** either by surgery or laser.

If the tension is not brought down, the eye passes into the next stage of chronic congestion.

3. *Chronic congestive stage*: On examination there is diminished vision but better than in acute attack phase. The eye is congested due to circumciliary congestion. AC is shallow. Pupil is dilated, large and sluggish. The tension is moderately raised.

   The fundus when visible may show glaucomatous change. The medical treatment fails to bring down the tension. The eye requires surgery to establish a passage between the AC and the subconjunctival space called **trabeculectomy**.
4. *Absolute glaucoma:* This is the end stage of all glaucoma's, congenital or acquired, primary or secondary. The eye is blind and painful. The tension is very high. There is mild congestion round the cornea. The cornea may show bullous keratitis. The anterior chamber is shallow. Pupil is dilated and fixed. The iris may show patches of iris atrophy. If the eye remain in this stage for few months, it develops ciliary staphyloma.

   No medical or surgical treatment is of any use at this stage. Retrobulbar injection (behind the globe) of absolute alcohol may abolish the pain. Otherwise the eye is removed by a method called enucleation.

Secondary Glaucoma

Secondary glaucomas are a group of intraocular disorders that produce changes in the angle, pupil or both and cause rise of intraocular tension. There are about forty causes of secondary glaucoma. They are seen in all ages from newborn to old age. Secondary glaucomas can be acute or chronic. They can be wide angle (like chronic simple glaucoma), narrow angle (like acute congestive glaucoma). They may be associated with pupillary block.

The common types of secondary glaucomas are due to:
1. Lens
2. Injury
3. Steroid
4. Uveitis
5. Neovascularization

Lens can cause glaucoma in the following cases:

i. Congenital – Microphakia
 – Spherophakia. The lens is like a small ball that closes the pupil, pushing the iris forward, closing the angle.
 – Dislocation of lens and subluxation of lens.

ii. Cataract – Change in size of lens.
Intumuscent cataract (swollen).
This can happen in senile cataract and traumatic cataract.
– Leak of cortex. The cortical matter blocks the angle.
– Allergy to cortical matter resulting in severe iridocyclitis and rise of tension.

Glaucoma Due to Injury (Traumatic Glaucoma)

This occurs more commonly in blunt injury. Tension may rise within few days due to following causes:

1. Swollen lens
2. Dislocated lens, blocking the pupil or obstructing the angle
3. Cortical matter blocking the angle
4. Large hyphema in the anterior chamber blocking the angle of the anterior chamber.

The management of lens induced glaucoma is surgical.

In the second type the tension rises weeks to months after blunt injury. The anterior chamber is deeper on the side of the injury. The angle is damaged. The condition is called **recession of the angle**. This is best seen on gonioscopy. The management is generally medical.

Steroid Induced Glaucoma

This glaucoma is very common but missed. This is commonly seen in children who are on strong local steroids for more than three to four times a day for more than three weeks. This is seen commonly in cases of spring catarrh, phlycten and iritis in children. However this can happen in adults also. Though local drops are most common cause of steroid induced glaucoma, it can develop in any person who is on oral steroid for many months. The glaucoma is open angle glaucoma. Association of steroids induced cataract in the same eye is common.

The tension comes down over weeks after stopping the steroids. Otherwise the patient may require local treatment or may require filtering surgery.

Hence, all children on steroids should be monitored for rise of ocular tension.

Glaucoma due to Intraocular Inflammation

About 10% of eyes with iridocyclitis develop rise of intraocular tension. The features of iridocyclitis may mask the glaucoma.

There are three types of glaucoma in inflammation of anterior uvea:

1. Open angle glaucoma
2. Closed angle glaucoma
3. Steroid induced glaucoma

1. The open angle glaucoma following iridocyclitis may be acute or chronic. The first is due to acute inflammation at the angle and second is due to scaring at the angle.
2. The closed angle glaucoma may cause either pupillary block glaucoma or the angle may be blocked. There may be a combination of the two.
3. Patients suffering from iridocyclitis are put on strong steroids very frequently for long period that may cause rise of intraocular tension. The glaucoma is open angle glaucoma.

Neovascular Glaucoma

In inflammatory glaucoma, the cause of glaucoma is in the anterior part of the uvea. In neovascular glaucoma the pathology lies in the posterior segment in the retina. The two common causes of neovascular glaucoma are **extensive diabetic retinopathy** and **central retinal vein occlusion**.

In both the conditions the iris develops new vessels on its surface that spreads to the angle and closes the angle.

The condition is painful. The vision is very low. The tension is high.

The treatment is treatment of vascular disorder by laser and lowering the tension by diamox orally.

Points to Remember in Glaucoma

1. Two percent of population above forty years of age suffer from some type of glaucoma.
2. A child may be born with glaucoma, may develop in first three years or between three to fifteen years. They do not respond to medical treatment.
3. Chronic simple glaucoma is nonpreventable but treatable glaucoma. Vision lost in chronic simple glaucoma can not be regained.
4. Acute congestive glaucoma is treatable as well as revertible. The vision lost in acute congestive glaucoma recovers after treatment by surgery or laser.
5. All patients on steroids should get there intraocular tension checked every three months.

CHAPTER

14

Disorders of the Retina and Optic Nerve

If we go back to the chapter on embryology of the eye (Development of the eye) we will see that:

1. The primary optic vescile is joined to the brain by optic stalk.
2. The optic nerve starts in the sensory retina and grows back to join brain as optic nerve.
3. The retina develops from the two layers of the secondary optic vesicle (Fig. 14.1).

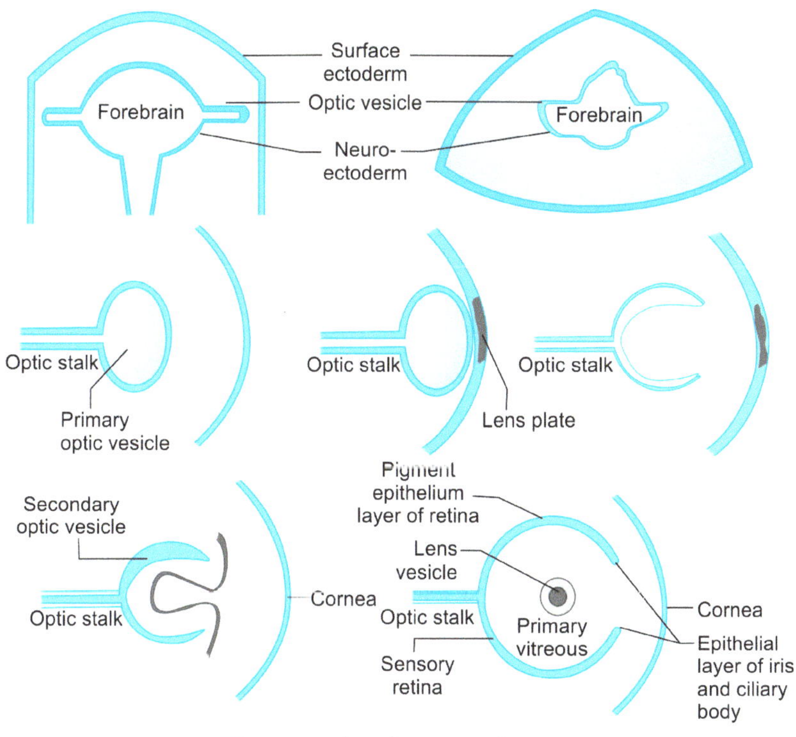

Fig. 14.1: Development of retina

4. The inner layer gives rise to nine layers of the sensory retina.
5. The ganglion cells of the sensory retina grow backwards in the optic nerve.
6. The outer layer of secondary optic vesicle gives rise to pigment epithelium of the retina and is attached strongly to choroids and weakly to sensory retina.
7. There is a narrow space between the sensory and pigment epithelium. This is called subretinal space.
8. The two layers of the retina can get separated if fluid develops in between the two layers and a condition of retinal detachment develops.
9. The pigment epithelium can not be separated easily from the choroids.
10. The optic nerve gets its blood supply from many sources.
11. The retina gets its blood supply from central retinal artery and the choroid.
12. Due to close relation of retinal layers to the optic nerve, inflammation and degeneration can pass in the optic nerve and inflammation of optic nerve can pass into the retina causing neuroretinitis.
13. The sensory retina at the future macula is thicker than rest of the retina up to eight months of pregnancy then it becomes thin but is not yet fully developed. The macula is not completely developed at birth. It continues to develop after birth. The macula needs a sharp image on it for its development up to first five years. If due to any cause the image is not sharp, the macula remains underdeveloped and amblyopia develops.

FEATURES OF RETINAL DISORDERS

The symptoms depend upon the part of retina involved:

1. Central
2. Peripheral

Disorders of central retina, i.e. the macula and area round the macula cause

1. Diminished distant vision
2. Loss of central field
3. Diminished vision in bright light
4. Distorted vision (metamorphopsia)

Disorders of **peripheral retina**:

1. Do not cause diminished distant vision
2. They cause diminished night vision (vision in dim light)
3. They cause peripheral loss of field of vision
4. Flashes of light

The Disorders of retina can be:

1. Congenital
2. Inflammatory
3. Trauma
4. Dystrophies and degeneration

5. Vascular
6. Detachment

Normal Fundus

It is helpful to know the normal appearance of retina before discussing its disorder.

The part of the retina, optic disc and retinal vessels that are visible through the pupil is called fundus of the eye. No part of the normal fundus is visible through the pupil by oblique illumination, i.e. torch light and slit lamp without special attachment.

The instruments that are used to see the fundus are:

1. Ophthalmoscope:
   i. Direct ophthalmoscope
   ii. Indirect ophthalmoscope
2. Slit lamp with special attachment
   i. Minus lens (Hruby lens)
   ii. Plus lens (+78 - +90 D)
3. Three mirror gonioscope
4. Fundus camera

Special methods used to see various pathologies of retina are:

1. Fundus fluorescein angiography
2. Ultrasonography:
   i. A scan
   ii. B scan
3. CT: Computed tomography
4. MRI: Magnetic resonance imaging
5. OCT: Optical coherence tomography

Out of all the instruments mentioned above, the most commonly used is direct ophthalmoscope. It is small, easy to handle, easy to use and cheap instrument. Its optics and power supply are incorporated in the instrument itself. It gives a vertical erect and fifteen times magnified image. The image is formed behind the retina.

The disadvantages of the instrument are:

i. It shows only a small area at a time.
ii. The illumination is poor.
iii. The periphery is not visible with the instrument.
iv. There is no depth sense.

Indirect Ophthalmoscope

It has a separate power supply, a separate illumination, separate focussing and magnifying system. The illumination system is worn on the forehead of the examiner. The magnifier also known as **condenser** is held in the right hand of the examiner. The power of the magnifier varies i.e. +15 D,

+20 D and +30 D. Lower the power, better is the magnification but smaller is the field. The +15 D gives five times magnification; +20 D has three time magnification and +30 D has only two times magnification but largest field.

The indirect ophthalmoscope gives a real, inverted and magnified image of the fundus. The image is formed in front of the eye of the patient. The magnification depends upon the power of the magnifier. Stronger is the magnifier (condenser), less is the magnification.

Ophthalmoscopic Appearance of Normal Fundus (Figs 14.2 and 14.3)

1. The area seen by an ophthalmoscope, direct or indirect is **circular**.
2. While seeing with direct ophthalmoscope, the disc is taken as center of the fundus.
3. While seeing with indirect ophthalmoscope, the macula is taken as center of the fundus.
4. The color of the normal fundus is **pink**. The retina is transparent. The color of the fundus is the color of choroids underneath. If the retina becomes opaque or translucent, the pink background becomes lighter or may become white.
   The causes of loss of transparency of the retina are:
   i. Retinal edema
   ii. Opaque nerve fibers
   iii. Exudates
   iv. Hemorrhages
   v. Retinal detachment
   vi. Retinal tumors
5. The optic disc:
   1. The term optic disc is used to denote the **visible part of the optic nerve**. The **normal disc** is circular in shape with clear-cut border and pink in color. The disc is oval in astigmatism. The disc is lighter

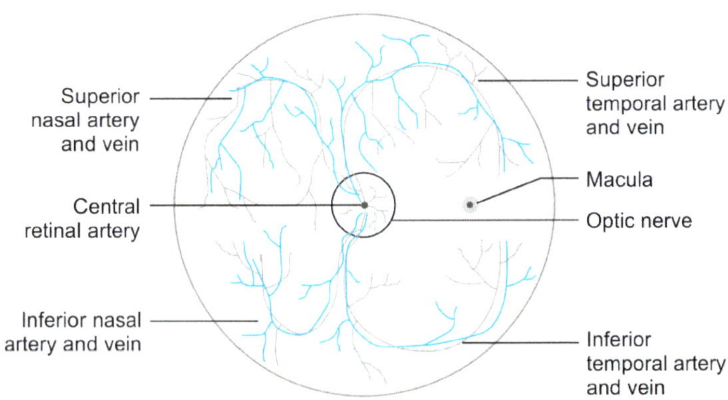

Fig. 14.2: Appearance of normal fundus by indirect ophthalmoscope

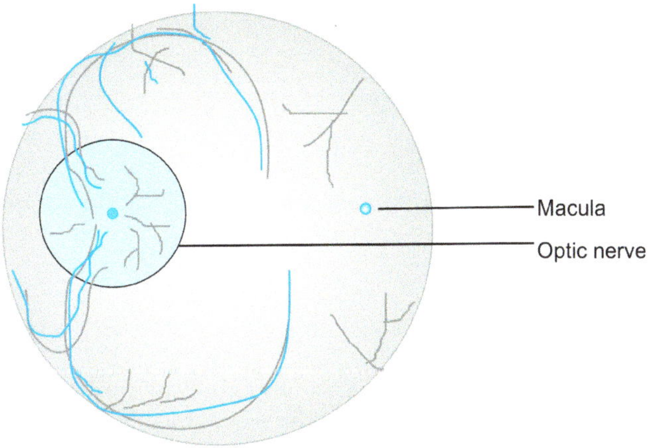

Fig. 14.3: Appearance of normal funds Fig 14.2 as seen by direct ophthalmoscope

than the rest of the retina. The color of the optic nerve due to small vessels on the surface of the disc. The color becomes more pink when there are more blood vessels (congestion) on the optic disc.

The causes of congestion of the disc head are:

i. Inflammation of the disc (optic neuritis)
ii. Papilldema (swollen disc)
iii. Pseudoneuritis (a congenital anomaly)
iv. New vessels on the disc, i.e. diabetic retinopathy
v. Central retinal vein obstruction
vi. The disc is small in hypermetropia and hypoplasia of disc. The disc looks smaller in aphakia. The disc is larger in myopia.
vii. If the blood supply is less, the disc looks pale. The paleness may range between mild pale to chalk white.

The causes of pallor of the disc are:

i. Anemia
ii. Optic atrophy
iii. Central retinal artery obstruction

6. **The cup of the optic disc**

The optic disc has a depression that extends from center of the disc to the temporal border of the disc. The cup represents the lamina of the disc. It is lighter than rest of the disc. Generally it occupies temporal one, third of the disc. It enlarges in glaucoma and myopia. In advanced glaucoma it may cover almost eighty to ninety percent of the disc and called a **glaucomatous disc**.

7. Swelling of the disc

The swollen disc is slightly raised from the surface of the retina. The optic cup is full and lamina not visible.

Causes of swelling of the disc are:

i. Pseudoneuritis
ii. Opticneuritis
iii. Papilledema
iv. Tumors of the disc
v. Drusen

8. The swelling of the disc is measured by direct ophthalmoscope. One millimeters of swelling is equal to +3 Dsph and one millimeter of depth is equal to –3 Dsph.
9. The macula
 The macula is the center of vision. A small lesion on it can cause great loss in vision.
 The macula is an ill defined area without clear cut border. The total area of the macula is larger than the disc which becomes visible only on fluorescein angiography and OCT.
 The macula is situated 3 mm away from the temporal border of the disc on the temporal side. A bright shinning area in the center of the macula is visible on direct ophthalmoscopy and is called **foveal reflex**. It is best examined by +78 D on slit lamp.
 The loss of brightness of the macula is an indication of marked diminished central vision.

The causes of dull foveal reflex are:

i. Hypoplasia of macula
ii. Edema (swelling) of the macula
iii. Exudates on the macula
iv. Hemorrhage on the macula
v. Central serous retinopathy
vi. Membrane formation on the macula
vii. Detachment of the macula
viii. Macular degeneration
ix. Scar on macula

10. Blood vessels
 The inner retina is supplied by the four branches of *central retinal artery*. The central retinal artery divides into two branches—the superior and the inferior branch. Each again divides into a nasal and a temporal branch. Each branch keeps on dividing till the branches reach the periphery where they are converted into capillaries. The distribution of the branches are not uniform on both sides. The temporal branches arch over the macula but do not reach the macula. Hence, the macula solely depends on blood supply from the choriocapillaries.
 The retinal veins accompany the retinal arteries. They start in the periphery as capillaries that unite to form venous branches. They have names corresponding to arteries. Thus each fundus has superior and inferior temporal and superior and inferior nasal veins.

The veins are wider than the arteries. They are darker than the arteries. The normal ratio of retinal artery to retinal veins is 2:3. The arteries are harder than the veins.

The veins may cross the arteries at some places either above or below the artery.

The arteries and veins have a common sheath (covering) at the crossing. If the arteries become harder than normal as is seen in raised blood pressure the arteries may press the vein.

Normally the arteries and the veins lie under the internal limiting membrane of the retina but in disease of the blood vessel and retina, they may grow in number and project on the surface of the retina or in the vitreous. This is called **retinal neovascularization**.

The common causes of retinal neovascularization are:

i. Diabetic retinopathy
ii. Central retinal vein obstruction
iii. Eales disease

Sometimes blood vessels grow under the retina, they are called **sub-retinal neovascularization**.

The causes of subretinal neovascularization are—Choroidal rupture, coloboma choroid, myopic degeneration, age related macular degeneration.

Congenital Anomalies of the Retina

1. *Coloboma of the retina*: This is always associated with coloboma of choroid. Both the retina and choroid are absent in the coloboma (Fig. 14.4). The floor of the coloboma is formed by the sclera, which is white in color. The retinal blood vessels are present over the coloboma. There is no vision in the area of coloboma. Hence it produces a field defect. A large coloboma may present as white reflex on plane mirror retinoscopy and may be mistaken as retinoblastoma.

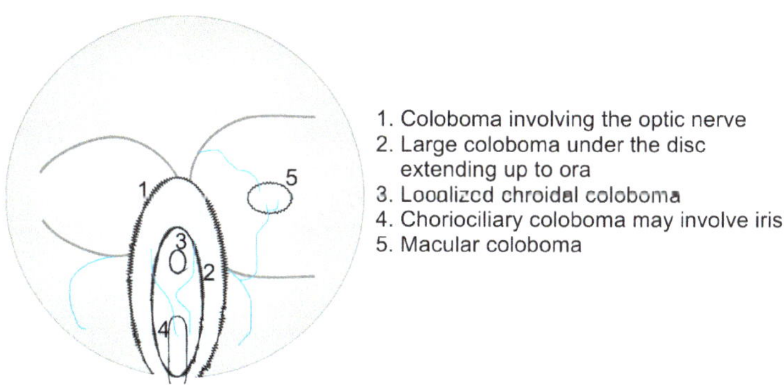

Fig. 14.4: Diagram showing various types of retinal and choroidal coloboma

2. *Opaque nerve fibers* (*medulated nerve fibers*): The retinal nerves are transparent up to the edge of the optic disc. Once they are incorporated in the substance of the nerve, they become opaque due to medulation. The medulation (the process of nerves becoming white) starts from the end which is towards the brain and stops at the border of the optic nerve. Sometimes the medulation fails to stop at the disc edge and continues on the surface of the retina as tongue shaped white feather like patch generally in one quadrant but sometimes it may develop all round the disc. In rare cases it develops away from the disc in patches. The condition is **symptomless**, is discovered on fundus examination. It produces field changes corresponding to the opaque nerve fiber. It does not require any treatment.
3. *Congenital retinal pigmentation*: This happens if the mother acquire some infection during first three months of pregnancy. The infections are **rubella**, **syphilis** and **influenza**. The pigmentation are small black granule like spots with white spots in between. This is called *pepper salt fundus*. This does not interfere with vision or night vision. No treatment is required for the condition.

RETINAL TRAUMA

Retina can be injured in following ways:
1. Mechanical
2. Radiation
3. Chemical

Out of these commonest type of injury is mechanical that can either be blunt injury or penetrating injury.

Blunt Injury of the Retina

The common effect of blunt injuries of the retina are:
- Retinal edema
- Rupture of retina
- Dialysis of retina
- Retinal hemorrhage

Retinal edema is caused by a blunt object like fist, cricket ball, tennis ball. Generally the objects are larger than the orbital diameter. The object compresses the eyeball from front which transmits the force of the injury to the retina just opposite the point of contact of the object to the cornea or sclera. This is called countercoup injury. The condition is called **commotio retinae**.

Commonest area to be involved is macula and the condition is called **Berlin's edema**. The Berlin's edema has typical picture of an edematous area with a pink center. The edematous area is a slightly raised white circular area. The central pink area represents the fovea. As the fovea does not have any nerve fibers, it is not capable of developing swelling, the fovea is thinner than the surrounding retina, hence the choriocapillaries shine through it as a **cherry red spot**.

Less common are the areas away from the macula. They do not have any pink area inside the swollen area.

The symptoms of Berlin's edema is blurring of central vision which gradually return to normal. Rarely this may be permanent loss of one or two lines on Snellen's chart due to pigmentation of the macula.

No active treatment is required.

Other Causes of Red Spot in the Macula

1. Central retinal artery occlusion (severe loss of central vision)
2. Tay-Sachs disease (rare, not seen in India)
3. Hemorrhage on the macula
4. Macular hole

Causes of macular hemorrhage

- Trauma
- High myopia
- Age related macular degeneration

Retinal Rupture

Rupture of retina without rupture of choroid is very rare. Retinal rupture is mostly associated with rupture of underlying choroid and the condition behaves like choroidal rupture.

Retinal Dialysis

When the counter coup is not directed towards the posterior pole (macula) but towards the ora serrata where the retina is loosely attached, the retina is torn from the attachment in a large area. This is called **retinal dialysis** or **disinsertion of the retina**. The detached area is biconvex in shape on the detached part and darker than normal retinal blood vessels. The detached retina lies between the optic disc and the dialysis. Generally the dialysis develops in the lower part and the detachment progresses very slowly but an upper dialysis spreads fast and ends in total retinal detachment. The dialysis is best seen by indirect ophthalmoscope.

Traumatic Retinal Hemorrhage

Isolated retinal hemorrhage due to blunt trauma is rare. It is generally seen in retinal edema choroidal rupture or dialysis of retina. However abnormal retinal vessels as in diabetic retinopathy, Eales disease, sickle cell retinopathy may bleed even with mild trauma. In such cases they are generally preretinal (in front of the retina). Occasionally traumatic retinal hemorrhages can be **interretinal** (in the substance of retina) or **retro retinal** (behind the sensory retina). These are called **subretinal hematoma** or **choroidal hematoma**.

Penetrating injuries of the retina are always associated with penetrating injuries of globe. It is associated with wound in the sclera and choroid. The choroid may prolapse through the scleral wound. It may be associated with retained intraocular foreign body. Penetrating injury of retina is a serious condition that requires repair in specialized vitreoretinal units. Generally multiple surgeries are required. Overall visual results are poor.

Inflammatory Disorders of the Retina

Inflammatory lesions are called **retinitis** but there are some conditions that are noninfectious, are also wrongly called retinitis. A few examples are—Retinitis pigmentosa which is a degenerative condition. Similarly solar retinitis is a chemical change due to infrared rays of the sun and retinitis proliferance is a vascular condition.

The word retinitis should only be used for infectious condition. The infection can be:

1. Viral
2. Bacterial
   Purulent—Streptococcal staphylococcal
   Nonpurulent—Tuberculosis, syphilis
3. Parasitic—Toxoplasmosis
   Out of these viral retina are more common than others.

The source of infection can be:

1. Blood
2. Choroid
3. Vitreous
4. Optic nerve

The retinitis can be limited to retina only without involving the other structures or may involve choroid, optic nerve or vitreous. The former is called primary retinitis and the second is called secondary retinitis.

Retinitis can be acute, subacute or chronic. Retinitis can involve the central part only or peripheral part (away from the macula). It can involve other part and known by various terms like **chorioretinitis**, **neuroretinitis**, **retinalvasculitis**.

Symptoms of Retinitis

Symptoms depend upon part of the retina and structure other than retina involved. Central retinitis is always associated with diminished central vision. A lesion between the disc and macula also cause diminished vision so does neuroretinitis.

Peripheral retinitis generally does not cause diminished vision but present as field defect corresponding to the lesion and floaters.

SPECIFIC TYPES OF RETINITIS

Rubella

This is a **congenital** type of retinitis. It develops in the **fetus** (unborn child) if the mother is infected by rubella during first three months of pregnancy. The retinal involvement is a mild form of peripheral retinitis that presents with typical **pepper and salt fundus** without causing any visual disturbance or night blindness. In severe form the child may have many birth defects, i.e. in heart, brain and eyes. The common defects in eye due to rubella are **microphthalmos**, **cataract** and **glaucoma**, all of which involve both the eyes. Congenital rubella is fully preventable disease by antirubella vaccine given to every girl at nine months of age.

Cytomegalovirus—Retinitis

This can be congenital or acquired. In congenital disease the virus is passed to the fetus during pregnancy. The acquired form has two methods of spread:

1. In new borne—From the birth passage during delivery.
2. In adults—From infected person by nasal droplet, sexually or by blood transfusion.

The condition can be very mild and the patient may not know about it or may be so serious as to involve whole of the retina except few areas of normal retina left in between.

The condition may involve the macula only and cause central chorio-retinitis. The cytomegalovirus retinitis becomes worse when present in a patient who also suffers from AIDS.

Retinitis in HIV

The word HIV stands for **human immunodeficiency virus**. It can infect any part of the body. The disease by it is called **acquired immunodeficiency syndrome** or in short AIDS. (The word immunity means ability of the body to fight infection while syndrome means a group of disorders). The body including the eye is involved in two different ways:

1. The effect of HIV itself.
2. The disease caused by organisms that generally do not cause disease as long as immunity is present. These organisms are called **opportunistic microorganism**.

The retinal involvement is bilateral. They are:

i. Cotton wool sports (white fluffy area)
ii. Deep and superficial hemorrhages
iii. Microaneurysm (small dilatation in the walls of the vessels)
iv. Retinal vasculitis

All the above diseases may be present alone or in combination. Other ocular disorders due to AIDS are—**Corneal ulcer, iritis, conjunctivitis, Kaposi sarcoma, squamous cell cancer (carcinoma) of conjunctiva.**

Bacterial Retinitis

Almost all bacteria can cause retinitis. They generally reach the retina through blood, may spread from choroid, vitreous or optic nerve.

The pus forming organisms can cause acute retinitis or subacute retinitis

Acute bacterial retinitis results in swelling of retina, superficial exudates and hemorrhages. If it involves the macula there is fall in vision otherwise there is corresponding field loss. Retinitis is not a painful condition. It does not cause redness of the eye. Acute bacterial retinitis if not treated passes into endophthalmitis and the eye may be lost.

Subacute Bacterial Retinitis

This is caused due to presence of pus forming mild microorganisms in retinal capillaries (finest retinal vessels). It consists of formation of **Roth's spot**. The Roth's spots are prominent white fluffy sports with red center specially seen in a disease of heart in children called **subacute bacterial endocarditis**. The other causes are leukemia (blood cancer) and purpura (a condition where bleeding even from very small vessels do not stop).

Chronic bacterial retinitis is seen in the form of retinal granuloma due to tuberculosis and syphilis.

Fungal retinitis is rare. It is seen in very ill patient who are on intravenous antibiotic in heavy dose for a long time. It is also seen in persons suffering from AIDS.

Parasitic Retinitis

Toxoplasmosis is the commonest parasitic infection of the retina. It is caused by a ***protozoa Toxoplasma gondii*** which is found in many animals out of which cat is the most important. Other animals are cattle, birds and rats. The humanbeings get the infection by eating food contaminated by stool of the cat or by handling beef (flesh of cattle) from where the organism reaches various parts of the body. The acquired disease is mild and not fatal (does not kill) unless the patient suffers from AIDS or is pregnant. In the **pregnant women** the protozoa reaches the fetus via **placenta** and infects many organs including the brain and the eyes of the fetus. In the eyes the retina is mostly involved. The **macula** is more involved than periphery. The macular involvement is **bilateral** and always **congenital**. As the lesion involves the macula the child has **poor vision** and the child develops **squint**. The diagnosis is made while examining the child for squint. The lesion may not progress for some years but can become active between ten to forty years.

The other lesion produced by toxoplasmosis are repeated **iridocyclitis** and **chorioretinitis**. Vitreous is also involved very often.

Retinal Vasculitis

This is a very common condition. In this disorder there are inflammatory changes in both **retinal arteries** and **retinal veins**. The veins are more frequently involved than arteries. The inflammation starts at the periphery (away from the disc) in finer branches and then spread towards the center. It is generally a **bilateral disease**. The causes of retinal vasculitis are:

1. **Ocular**—Retinitis, pars planitis, choroiditis
2. **Systemic**—Secondary to tuberculosis, syphilis, herpes zoster, cytomegalovirus
3. **Idiopathic**—When no definitive cause can be found out, most probably there are **autoimmune diseases**.

The idiopathic retinal vasculitis is commonly known as **Eales' disease**.

Eales' disease is a **bilateral** disease of retinal vessels. One eye may be involved more than the other and the patient may not know about the involvement of the other eye, which may even be more affected.

It is seen more commonly in **healthy males** between **thirty years to forty** years of age.

The commonest form of presentation is **sudden painless loss** of vision in a non-congested eye. The loss of vision may be as small as loss of few lines to hand movement depending on amount of hemorrhage and part of the retina involved. A small hemorrhage on the macula causes more loss of vision than a large hemorrhage away from the macula.

On examination the eyes are **white** (not red). There is **no pain** in the eyes, **no tenderness** (pain on pressing the eyeball) of the eyeball.

The **vision is diminished**.

The **pupillary reaction** is **brisk** both direct and indirect.

The real finding lies in the fundus:

1. A large fresh hemorrhage may be visible behind the clear lens on torch examination.
2. The changes can be divided in two groups:
   i. Those in the retina
   ii. Those in the vitreous

   The retinal changes in Eales' disease are:
   i. The vessels show evidence of peri vasculitis
   ii. There may be new vessels on the surface of the retina
   iii. The vessels may grow in the vitreous
   iv. Superficial hemorrhages and inter retinal hemorrhages

   The vitreous changes in Eales' disease:
   i. There may just be a few new vessels growing into the vitreous from the retinal vessels.
   ii. There may be frank hemorrhages in the vitreous.
   iii. There may be vitreous bands.

In case of Eales' disease the other eye should always be examined even when it has normal vision. The other eye may show more advanced stage of the disease without symptoms when the lesions are away from the macula.

Generally the first episode of hemorrhage clears even without treatment and vision returns to normal but recurrences are very common. There may be a gap of months before the next episode. Gradually the gap between two episodes get reduced and the time taken to clear the hemorrhage is increased until a stage is reached when the vision does not improve at all.

Common Causes of Nonimprovement of Vision in Eales' Disease

1. Large nonabsorbed hemorrhage called **hemophthalmos**
2. Traction detachment of retina
3. Complicated cataract
4. Neovascular glaucoma

Diagnosis of Eales' disease is easy if following features are present.

1. Age—Between 20 to 40 years
2. Sex—Male
3. Symptoms—Sudden painless loss of vision in one eye without redness of the eye.
4. No history of diabetes, sickle cell anemia, hypertension
5. Satisfactory projection of light from all quadrants
6. Normal pupil
7. Intraocular tension within in normal limits
8. Fundus changes of retinal vasculitis

Other Causes of Retinal Haemorrhages

1. Diabetic retinopathy
2. Hypertensive retinopathy
3. Sickle cell anemia
4. Central retinal vein occlusion
5. Branch retinal vein occlusion
6. Trauma
7. High myopia
8. Congenital anomalies of retinal vessels

Management

The first step is to exclude any systemic cause and treat it. If no cause is found out, the case is confirmed as Eales' disease.

Treatment

1. Medical—Oral steroid for weeks.
2. Photocoagulation of newly formed blood vessel by Laser.
3. Vitrectomy with repair of retinal detachment.

Retinal Dystrophies and Degeneration

Dystrophies are those conditions that are **genetic**, may be seen **in many members of the same family**, they may be **congenital** or **develop** later. When acquired they involve the body few years after birth. They are generally **bilateral**, **slow progressive**. There are no evidence of other disease. The two parts of the eyes that are generally involved are **retina** and **cornea**. There is no known treatment for ocular dystrophies. However the dystrophied cornea may be replaced by healthy cornea by a surgical procedure called keratoplasty. No such treatment is available for retinal dystrohies.

Degeneration are **acquired**. They may be unilateral, they are nongenetic, do not run in families. They generally do not progress. The management is management of ocular disease that is responsible for the degeneration. Here also there is no known treatment for retinal degeneration but corneal degeneration may also improve keratoplasty.

Retinal Dystrophies

Retinal dystrophies may involve any part of the retina. However, it is divided into two broad groups they are:

1. Central also known as macular dystrophies
2. Peripheral

The two types differ vastly in their symptoms and signs.

As the macular dystrophies involve the macula which is rich in cones. They cause:

- Diminished, uncorrectable distant vision
- Poor vision in bright light
- Better vision in dim light
- Distorted vision
- Reduced color sense
- Temporal pallor of the disc

The peripheral dystrophies involve the rods mostly, hence, they cause

- Diminished night vision
- Ring scotoma
- Central vision is retained for long time
- The disc develops pale yellowish white appearance after many years.

The common macular dystrophies are:

1. Best's disease (Vitelliform macular dystrophy)
2. Stargardt's disease
3. Cone dystrophy
4. Sorsby macular dystrophy

> All patients with macular dystrophy and degeneration may benefit from low vision aid.

Peripheral Retinal Dystrophies

The commonest form of retinal dystrophy is **retinitis pigmentosa,** which is a dystrophy of photoreceptors and pigment epithelium.

> There are two types of photoreceptors in retina, i.e. cones and rods. The first are mostly found in macula and are involved in central vision they are responsible for vision in bright light and color vision such lesions cause central scotoma. The rods are found in the retinal periphery and are involved in night blindness and peripheral vision.

Retinitis Pigmentosa

This is the commonest retinal dystrophy. The commonest **symptom** of retinitis pigmentosa is diminished vision in dim light, called **night blindness**. The dystrophy mostly involves rods and less frequently cones, when cones are also involved the condition is called **rod cone dystrophy**. According to fundus picture the retinitis pigmentosa is divided into two types—a. Typical retinitis pigmentosa and b. Atypical retinitis pigmentosa.

Features of typical retinitis pigmentosa are:

1. It is a hereditary disease. Generally more than one member of family are involved. It is more common in males. It is a bilateral progressive disease. The patient first becomes aware about diminished vision in teens. The night blindness becomes worse as time passes.
2. Central vision is good for many years but is lost ultimately in most of the cases.
3. The patient has poor peripheral field of vision. He has to move his head to see on the sides.
4. Fundus examination shows very thin retinal vessels with black star like pigments around the vessels between the macula and ora.
5. The disc is waxy pale.

The causes of diminished central vision in retinitis pigmentosa are:

1. Involvement of macula:
   - Cone rod dystrophy
   - Cystoid macular edema
   - Atrophy of macula
2. Other causes are:
   - Associated myopia
   - Posterior subcapsular cataract
   - Chronic glaucoma

Atypical Retinitis Pigmentosa

The number of persons suffering from atypical retinitis pigmentosa is less than typical retinitis pigmentosa.

The atypicallitis may be in:

- Pigmentation
- Associated systemic disorders

Atypical Pigmentation

1. Only on eye is involved.
2. Only one sector of retina is involved.
3. The central retina is involved extensively.
4. There are no visible pigmentation but other signs and symptoms of retinitis pigmentation are:
   i. Diminished night vision
   ii. Thin retinal vessels
   iii. Peripheral field changes
   iv. Abnormal ERG (A method to record function of photoreceptors).

Systemic conditions associated with retinitis pigmentosa:

1. Obesity (fatness) polydactyly (more than five fingers and toes), hypogonadism (nondeveloped genitals), mental retardation (dull mind).
2. Premature old age, deafness, mental retardation, skin sensitive to sun rays.
3. Deafness, ataxia (unable to maintain balance), salt pepper fundus.
4. Deafness, microcephaly (small head).

Differential Diagnosis

1. Separating other causes of night blindness from retinitis pigmentosa and peripheral field defect.
2. Separating retinitis pigmentosa from other causes of retinal pigmentation.

The first group consists of:

1. Vitamin A deficiency
2. Choroidal dystrophies
3. Advanced chronic simple glaucoma

Night blindness due to vitamin A deficiency requires special mention in relation to retinitis pigmentosa. Both cause night blindness. Retinitis pigmentosa is often mistaken as vitamin A deficiency and the patient is put on large dose of vitamin A and food rich in vitamin A without any improvement.

Simple Rule of Night Blindness

If a child under fiver years presents with night blindness, it is most probably due to vitamin A deficiency. A single dose of 200000 IU of water soluble vitamin A given intramuscular will improve night vision within 48 hours. If an adult or person in teens presents with night blindness, chances are that he is not a case of vitamin A deficiency but a case of retinitis pigmentosa and will not improve with an injection of vitamin A.

Treatment of Retinitis Pigmentosa

1. There is no successful treatment of retinitis pigmentosa.
2. If diagnosed in teens the child should be treated as visually handicapped and rehabilitated.
3. Some patients benefit from low vision aids. Persons with retinitis pigmentosa have two main problems:
   a. Diminished night vision
   b. Constricted field

Both are generally not corrected by usual low vision aids. Diminished night vision is improved by using strong torch light with halogen bulb.

Patients with constricted peripheral field are trained to use canes to maximum benefit.

Usual magnifier and telescopes are good for macular and optic nerve disorders. They are of no use in restricted field because part of the magnified image falls in the ring scotoma.

Computers and closed circuit television are of some help because the size of the image can be changed according to field available.

COMMON MACULAR DISORDERS

Central Serous Retinopathy

This is also known as **central chorioretinopathy** because the choroidal vessels under the sensory retina at the macula are involved. There is a leak in the retinal pigment epithelium that is visible on fluorescein angiography. In some cases the leak is away from the fovea.

The exact cause of the condition is not known. It is seen in young adult males as unilateral loss of central vision. The patient complains of a circular black spot in front of the eye. Otherwise the eye is extremely normal including pupillary reaction.

The vision may be just loss of two to three lines on Snellen's chart. Vision does not improve pinhole but comes to almost 6/6 with +1.0 Dsp to +2.0 Dspl.

The patient has metamorphopsia (distorted vision).

The patient takes longer time to recover from glare.

On retinoscopy there is shift towards hypermetropia.

On fundus examination there is an elevated circular area of macula. The circular area may be many times more than the diameter of normal optic disc.

On fluorescein angiography there is a visible leak at the level of retinal pigment epithelium.

Management

The condition is self-limiting. The vision returns to normal even without treatment after 3 to 4 months unless there is a leak which should be closed by laser.

Role of steroid is not well established. Recurrences in the same eye or in the other eye is known.

Cystoid Macular Edema

There are two types of macular edema
1. Commotio retinae (Berlin's edema)
2. Cystoid macular edema

Cystoid macular edema (CME) is one of the major causes of non-improvement of vision next to posterior capsular opacfication (PCO) after lens extraction by any method with or without IOL.

Besides aphakia CME is seen in following case:
1. Diabetic retinopathy
2. Central retinal vein thrombosis
3. Posterior uveitis
4. Retinal dystrophies
5. Local and systemic drugs
6. Idiopathic (no cause can be detected)

The commonest cause is accumulation of fluid in the outer plexiform layer and inner nuclear layer of the retina near the macula. The macula is thickened. It takes three to four months for CME to develop after lens extraction.

The diagnosis is confirmed by fundus fluorescein angiography which gives an appearance of flower petals radiating from the macula.

There is no definite treatment. Local and systemic steroids and non-steroidal antiinflammatory drugs given many time a day for month may arrest the progress.

AGE-RELATED MACULAR DEGENERATION (ARMD)

This is also known as **senile (old age) macular degeneration**.

It is a very common cause of nonpreventable and nontreatable causes of blindness in old persons. It is a bilateral, progressive, painless cause of loss of vision over fifty years of age in both the sexes as the age increases more and more people get this disorder.

The symptoms of ARMD consist of:
1. Noncorrectable diminished vision
2. Metamorphopsia (distorted vision)
3. Central scotoma
4. Fairly good peripheral vision

There are two types of age-related macular degeneration:
1. Dry type
2. Wet type

The dry ARMD is more common, less troublesome condition caused due to development of **drusen** in the macula and atrophy (death) of retinal pigment epithelium.

Drusens are small white yellowish deposits. They can be soft or hard. They develop between the Bruch's membrane and the retinal pigment epithelium. They are present in ARMD even before the blindness sets in but are not visible with ophthalmoscope. By the time they become visible, the vision is generally reduced. They do not require any treatment unless they cause diminished vision. On fundus fluorescein angiography they give a typical picture called **window defect**. They are visible on ocular coherence tomography (OCT).

Wet ARMD is less common than dry type. Only 10% of ARMD are wet in nature but 90% of them will have severe loss of vision. It is more common in women. It is thought that some dry ARMD may be converted into wet ARMD on long run. The wet ARMD is also called **exudative** ARMD or **neovascular** ARMD. It is due to development of new blood vessels in the choroid under the macula which leads to bleeding under the macula, exudative retinal detachment and scar formation. It is best seen in **fluorescein angiography** and **OCT**.

The condition is difficult to treat. There are some costly specialized treatments available but the results are not very good.

Other causes of choroidal neovascularization are:
1. High myopia
2. Rupture choroid
3. Drusen of optic nerve

Vascular Disorders of Retina

The important vascular disorders are:
1. Vascular retinopathies
   i. Diabetic retinopathy
   ii. Hypertensive retinopathy
   iii. Retinopathy of pregnancy
   iv. Retinopathy of prematurity
   v. Sickle cell retinopathy
2. Obstruction of retinal vessels
   i. Retinal artery occlusion (closure)
   ii. Retinal vein occlusion (closure)

Diabetic Retinopathy

Diabetic retinopathy is a common cause of diminished vision and loss of vision. This is due to a common disease called diabetes mellitus that cause a rise of sugar level in the blood which is passed in the urine (persons without diabetes do not pass sugar in urine) . It is caused either due to less of **insulin** in the body or inability to use insulin present in the body. **Insulin is a hormone produced by an organ called pancreas**.

About 10% of population suffer from diabetes. The number of diabetic is increasing every year, hence the number of persons suffering from diabetic retinopathy will also increase.

There are two types of diabetes:

1. *Type I*: This is also known as insulin dependent diabetes. This is seen due to low level of insulin in the body and is treated by insulin injection. This is seen under twenty years of age and causes loss of weight, excess of thirst, hunger, increased frequency of urination. Type I diabetics develops diabetic retinopathy less frequently than type II diabetes but develop other complication more frequently.
2. *Type II*: Diabetes develops in elderly persons who are obese (heavy weight). Positive family history is common. The disease may be present for long time without any symptom. They cause diabetic retinopathy more commonly than type I diabetes. The disease is mostly treated by drugs other than insulin.

Some of the factors that cause diabetes retinopathy are:

1. Uncontrolled or poorly controlled diabetes.
2. Diabetes present for more than 15 years.
3. Presence of hypertension.
4. Raised lipid (fat) in blood.
5. Pregnancy.

Diabetes retinopathy can be divided in two types

1. Background Retinopathy
2. Proliferative retinopathy

Background Retinopathy

The retinopathy develops in the posterior pole with mostly small dots of hemorrhage, few flame shaped of hemorrhage and deep exudates. There may be associated macular edema.

Proliferative Retinopathy

This develops months or years after background retinopathy. The fundus findings are: Superficial and deep hemorrhages all over the fundus with new vessels on the periphery of the disc. The macula is generally edematous and vision is reduced. There may be some vitreous hemorrhages.

On long standing proliferative diabetic retinopathy traction bands may develop which in turn cause traction retinal detachment.

Management of Diabetic Retinopathy

The treatment depends on stage of retinopathy:

1. Background diabetic retinopathy
   All cases of background retinopathy do not require ocular treatment. They should be examined every six months for evidence of macular edema and conversion to proliferative retinopathy.
   Both the conditions require laser photocoagulation.
2. Proliferative retinopathy is treated by extensive laser photocoagulation. If vitreous bands are present, they are cut along with vitrectomy and any detachment is corrected by suitable methods.

Ocular Manifestations of Diabetes

All parts of the eye are prone to be effected by diabetes. Uncontrolled diabetes causes acute diseases while controlled diabetes develop slow changes.

The common diabetic disorders of the eyes are:

Part	*Disorder*
1. Lids	Boils, abscess, cellulitis, stye, infected chalazion, diabetic ptosis
2. Sac	Dacryocystitis
3. Conjunctiva	Acute and chronic conjunctivitis, sub-conjunctival hemorrhages
4. Cornea	Diabetes are more likely to develop corneal ulcers
5. Sclera	Episcleritis, scleritis
6. Uvea	Anterior uveitis, neovascular glaucoma
7. Lens	Cataracts develop early and progress fast
8. Vitreous	Vitreous hemorrhages and vitreous band
9. Macula	Macular edema
10. Retina	Retinopathy, traction detachment
11. Optic nerve	Optic neuritis
12. Glaucoma	Chronic simple glaucoma is more common in type II diabetic while neovascular glaucoma is more common the proliferative retinopathy
13. Cranial nerve palsy	Painful third nerve palsy, 4th and 6th nerve palsy

All diabetic patient undergoing any surgery should get their blood sugar controlled before surgery and keep blood sugar under control after the surgery.

HYPERTENSIVE RETINOPATHY

About ten percent of population suffer from hypertension (raised blood pressure). Hypertension leads to increased pressure of blood on the wall of the arteries all over the body including the retinal arteries. Arteries in places other than retinal arteries are not visible. The retinal arteries and veins are visible with ophthalmoscope. The changes in retinal vessels are similar to changes in brain, heart and kidney, which are all effected by hypertension. Hence, the changes visible in the retinal vessels indirectly reflect the changes in other organs.

There are two types of changes in the retinal vessels:

1. Hypertensive changes with sclerosis (hardening) of arteries. These are generally seen in older persons with moderate rise of blood pressure of many months.
2. Hypertensive changes without sclerosis. This is generally seen in young person with very high blood pressure generally of short duration.

The common changes in the first group are:

1. The vessels look tense, straight and pale.
2. The arteries press the veins, which are dilated beyond the crossing of the vein by hard arteries.
3. The color of the artery shifts toward brown and the arteries look as if they are made of copper called copper wire appearance.
4. Some flame shaped hemorrhages and cotton wool exudates.

The changes in second group are:

1. Increased tone of arteries
2. Veins are concealed (hidden) by arteries
3. Retinal edema
4. Many flame shaped hemorrhages and cotton wool exudates
5. Silver wire appearance of retinal arteries
6. Blurring of disc margin

RETINOPATHY OF PREGNANCY

This is also called retinopathy of toximaea in pregnancy.

Toximaea in pregnancy is a late feature of pregnancy where there is high blood pressure, swelling of limbs, fits and the patient passes albumin in urine.

The fundus changes are bilateral and the condition is brought to notice due to fall in vision.

The retinal changes consist of:

1. Narrowing of arteries
2. Swelling of retina
3. Superficial hemorrhages and exudates
4. Exudative retinal detachment

The causes of diminished vision is retinal edema and exudative retinal detachment.

The detachment subsides with termination of pregnancy normal or artificial and vision returns to normal.

Retinopathy of Prematurity (Retrolental fibroplasia)

This occurs in children who are born before full term, when birth weight is less than 1200 gm and have been put on oxygen for long time. The condition is bilateral.

The retinal vessels are not fully developed before eight months and these under developed vessels when exposed to oxygen for long time, start growing fast in irregular manner. In severe cases they grow in the vitreous and cause traction retinal detachment.

The disease can be divided into two forms:
1. A common regressive disease which does not require active treatment and does not cause much visual damage.
2. A rare form that causes extensive traction detachment and blindness.

To prevent such damage all preterm children (born before 36 weeks of pregnancy) with birth weight less than 1200 gm who have been on prolonged oxygen therapy should be examined by vitreoretinal surgeon and treated.

Sickle Cell Retinopathy

Sickle cell disease is caused due to deformed red blood cells. The normal red blood cells are round, disc like structure. In sickle cell disease, the red blood cells become curved and look like crescent of moon or sickle.

The main symptoms are anemia and obstruction of small vessels. The normal hemoglobin is replaced by an abnormal hemoglobin.

This is a genetic disorder. The ocular involvement are comma-shaped conjunctival vessels and various grades of proliferative retinopathy, which cause vitreous hemorrhage and traction detachment.

Obstruction of Retinal Vessels

There are two types of obstruction of retinal vessels:
1. Retinal artery obstruction
2. Retinal vein obstruction

They always happen separately. The central vein obstruction is more common than central artery obstruction. Chances of retaining some vision is better in venous obstruction. Generally both are unilateral. Both cause sudden painless loss of vision.

Retinal artery obstruction can be complete or partial. It is said to be complete or central, when the obstruction occurs before the central retinal artery divides. In partial obstruction any of the four branches may be obstructed. The central retinal artery obstruction is seen generally in elder persons who suffer from hypertension, diabetes or narrowing of main artery to the brain (internal carotid artery).

There is sudden profound painless loss of vision in one eye. The loss of vision depends upon the location of the obstruction. If the obstruction is in the central retinal artery, the vision may be lost totally, i.e. patient is not able to see light even (NOPL) but if only branch is effected. Some vision is lost in the area supplied by the effected branch.

On Examination

There is no redness, pain or watering in the effected eye. Only finding is **dilated sluggish pupil**. The direct light reflex is lost but indirect is present. The findings of central retinal artery block are seen in the fundus. They are:

1. The retina is pale white.
2. The retinal arteries are very thin and pale.
3. There are no exudates or hemorrhages on the retina.
4. The macula stands out prominently as a red spot (**cherry red spot**) in the center of white retina.
5. The optic disc is pale.

In case of branch artery block the findings are seen around the obstructed branch. There is no cherry red spot.

There is no known treatment for central retinal artery obstruction. The vision is lost due to atrophy of the retina and primary optic atrophy.

Central Retinal Vein Obstruction (Central Retinal Vein Thrombosis)

This also presents with sudden painless loss of vision in one eye in hypertensive and diabetic patients over forty years of age.

There can be obstruction of central retinal vein or its branches.

The symptoms and external signs are similar to those seen in artery obstruction, i.e. no redness, watering or pain in the effected eye. The vision is reduced to hand movement.

The findings are in the fundus. They are:

1. The veins are dilated and congested (more red than normal).
2. Whole of the retina is splashed with large patches of bright hemorrhages.
3. The disc is more red than normal. It's borders are blurred.
4. The macula is not visible.
5. Details of fundus are not visible.

One of the complications of central retinal vein thrombosis is development of thrombotic (**neovascular glaucoma**) in which there is very high rise of tension with pain and redness of the eye.

The treatment of central retinal vein obstruction is pan-retinal photocoagulation where large area of retina is destroyed by laser.

Causes of sudden painless loss of vision:

1. Central retinal artery occlusion
2. Central retinal vein thrombosis
3. Vitreous hemorrhage
4. Hemorrhage on the macula
5. Retinal detachment
6. Cystoid macular edema

RETINAL DETACHMENT

The retina develops from two layers of optic cup. The outer layer gives rise to the pigment layer that is firmly attached to the Bruch's membrane of choroid. The inner layer develops from the inner layer of the optic cup. The two layers are very near each other with a very thin empty space between the two layers. If some fluid or solid get into this space, the two layers separate from each other and this is called retinal detachment.

Retinal detachment is partly preventable and treatable. The retinal detachment can occur at any age. In 10% of cases it is bilateral. It has some hereditary tendency. The following cases are more likely to develop retinal detachment.

1. Positive family history
2. Myopia
3. Aphakia
4. Pseudophakic
5. Blunt injury
6. Fluid vitreous
7. Peripheral retinal degeneration

There are three types of retinal detachment:

1. Rhegmatogenous (with hole) retinal detachment
2. Tractional retinal detachment
3. Exudative retinal detachment

In rhegmatogenous retinal detachment, it is essential to have at least one full thickness hole in the sensory retina. **In traction detachment** the hole is caused due to bands between the vitreous/blood vessels and the retina. An eye can have both the types of detachment at the same time.

In exudative retinal detachment, it is not necessary to have a hole. Fluid develops between the pigment epithelium and the sensory retina lifting the sensory retina away from the pigment epithelium. The retina settles down once the fluid is absorbed or drained.

The **retinal holes** may develop at any place on the retina but generally develop on the periphery of the retina, they may be located anywhere on the circumference.

According to shape, the holes are called—Round, horseshoe (arrowhead) and dialysis. It is possible to have more than one hole in the same retina and also have different shapes of holes in the same eye. All holes do not lead to retinal detachment. To develop a detachment, it is essential to have a hole and some fluid should get into the space between the two layers of the retina. The commonest liquid to cause retinal detachment is fluid vitreous. Once the retina is separated the detachment starts growing. The upper detachments grow faster than lower detachments.

Symptoms of Retinal Detachment

1. Flashes of light on the retinal periphery.
2. Loss of field corresponding to detachment. The lower detachment causes upper field loss and nasal detachment causes temporal field loss.
3. Sudden loss of vision: This happens when the detachment involves the macula. The upper detachments cause more visual loss than lower detachment. Temporal detachment causes more visual loss than nasal detachment.
4. If the detachment is not treated, whole of the retina gets detached.
5. On long run a total detachment lead to chronic uveitis, complicated cataract and glaucoma.

Diagnosis

Diagnosis of a fully established retinal detachment is easy. The difficulty arises in locating the holes especially in hazy media and aphakia. To find out the holes and extent of the retinal detachment, it is essential to dilate the pupil by strong mydriatic cum cycloplegic and use an indirect ophthalmoscope. The detached retina looks white, its surface is uneven. The blood vessels over the detachment look darker than normal. The holes look bright red.

Management

1. Prophylaxis:
   i. All persons with history of ocular trauma, intraocular surgery myopia, positive family history should get their retinal periphery examined by a trained retinologist who will examine the fundus with indirect ophthalmoscope every year.
   ii. Whenever there is a retinal detachment in one eye, the other eye should be examined by indirect ophthalmoscope.
   iii. If holes are detected even without detachment, they should be closed by laser photocoagulation.

Treatment

There is no medical treatment for rhegmatogenous and traction retinal detachment. The detachment is treated by surgery. The aim of the surgery is to:

1. Search for the hole/holes
2. Locate the hole/holes
3. Close the holes
4. Drain the fluid under the sensory retina
5. Keep the two layers of the retina pressed against each other

TUMORS OF RETINA

Retinoblastoma

Retinoblastoma is commonest type of malignancy (cancer) of the eye in children. It can be successfully treated in early stages but can cause death of the child in late stages even with treatment.

It is seen in both the sexes equally. The commonest age of presentation is three years. It becomes rare after six years of age. There are two types of retinoblastoma—(1) Sporadic (without family history), (2) Heritable (with family history).

Ninety percent are sporadic and only ten percent are heritable. Sporadic cases are unilateral and thirty percent of heritable cases are bilateral.

The retinoblastoma can be divided into two main groups:

1. Without visible white reflex in pupillary area and
2. White reflex in pupillary area

The second group passes into following stages if not treated –

i. Stage of glaucoma
ii. Stage of extraocular extensive (the tumor comes out of sclera)
iii. Metastasis—The tumor spread to other parts of the body.

Symptoms and Signs of Retinoblastoma

Symptoms depend on stage of the diseases. In the stage of no visible white reflex the only symptom may be squint or diminished vision for which the child is brought to ophthalmologist and on fundus examination a white raised mass is detected in the posterior pole.

The second symptom is that when the child moves the eye, a white reflex is visible in the pupil.

In the stage of white reflex in pupillary area, the most important finding is a white reflex in the pupillary area even when the child is looking straight but there is no pain or redness. The vision is diminished and the eye may squint.

In the next stage, the white reflex present but the eye is red and painful. The pupil is dilated and fixed. There is gross loss of vision.

In the next stage, the eye bulges forward (proptosis) with all the findings of the previous stage.

In stage of metastasis, there are symptoms of involvement of other organs.

Differential Diagnosis of Retinoblastoma

These are the conditions that present with white reflex in the pupillary area but are not retinoblastoma. Some of them cause blindness but none cause death.

They are:
1. Congenital cataract
2. Traumatic cataract
3. Chronic iridocyclitis
   i. Exudate over the lens
   ii. Exudate behind the lens
4. Retrolental fibroplasia
5. Intraocular parasitic cyst

All cases with white reflex on the pupillary area should undergo following tests:
1. Recording of vision
2. Refraction under cycloplegia
3. Fundus examination by
   i. Direct ophthalmoscope
   ii. Indirect ophthalmoscope
4. Ultrasonography
5. CT and MRI

Treatment

In stage 1: White reflex without pain or redness is treated by removal of the eye by cutting the extraocular muscle and optic nerve without puncturing the globe. This process is called enucleation.

In stage 2: Eye is red and painful, treated by enucleation and chemotherapy.

In stage 3: When the tumor comes out of the globe.-The condition is treated by Chemotherapy and radiation. (treatment by anti cancer drug is called chemotherapy).

DISORDERS OF THE OPTIC NERVE

Optic nerve is the second cranial nerve, it is responsible for vision, color vision, and contrast. It also carries pupillary fibers. The optic nerve joins the retina to the brain. In fact the optic nerve is backward extension of retinal ganglion cells, extending from the retina up to the chiasma. The ganglion cells in retina are transparent and not visible by ophthalmoscope. Once they reach the disc they become medulated (myelinated) and become white and hence visible by ophthalmoscope. Optic nerve is covered by dura from back of the globe to the optic foramen (Fig. 14.5).

The part of the optic nerve visible by ophthalmoscope is called optic **nerve head** or **optic papilla**. The rest of the optic nerve is not visible by ophthalmoscope and called retrobulbar optic nerve. The two optic nerves are from each eye join to form a structure called **chiasma**. Each chiasma contains fibers from both the sides.

Each chiasma ends in **optic tract** that reaches the **lateral geniculate body** from where the **optic radiation starts**. The optic radiation ends in **visual cortex** at the back of the brain.

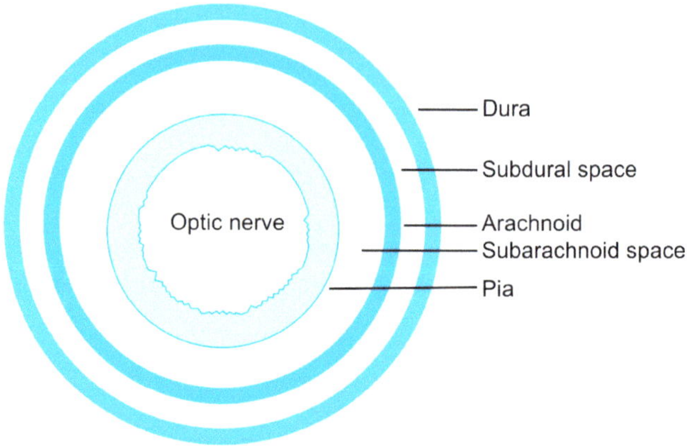

Fig. 14.5: Section of optic nerve showing its convering

The structure starting at the optic nerve head and ending at visual cortex constitute the **visual path.**

The visual path from optic nerve head to the end of the optic tract contain both visual as well as pupillary fibers hence lesion at this level will cause defect, both in vision as well as pupillary reaction.

The visual fibers continue up to visual cortex and any lesion in the region will have only visual finding in the form of field defect on both sides. The pupillary fibers leave the visual path at the lateral geniculate body so lesion beyond lateral geniculate body will not have pupillary defect.

The features of disorders of the optic nerve are both—visual as well as pupillary.

The optic nerve gets its blood supply from the central retinal artery and pial plexes. The optic nerve head gets its blood supply from central retinal artery as well as ciliary circulation (Fig. 14.6).

The visual features of optic nerve discorders are:
1. Diminished central defect
2. Central field defect
3. Diminished color sense
4. Diminished brightness

The pupillary features are:
1. Faulty direct pupillary reaction
2. Faulty indirect pupillary reaction

The disorders of the optic nerve can be:
1. Congenital
2. Hereditary
3. Traumatic
4. Inflammation

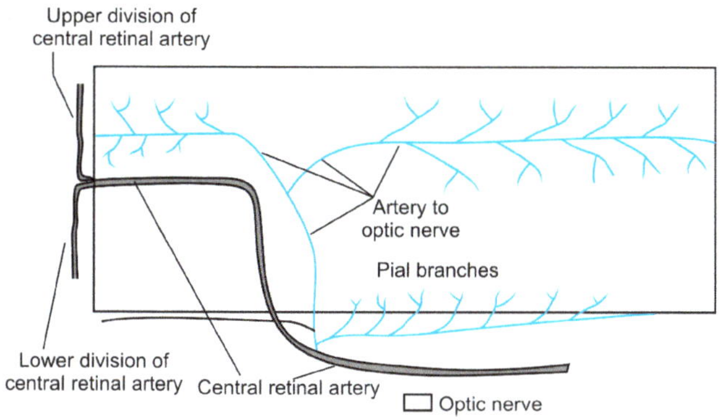

Fig. 14.6: Diagram showing origin of the central retinal artery and blood supply to the optic nerve

5. Swelling (papilledema)
6. Optic atrophy
7. Vascular
8. Tumors

Congenital Anomalies of Optic Nerve

The common congenital anomalies of optic nerve are:

- Opaque nerve fiber
- Pseudoneuritis
- Hypoplasia of optic disc
- Coloboma of the disc

Opaque Nerve Fibers

The ganglion cells are transparent in the retina up to the margin of the disc than they become opaque (white). Sometimes this opacity spreads over the retina as white irregular area visible on ophthalmoscopy. The condition is symptomless and does not require any treatment.

Pseudoneuritis is a congenital condition where the posterior scleral foramen (the hole at the back of the sclera through which the optic nerve passes) is very small. It is so small that the fibers of optic nerve are crowded in a small place. This gives an appearance of swelling of the disc. The margins are blurred and the lamina is not present. All the findings are suggestive of two conditions—(1) Papillitis, (2) Papilledema which the condition is not. Hence, it is also called as pseudopapillitis or **pseudoneuritis**. The condition is **bilateral**. The eyes are generally **hypermetropic**. The condition is stationary without any complication. The only treatment required is treatment of associated hypermetropic.

Hypoplasia of Optic Disc

This is much rare than opaque nerve fiber and pseudoneuritis. Here the disc is very small. In about 2/3 cases the condition is bilateral. The eyes have greatly reduced vision and afferent pupil. It may be associated with other congenital anomalies of the eye. **Nystagmus is common**. There is no known treatment. Associated error of refraction should be corrected.

Coloboma of the Optic Disc

This is also a rare condition. It may be associated with coloboma of uvea that may include the disc or may be localized in the disc only. In such cases the normal cup extends more on the lower side causing narrowing of the rim of the disc. In severe form there may be a retrobulbar cyst related to the disc.

These eyes have poor uncorrectable vision and the milder forms are confused as glaucomatous disc.

Hereditary Disorder of Optic Nerve

There are many hereditary disorders of optic nerve. Some are seen in childhood and others are seen in adults. Some of the them present as optic neuritis and end in optic atrophy. Others present as optic atrophy of childhood. All are bilateral, some cause blindness. Other causes diminished uncorrectable vision. All of them end in partial or total optic atrophy.

The commonest of heredofamilial optic neuropathy is **Leber's optic neuropathy**, which starts between fifteen to twenty five years of age in healthy males as sudden painless diminished vision in one eye. The other eye gets involved within few months. The vision may be reduced to 6/60 with normal pupillary reaction. The disease is transmitted through the mother who may not be effected. There may be some improvement in vision even without treatment. There is no effective treatment for the condition.

Trauma to Optic Nerve

The optic nerve is well protected in the orbit from all sides by extraocular muscles and retrobulbar fat. It lies loose in the orbit, so it can be stretched to some extent without harm.

The optic nerve can be injured by:

1. Direct trauma (injury) to the nerve by sharp penetrating object
2. Indirect trauma

Indirect trauma leads to stretching of the optic nerve that results in tearing of small vessels that supply blood to the optic nerve and formation of hematoma (collection of the blood under the covering of optic nerve) of the optic nerve. These are associated with loss of vision, and afferent pupillary reaction. It is difficult to treat injury to optic nerve.

Inflammation of the Optic Nerve

The inflammation of optic nerve is called **optic neuritis**. According to location of the condition, it is called:

i. **Papillitis**, when the visible part of the nerve (the disc) is involved and the condition is visible by ophthalmoscope.
ii. **Retrobulbar neuritis**, when the nonvisible part of the nerve is involved. The papillitis is generally acute (sudden onset) and retrobulbar neuritis may be acute or chronic (gradual onset). The papillitis is generally unilateral and the retrobulbar neuritis is bilateral.

Papillitis is seen in young adults. In children it occurs many a times after undergoing immunization. Some of the virus infections also cause papillitis in children.

The symptoms are very typical in all ages:

1. Visual—There is fall of vision over first twenty four hours. The vision may fall from 6/6 to hand movement within hours. The vision remains low for next seven to ten days and is not correctable by lenses, then the vision starts improving to original level. This can happen without treatment. There may be similar episodes within months.
2. Central scotoma
3. Pain in movement of the eye upward and outwards
4. Tenderness on the globe
5. Diminished color vision
6. There is no redness or watering from the eye. The only external findings are moderately dilated pupil with afferent pupillary reaction. The real findings are in the disc on fundus examination. They are:
   i. Hyperemia (increased redness) of the optic disc.
   ii. The lamina is not visible.
   iii. The cup is full.
   iv. The disc margin is blurred.
   v. The whole of the disc is swollen but not more than +3 D. There may be few superficial exudates or hemorrhages near the disc.

The exact cause of the condition is not understood. In 30% cases no cause can be found out. The commonest cause is an autoimmune disorder. This leads to demyelination of the optic nerve fibers. Other causes are systemic diseases like tuberculosis, syphilis. The third group consists of infection spreading to the optic nerve from retina, choroid or from the covering of the optic nerve.

Treatment

i. If there is definitive infective disease like tuberculosis or syphilis than the primary cause should be treated along with steroid.
ii. Only steroids have no definite role in treating papillitis.
iii. Recurrences are common. Steroids delay recurrence and shorten the period of recovery.

The end result of recurrent papillitis is postneurotic optic atrophy.

Retrobulbar Neuritis

Retrobulbar neuritis is inflammation of the orbital parts of the optic nerve (The part that is behind the globe and not visible by ophthalmoscope). It can be acute or chronic.

The signs, symptoms and causes of acute retrobulbar neuritis is same to papillitis. Only difference is that there are no visible finding on the disc.

Chronic Retrobulbar Neuritis

This is also called **toxic amblyopia**. This is due to effect of external toxins and chemical taken by the patient, i.e. alcohol, tobacco. Many drugs also cause chronic retrobulbar neuritis. The disease is most of the time due to death of the ganglion cells in the retina and less commonly due to direct effect on the optic nerve. The common toxic substances are tobacco and alcohol, both ethyl and methyl alcohol can cause retrobulbar neuritis. Methyl alcohol causes acute lesion of the retina and cause severe irreversible blindness and primary optic atrophy. Methyl alcohol poisoning can cause death. Ethyl alcohol along with tobacco cause chronic retrobulbar neuritis where. There is gradual painless loss of vision with central scotoma in both the eyes. There is no specific treatment. Stopping consumption of alcohol and tobacco may stop further progress.

PAPILLEDEMA (SWOLLEN DISC)

This is noninflammatory bilateral painless condition caused due to rise of *intracranial pressure*. *Cerebrospinal fluid* is a clear fluid formed inside the brain and circulates round the brain and spinal cord. The brain has three coverings, i.e. the dura, arachnoid and pia. The space under the arachnoid is called subarachnoid space. These three covering extend round the optic nerve as well. If there is rise in pressure in the subarachnoid space it presses over the central retinal vein. This leads to swelling of the optic nerve head.

The commonest cause of papilledema is brain tumor. Other causes are brain abscess, meningitis and hypertension.

The vision is normal in papilledema unless very late.

The findings are in the fundus.

They are:

- Hyperaemia of the disc
- Swelling of disc more than 3 D
- No cup visible
- Blurring of disc margin
- Exudates and hemorrhages round the disc
- Exudate over the macula

After few months the optic nerve passes into postpapilledematous optic atrophy and blindness.

The early papilledema should be differentiated from late papillitis and pseudoneuritis of the disc. In papillitis there is fall of vision in early stages which is absent in early papilledema.

The papilledema is a serious blinding, crippling condition. It is treated by removing the main cause like brain tumor.

OPTIC ATROPHY

Optic atrophy is the end result of all disorders of the optic nerve. There is degeneration of optic nerve fibers and the fibers die down. The blood vessels of the disc are obliterated (becomes very thin). The result is change in color of the disc from pink to white. Depending upon the type of atrophy, the color of the disc ranges between pale yellow to chalk white. The optic atrophy is never acute in onset.

According to ophthalmoscopic appearance, optic atrophy is classified as:

1. Primary
2. Secondary

Primary Optic Atrophy

Primary optic atrophy is generally bilateral except in trauma and central retinal artery occlusion. The commonest cause is neurosyphilis (syphilis of brain).

Generally, there is loss of vision which may be loss of few lines on Snellen's chart to total absence of light.

The condition is painless. There is no congestion. Only finding is semi-dilated pupil with sluggish direct and indirect pupillary reaction.

The diagnosis depends on the fundus examination.

The disc is pale. The lamina is visible. The cup is present. The disc margin is clear. The blood vessels are thin. There are no exudates or hemorrhages. Overall result is bad.

Secondary Optic Atrophy

Whenever a cause can be found for optic atrophy, it is called secondary optic atrophy. The secondary optic atrophy can be:

- Postpapilledematous, this follows papilledema
- Postneuritic, this follows optic neuritis
- Central retinal artery obstruction
- Acute ischemic optic neuropathy
- Consecutive optic atrophy is due to inflammation or degeneration of retina archanoid

Common causes of consecutive optic atrophy are:

- Retinitis pigmentosa
- Choroidal dystrophy
- Extensive choroiditis

Glaucomatous optic atrophy is due to prolonged rise of intraocular pressure. The disc is pale, the cup is large and deep.

The diagnosis of secondary optic atrophy is based on fundus appearance of the disc and retina. The color of the disc is yellowish white, the lamina is not visible. The cup is full and the margin is blurred. The vessels may show sheathing. The rest of the fundus show evidence of degeneration or previous inflammation.

Tumors of the Optic Nerve

There are two types of tumors of the optic nerve, both are not cancerous. They are **glioma of optic nerve** and **meningioma of optic nerve**.

Glioma of the Optic Nerve

Glioma is the commonest tumor of the optic nerve. It is seen in children, is unilateral, slow growing, develops in the orbital part of the substance of the optic nerve. It may grow forward or backward. It is a diffuse growth. It causes early loss of vision and late proptosis. If it spreads back, it causes enlargement of optic foramen that is visible on X-ray.

The treatment is excision if there is too much of proptosis.

Meningioma of optic nerve is seen in elderly person. It develops from the meningial covering of the optic nerve. It is slow growing tumor. It causes early proptosis and late loss of vision. There is no satisfactory treatment. The tumor may be removed surgically.

CHAPTER

15

Squint (Strabismus)

Squint is a very common ocular disorder. There is hardly any person who does not have squint sometimes or other in life. It is seen in all ages from *new born* (congenital) to *ripe old age*. (paralytic)

Both the sexes are involved equally. It can be *unilateral*, i.e. only one eye squints always. Alternate, both eyes squint but one at a time. It can be bilateral, simultaneously both eyes squint at the sametime (rare).

To understand squint we should know some of the terms used commonly:

1. *Orthophoria*: For all practical purposes, this means absence of deviation of eyes under all conditions.
2. *Binocular single vision*: Two separate images of a single object are formed, one the macula in each eye. They are coordinated in the brain to give a single image in three dimensions, i.e. the object has height, width and depth. This is called binocular vision.

In absence of binocular single vision a person will see everything in duplicate. This is called *diplopia*.

It is essential to have binocular single vision to avoid diplopia.

Binocular single vision is acquired, i.e. it develops after birth.

The following things must be present to have binocular single vision:

1. Sharp image on the macula
   i. This is brought about by a clear media (no opacity in the cornea or lens) and absence of error of refraction.
   ii. Intact conduction system (normal retina and optic nerve).
   iii. Straight eye—The image is formed on the macula.
   iv. No physical obstruction, i.e. ptosis.
2. Balance (coordination) between movement of both eyes in all direction.
3. The brain should be able to overlap (fuse) two images.

The brain tries to overcome this by following methods:

1. Suppression—Image formed by one eye dominates over the other eye.
2. Amblyopia—Diminished vision without any visible cause.
3. Deviation.

DIPLOPIA

Diplopia can be:
1. Binocular (common)
2. Uniocular (rare)

A diplopia is called binocular when it is present with both eyes open but disappear as soon as any of the two eyes is closed. The commonest cause of binocular diplopia is **paralytic squint**. Other causes are displacement of the eye ball by an orbital growth or restriction of movement of a muscle by injury or its being caught in fracture or by changes in muscle as in dysthyroid condition and myasthenia.

In case of binocular diplopia the patient tries to overcome diplopia in following ways:
1. Closing an eye.
2. Turning up head towards the action of paralyzed muscle. For example in case of right lateral rectus palsy the diplopia will disappear if the patient turns his head towards the right side.
3. Develops amblyopia.
4. Diplopia can also be avoided by using suitable prism.

Presence of diplopia is confirmed by diplopia charting and Hess screen test.

A diplopia is said to be uniocular when the diplopia disappear only when the eye with the lesion is closed and not the other eye, i.e. if the right eye has the lesion, the diplopia will disappear when the right eye is closed. This is in contrast to binocular diplopia where diplopia will disappear on closing any of the eyes, for example, if right lateral rectus is paralyzed the diplopia will disappear even when the left eye is closed.

The causes of uniocular diplopia are:
1. Subluxated lens
2. Iridodialysis
3. Large iridectomy
4. Recent corneal opacity

Polyopia

In case of polyopia all things look more than two, it may be uniocular or binocular. Commonest cause incipient immature cataract.

Amblyopia

Amblyopia is a state of diminished vision that is not correctable by glasses, medicine or surgery without any anatomic lesion is detected in the visual path. Amblyopia is generally unilateral, most commonly seen in squinting eye but can be bilateral also and develop in nonsquinting eye. The most important period to develop amblyopia is before six months of age when the macula is still developing. Amblyopia rarely develops after six years of age and must be treated before eight years of age.

Common Causes of Amblyopia

Congenital: Cataract, ptosis, corneal opacity, refractive error, unilateral error of refraction. Difference in refraction more than 2.5 D in two eyes.

Squint: Squinting eyes develop amblyopia commonly. The amblyopia persists even after surgical correction of squint if amblyopia has not been treated before correction of squint.

Treatment of Amblyopia

1. Amblyopia should be diagnosed before six years of age. Hence it is mandatory to have compulsory school health check-up in preprimary age.
2. If amblyopia is detected, treatment should be started before six years of age and continued till vision is equalized in two eyes.
3. Removal of cause whenever possible by lens extraction, keratoplasty, and ptosis.
4. Correction of refractive error.
5. Occlusion.

Occlusion is closing the **better eye** completely or partially and forcing the amblyopic eye to see throughout the waking hours. Occlusion therapy should be undertaken under the supervision of a trained person. They are called orthopticians.

SQUINT

It is a condition where one eye is directed towards point of fixation and the other eye deviates.

In normal conditions when the head is kept erect and a far object is seen, the axis of the two eyes are parallel and remain parallel in all direction except in convergence and divergence where the two eyes either turn in (convergence) or move out (divergence).

The most convenient classification of squint is given below:

Pseudosquint is when the child seems to have squint without having squint. None of the eyes deviate under cover. The movements are normal in all direction. The commonest cause is **epicanthic fold**. The epicanthic fold is a fold of skin that starts in the upper lid, covers the medial canthus and merges below (Fig. 15.1).

The squint disappears if the epicanthic fold is pushed towards the nose. The mild epicanthus generally disappears with age but if it persists after 7 to 8 years of age it should be corrected by surgery. Epicanthus is commonly associated with congenital ptosis.

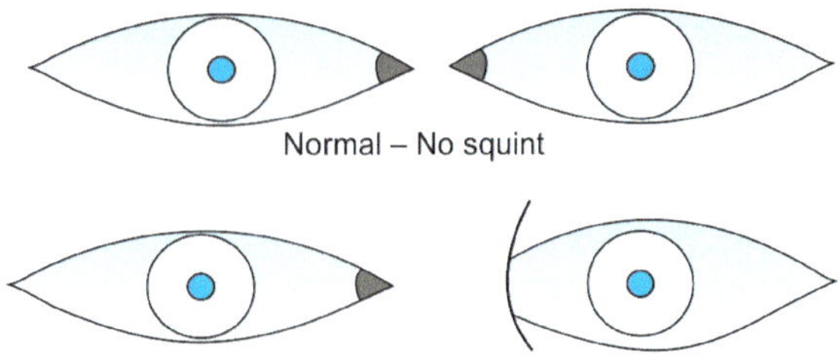

Fig. 15.1: Left pseudosquint due to epicanthus, the cornea looks deviated towards the nose (medially)

LATENT SQUINT (HETEROPHORIA)

Latent squint is a squint of which the patient is not aware and an observer can not see unless the fusion is broken (Figs 15.2 and 15.3).

The commonest method to break the fusion is to cover any of the eye for a short period and observe the movement of the eye behind the cover. If there is latent squint the eye behind the cover deviates. As soon as the cover is removed the eye will be back to the normal position. The movement towards the same side and equal when the other eye is covered. If the eye under cover deviates towards the nose, this is called **esophoria**. If the eye deviates towards the lateral side (towards the ear), it is called **exophoria** and shift upwards is called **hyperphoria**.

Causes of Heterophoria

Phorias develop commonly following fever, fatigue, anxiety and in those who perform close work.

In childhood when binocular fixation has not developed fully, the eye may go for exophoria. In school-going children excess of convergence

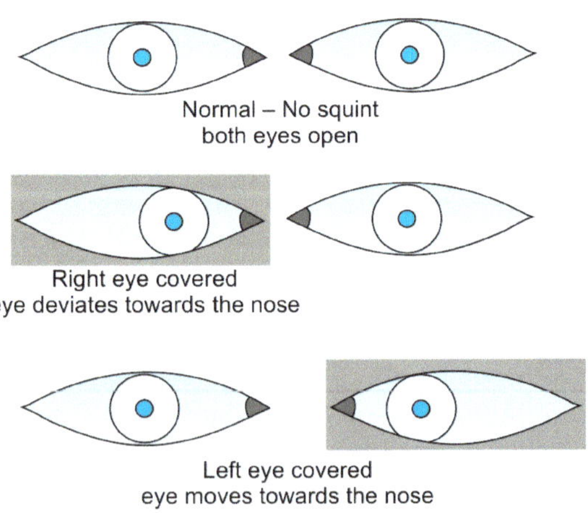

Fig. 15.2: Cover test in esophoria

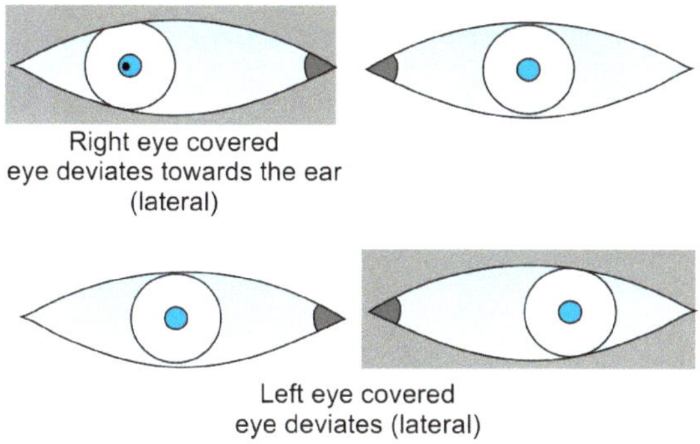

Fig. 15.3: Cover test in exophoria

Note: The deviation is equal in both eyes under cover in all types of phoria.
The eyes come to straight position on removal of cover.
The movements are normal.

cause esophoria. After forty years if near correction is not used, exophoria develops. Myopia causes esophoria. Hypermetropia causes exophoria.

Symptoms of Heterophoria

The patient may overcome breakdown of fusion and be symptom-less. Once fusion breaks the person develops **asthenopia** that is tiredness after prolonged visual activity it causes:-

Running of letters while reading.

Headache after day long work.

Diplopia in the evening and after prolonged near vision.

The phorias may be converted to tropias, before constant tropia develops, there may be intermittent tropias.

Diagnosis

Diagnosis is easy. All cases of asthenopia should be suspected to have phoria and a cover test should be done. In fact cover test should be performed on every patient that consults an ophthalmologist.

Treatment

The aim of the treatment is to give relief from asthenopia and prevent phoria to be converted to tropia.

The treatment consists of:

1. Correction of refractive error
2. Correction of presbyopia after forty years of age
3. Orthoptic treatment:

This consist of a series of movements of the eye by a special instrument called **synoptophore**. Prisms have limited role in few selected cases.

MANIFEST SQUINT (HETEROTROPIA)

This type of squint is visible to the onlooker and the patient becomes aware of it. It is visible on photographs. Besides causing diminished vision and amblyopia the visible deformity results in a social complex.

The manifest squint can be divided into following groups:

1. Concomitant squint
2. Paralytic squint
3. Restrictive squint

Out of the three, the first is commonest and the third is least frequent.

Concomitant squint is a manifest squint that remains the same in all directions of gaze. Concomitant squint may develop in infancy (infantile) or may develop late. It is seen equally among boys and girls. It may be confined to one eye only and the other eye is straight and the patient fixes with the straight eye. Hence, the straight eye is called **fixing eye**. The uniocular squint may be present always and called **constant squint** or may be **intermittent**, i.e. the eye squints only during a limited period and in between both the eyes are straight. The intermittent squints may remain intermittent throughout the life or may be converted to constant squint.

The squint may **alternate** between the two eyes. In this case the fixation is alternated between the two eyes when one eye fixes the other eye deviates. The angle of the squint is same in two eyes.

The causes of heterotropia are:

1. Conversion of heterophoria to tropia.
2. Abnormal relation between accommodation and convergence.
3. Failure to develop binocular single vision:
   - i. Uncorrected error of refraction
   - ii. Anisometropia
   - iii. Opacities in media:
     - a. Corneal opacity
     - b. Cataract
   - iv. Diseases of macula and optic nerve
4. Congenital anomalies of orbit
5. Congenital anomalies of muscles
6. Inability to fuse two images in brain

Symptoms of Heterotropia

Squints in children are detected by parent. The child becomes aware of squint in school-going age. Adults are always aware of squint and are embarrassed about it.

There may be diminished vision in the squinting eye which may or may not be correctable by glasses. There is no diplopia.

There is no binocular single vision.

There is no abnormal head posture.

The movements are normal in all directions.

Signs

One of the eyes is deviated. If the eye is deviated inwards, it is called **esotropia**, when deviated outwards it is called **exotropia**. If one of the eyes is higher than the other it is called **hypertropia** (Figs 15.4 to 15.6).

Once it has been confirmed that the person has squint, it should be found out if it is unilateral or alternate

For this a cover test is done.

Cover Test

The patient is asked to fix a distant object and the fixing eye is covered. As soon as the fixing eye is covered the squinting eye takes up fixation and becomes straight. At the same time the covered eye squints behind to cover and moves towards the same direction by same amount. Now the cover

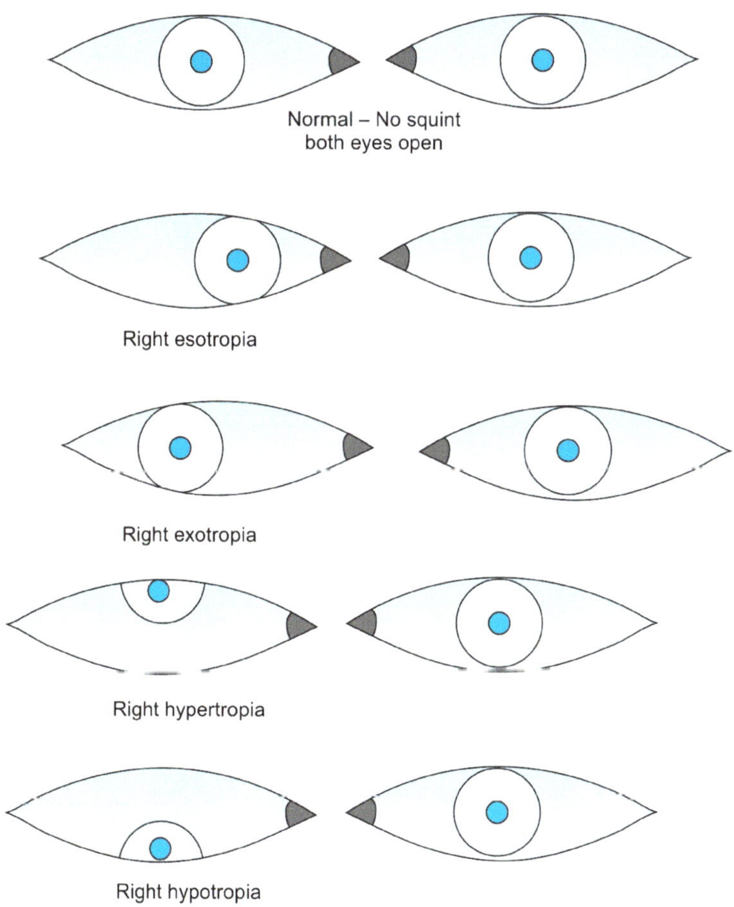

Fig. 15.4: Various types of tropia

is removed, the eye behind the cover becomes straight to take up fixation and the originally squinting eye starts squinting again (Figs 15.6 to 15.9). This happens in uniocular squint.

In alternate squint the eye under cover remains deviated when the cover is removed.

The next step is to find out the degree (amount) of squint.

To measure the degree of squint the patient is asked to look straight, keeping both eyes open. A pinpoint light is held in front of the eye about half a meter away. The light forms an image on both the corneas. If there is no squint the images in both the eyes will be formed at the center of the pupil. If the eye is deviated the image on the deviated side will be shifted. If the eye is deviated in, i.e. esotropia, the image is formed on the lateral side and if the eye is deviated out, i.e. exotropia the image moves upwards (Figs 15.10 and 15.11).

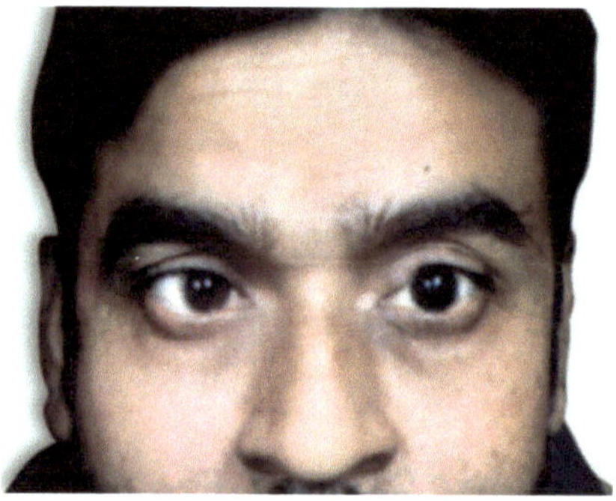

Fig. 15.5: Right esotropia

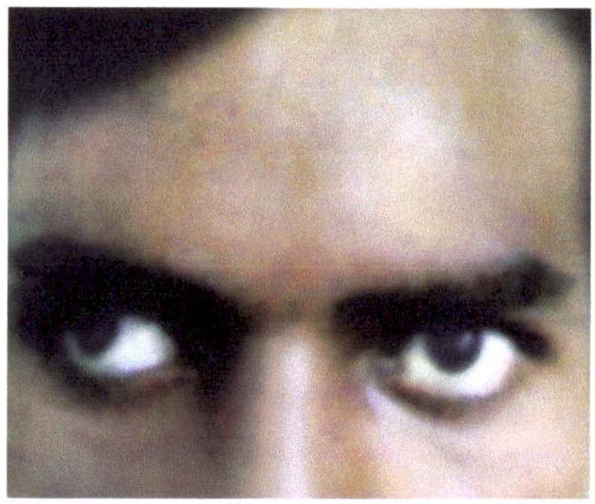

Fig. 15.6: Right exotropia

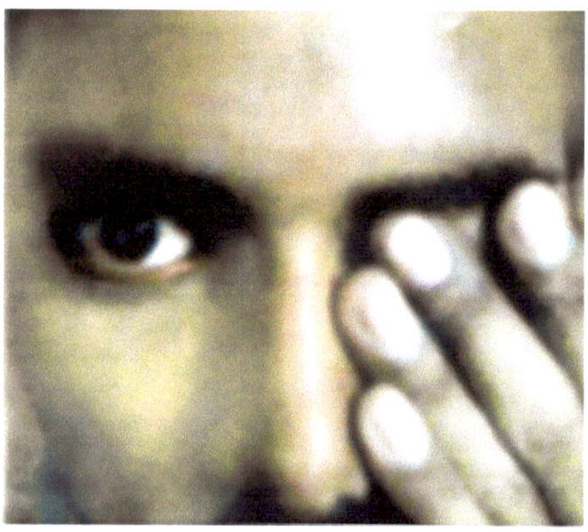

Fig. 15.7: Right eye straight, left eye covered

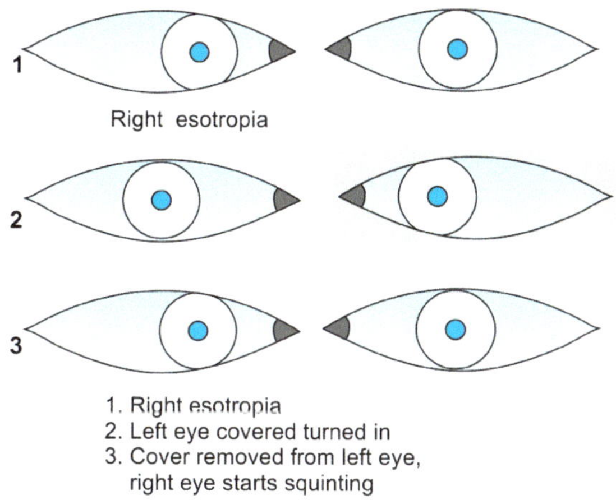

Fig. 15.8: Cover test in tropia

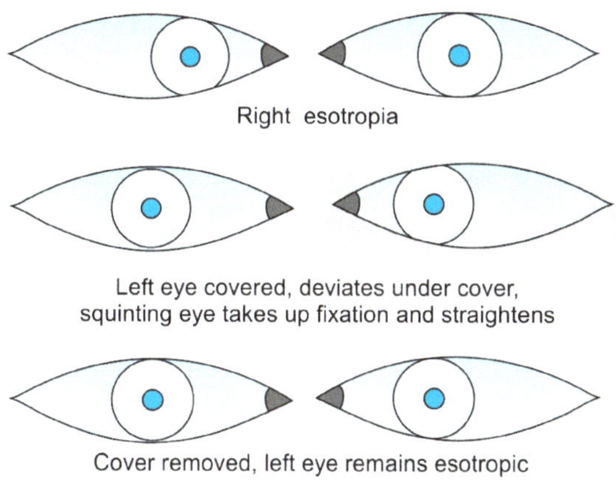

Fig. 15.9: Cover test in alternate squint

Measurement of the Deviation

If the image is formed in the center of the pupil, the eye is straight. If the image is on the pupillary margin the eye is deviated by 20°. If the image is on the limbus, the eye is deviated by 45° (Figs 15.10 and 15.11).

The best method to measure the deviation is on **synoptophore**, which is a multi-purpose instrument in diagnosis and treatment of squint.

Once degree of squint has been found out, it is essential to find out if the squint is concomitant or paralytic (Fig 15.12). This is required to decide the management of squint. The two types require different treatment.

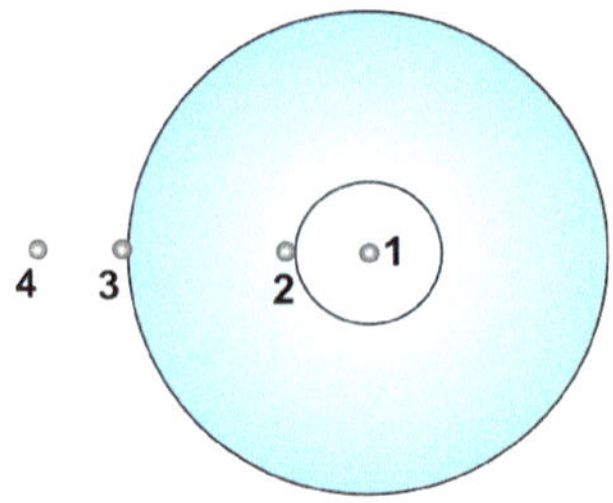

1. Corneal reflex in the center = no squint
2. Corneal reflex at the pupillary margin - 20° squint
3. Corneal reflex at limbus - 45° squint
4. Corneal reflex away from limbus - squint >45°

Fig. 15.10: Measurement of deviation by Hiershberg test

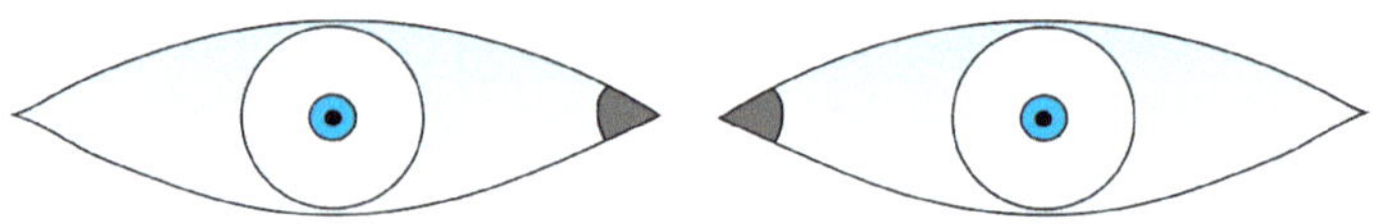

Light reflex in the center of the pupil – No squint

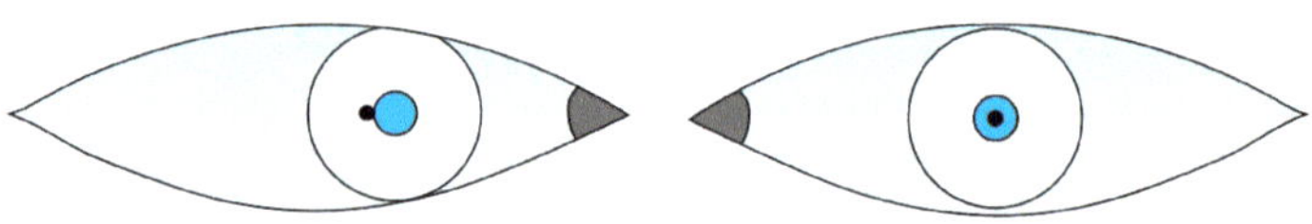

Light reflex at the pupillary margin of the right eye 20° esotropia, left eye straight

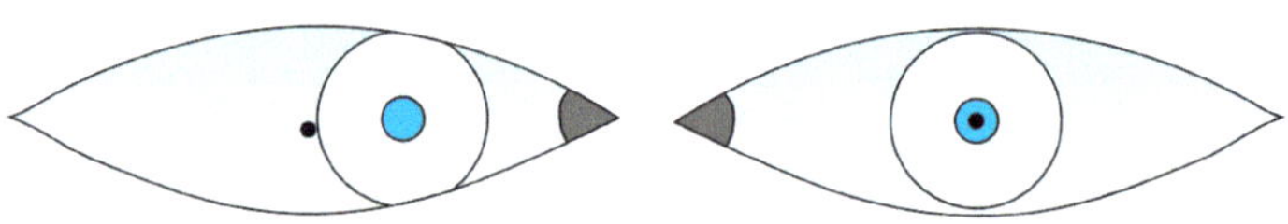

Light reflex at the limbus of right eye 45° esotropia, left eye straight

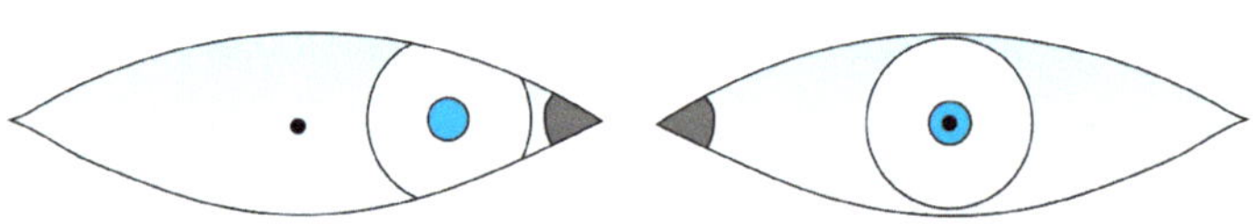

Light reflex away from the limbus, right eye esotropia > 45° left eye straight

Fig. 15.11: Measurement of deviation by light reflex

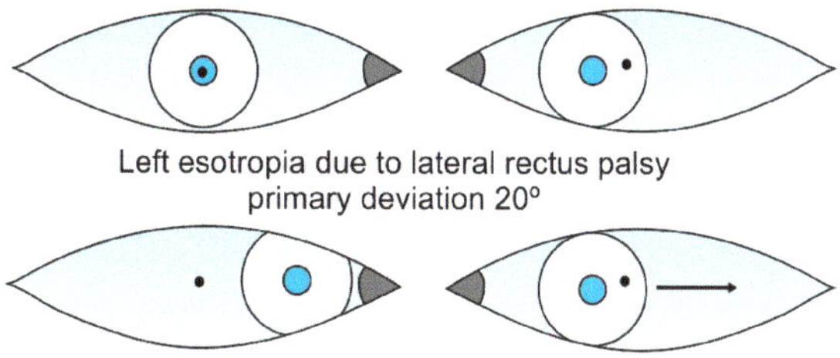

Fig. 15.12: The left eye does not move laterally, the right eye moves medially and develops esotropia more than left when the eyes look left laterally, secondary deviation of the right eye >20°

Difference between concomitant and paralytic squint

Concomitant squint	*Paralytic squint*
1. No diplopia	Diplopia is constant feature
2. No nausea, vomiting or vertigo	Generally present
3. May have diminished vision in the squinting eye and the diminished vision is the cause of squint	Diminished vision when present is not the cause of squint
4. No abnormal head posture	Abnormal head posture is always present
5. Angle of squint is same in all direction	Angle of squint changes with direction of eye
6. Ocular movements are normal	Ocular movement is less in the direction of action of paralyzed muscle
7. Primary and secondary deviation are equal	Secondary deviation is greater than primary deviation (Fig. 15.12)
8. No neurological defect is present	Some neurological disorders can be present
9. They generally develop over months	Have sudden onset

Primary deviation is the deviation of the squinting eye. **Secondary deviation** is the deviation of the sound eye when the squinting eye is forced to fixate.

Management of Concomitant Squint

1. There is no medical treatment.
2. Squints do not get corrected with age.
3. The aim of treatment is to give straight eye with binocular single vision.
4. The treatment consists of—Four O's
   a. Optical (spectacle)
   b. Occlusion (closing one eye)
   c. Orthoptics (exercise)
   d. Operation (surgery)

Correction of error of refraction: Before prescribing glasses the eyes should be refracted under cycloplegic. Children under five years should be refracted under atropine. Slight over correction or under correction of spherical error does not harm much but astigmatism should be corrected fully in dioptre (strength) and axis. Children may be required to be refracted on automated computerized refractometer to get correct axis. Children with accommodative esotropia may require bifocals for near vision. Correction of error of refraction will not only improve vision but also prevent amblyopia if not yet present.

Management of amblyopia by occlusion: Both the eyes are given glasses when error of refraction is present. **The eye with better vision is occluded** completely and the squinting eye is forced to see. There are many protocols to occlude the eyes. If vision in the amblyopic eye does not improve within three months, treatment for amblyopia is given up and the patient is advised to undergo surgery, to correct deviation. Surgery will neither cure amblyopia nor correct vision. It only corrects the deviation.

> If the child has error of refraction, he will be required to use them even after surgery In higher degree, both eyes may have to be operated.

Alternate Squints

Characteristics of alternate squint:

1. Alternate squints are generally large angled squint.
2. They have good vision.
3. Error of refraction when present is small.
4. They do not have binocular vision.
5. Alternate squints are not corrected by glasses or occlusion.
6. They are corrected by surgery only.

Paralytic Squint

Paralytic squints can be congenital or acquired. The second is more common persons in any age can develop acquired paralytic squint. It is more common in old age due **to diabetes**, **hypertension** or **brain tumors**. It may be localized to the eye only without any other defect in the limbs or may have both. Paralytic squint may involve **only one muscle,** i.e. lateral rectus or superior oblique as in sixth nerve palsy and fourth nerve palsy. Third nerve palsy involves **more than one muscle**. There may be third nerve palsy without involvement of pupil in diabetes. When all **the six muscles, iris and ciliary muscles are** paralyzed, it is called **total ophthalmoplegia**, when only extraocular muscles are paralyzed, it is called **external ophthalmoplegia**, when only iris and ciliary muscles are involved, it is called **internal ophthalmoplegia**. Paralysis of iris is called **iridoplegia**. It causes mydriasis (dilatation of pupil). Paralysis of ciliary body is called **cycloplegia**. In case of third nerve palsy it is common to have ptosis. Sixth nerve palsy may be associated with seventh nerve palsy and loss of corneal sensation (Figs 15.13 to 15.15).

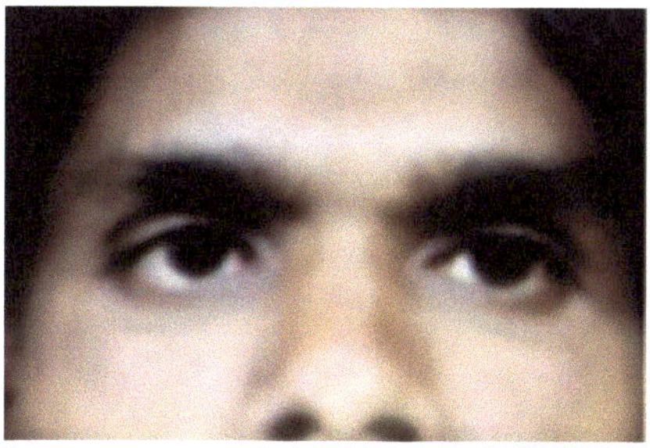

Fig. 15.13: Right lateral rectus palsy, primary position

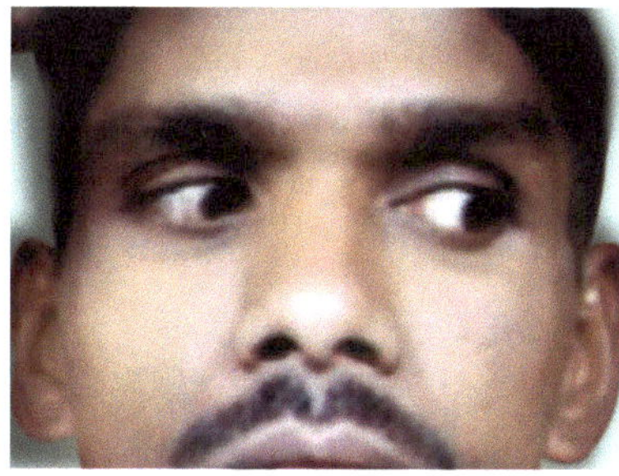

Fig. 15.14: Right lateral rectus palsy, looking left

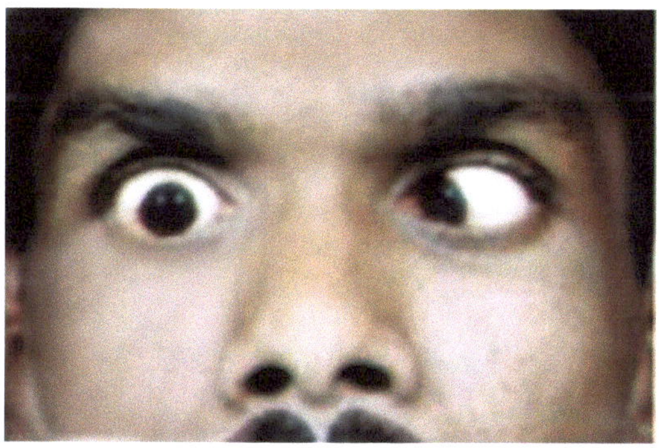

Fig. 15.15: Right lateral rectus palsy, looking right

Treatment

Ophthalmologists have limited role in treatment of paralytic squint. It is treated by neurologists. The ophthalmologist only manages diplopia by asking the patient to patch the effected eye or prescribing suitable prism.

No attempt should be made to correct paralytic squint by surgery unless the squint is stabilized for at least sixth months.

NYSTAGMUS

Nystagmus is an abnormality of eyeball that has rapid to and fro movement of the eye in all positions of gaze. It is mostly horizontal, i.e. the eyeballs move from side to side, rarely it can be vertical, i.e. the eyes move up and down. Least common are the cyclic (circular) where the eyes turn in or out.

Nystagmus is generally bilateral and equal in both eyes. It has two components; a rapid component and a slow component. The extraocular muscles have full range of movement.

Nystagmus can be **latent** or **manifest**. In latent nystagmus movements are not present when both eyes are open but movements develops when any of the eyes is closed. In such cases one eye has poor vision.

The **causes** of nystagmus can be divided into two broad groups, i.e. **ocular** and **nonocular**. Most of the time a patient is aware of nystagmus except in very small children.

Ocular Causes of Nystagmus

It can be congenital when the child is born blind.

A nystagmus is called amblyopic when vision is poor in both eyes due to non-development of macula with in six months of birth. Such cases are very common in albinism and congenital coloboma of macula.

Nonocular Causes of Nystagmus

1. Due to lesions of eighth cranial nerve.
2. Due to lesions of brainstem, cerebellum and spinal cord.
3. Idiopathic. It is genetic, the eyes are normal with good vision, normal nervous system. The exact cause is not known.

Treatment

There is no treatment for nystagmus except for brain lesion which may benefit with treatment. The aim is to give best corrected vision. Those with uncorrectable diminished vision should be rehabilitated. There are some surgeries to correct nystagmus, but none of them give satisfactory result.

Index

Page numbers followed by *f* refer to figure and *t* refer to table

B

C

D

E

F

L

M

N

P

Q

R